GIFT OF LIFE

HEALTH, MEDICINE, AND SOCIETY:
A WILEY-INTERSCIENCE SERIES

DAVID MECHANIC, Editor

Evaluating Treatment Environments: A Social Ecological Approach
by Rudolf H. Moos

Human Subjects in Medical Experimentation: A Sociological Study of the Conduct and Regulation of Clinical Research
by Bradford H. Gray

Child Health and the Community
by Robert J. Haggerty, Klaus J. Roghmann, and Ivan B. Pless

Health Insurance Plans: Promise and Performance
by Robert W. Hetherington, Carl E. Hopkins, and Milton I. Roemer

The End of Medicine
by Rick J. Carlson

Humanizing Health Care
edited by Jan Howard and Anselm Strauss

The Growth of Bureaucratic Medicine: An Inquiry into the Dynamics of Patient Behavior and the Organization of Medical Care
by David Mechanic

The Post-Physician Era: Medicine in the Twenty-First Century
by Jerrold S. Maxmen

A Right to Health: The Problem of Access to Primary Medical Care
by Charles E. Lewis, Rashi Fein, and David Mechanic

Gift of Life: The Social and Psychological Impact of Organ Transplantation
by Roberta G. Simmons, Susan D. Klein, and Richard L. Simmons

GIFT OF LIFE:

THE SOCIAL AND PSYCHOLOGICAL IMPACT OF ORGAN TRANSPLANTATION

Roberta G. Simmons, Ph.D.
Susan D. Klein, Ph.D.
Richard L. Simmons, M.D.

A WILEY-INTERSCIENCE PUBLICATION

JOHN WILEY & SONS, New York · London · Sydney · Toronto

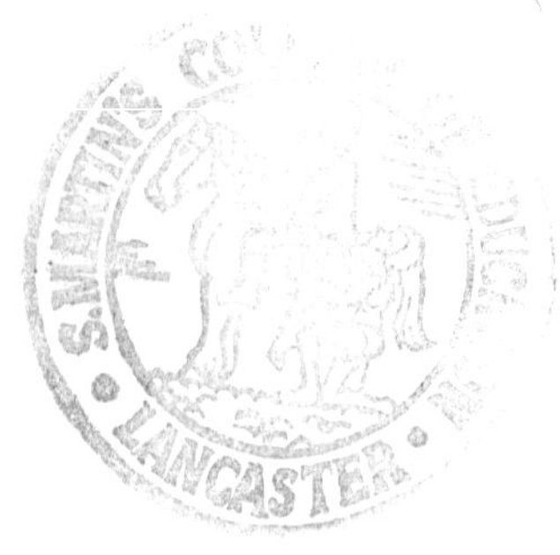

Library of Congress Cataloging in Publication Data

Simmons, Roberta G.
Gift of life.

(Health, medicine, and society)
"A Wiley-Interscience publication."
Bibliography: p.
Includes index.
1. Kidneys—Transplantation—Social aspects.
2. Kidneys—Transplantation—Psychological aspects.
I. Klein, Susan D., Joint author. II. Simmons, Richard Lawrence, 1934– joint author.
III. Title. [DNLM: 1. Transplantation.
2. Socioeconomic factors. W0690 S592g]

RD575.S55 301.24'3 77–2749
ISBN 0–471–79197–0

Printed in the United States of America

10 9 8 7 6 5 4 3 2 1

To our parents with appreciation

ANN and BURTON
IMOGENE and HARRY
ANNE and NATHANIEL

and to

JOHN S. NAJARIAN, M.D.

without whose cooperation and encouragement
this study would have been impossible

ACKNOWLEDGMENTS

We are gratified to be able to thank all those people who have aided in this study since 1970. The cooperation of the Transplant, Dialysis, and Pediatric Nephrology services and the follow-up clinics at the University of Minnesota Transplant Center was excellent and indispensable. To John S. Najarian, M.D.; Carl Kjellstrand, M.D.; Ted Buselmeier, M.D.; Alfred Michael, M.D.; Alfred Fish, M.D.; Robert Vernier, M.D.; Justine Willmert, R.N.; Audrey Boyd; Cindy Forsman, R.N.; Rhonda Meyer, R.N.; and Carol Paulini, R.N. we express special gratitude both for their cooperation and for the knowledge they imparted to us. The other physicians, nurses, and secretaries on these services also were exceedingly helpful during the data-collection stages.

On the sociology staff itself, there is no way adequately to express appreciation to Barbara Bailey who, as the major secretary to the project for several years, has often played the role of major collaborator. Some members of the research staff—Kathleen Schilling, Linda Kamstra, and Kenneth Thornton in particular—were integral parts of the study from beginning to end, and their work is an invaluable part of the total effort. In addition, Ann Moore played a major part in organizing and participating in the data collection of the cadaver-donor study; and Diane Bush was responsible for much of the computer processing and analysis of the larger study. Others were important to various stages of data collection, data processing, or data analysis: Elaine Bolland, Paul Feiss, Tom Byrne, Sue Cogdill, John Cogdill, Kati Miller, Connie Stapleton, Lynn Abrahamsen, Jana Adair, Louanne Ditchett, Pam Farkas, Doris Covill, Bruce Fisher, Tony Norcia, Jeff Nelson, Debbie Ferguson, Jane Lanctôt, Terri Erickson, and Wanda Miszkiewicz. Sociology department secretaries aided in typing various manuscript drafts, and we are in their debt as we are in the debt of Kathi Zubrod, secretary to Richard L. Simmons.

The social work staff on the transplant service have throughout the data-collection years provided valuable information and insights. We wish to thank Kathy Hickey Read, M.S.W., Gerry Moquin, M.S.W., and Marvin Haymond, M.S.W. for their help.

Professional advice from social scientists such as Reuben Hill, Ph.D.; Jeylan Mortimer, Ph.D.; Paul Reynolds, Ph.D.; James Butcher, Ph.D.; Steven McLaughlin, Ph.D.; Dale Blyth, Ph.D.; Martin Peterson, Ph.D.; John Brantner, Ph. D.; Shalom Schwartz, Ph.D., and David Mechanic, Ph.D. is also greatly appreciated, although all shortcomings of the present analysis are the responsibility of the authors alone. The basic interest in the self-image and the conceptualization and measurement in this area have been a direct outgrowth of the work of Roberta Simmons with Morris Rosenberg, Ph.D., and his influence is highly valued.

This study has been funded by the following grants from the Public Health Service: 2KO2 MH 41688; MH AM 18135; 2R01 MH 18134; AM 13083; and several grants from the Kidney Foundation of the Upper Midwest and by the Center for Death Education and Research, University of Minnesota.

Finally, the patients and their families have cooperated with the study to contribute to an understanding of the social-psychological aspects of this new and unique therapy. They are indeed the unnamed collaborators in the research effort. It is important to us to be able to express here our admiration for their strength in the face of crisis, our sympathy for the losses many of them had to incur, and our gratitude for their help.

Minneapolis, Minnesota
Denver, Colorado
Minneapolis, Minnesota
April 1977

Roberta G. Simmons
Susan D. Klein
Richard L. Simmons

CONTENTS

GIFT OF LIFE

I

INTRODUCTION

1

INTRODUCTION

Modern medical technology raises unprecedented and fundamental social questions. Can the United States, the wealthiest nation in existence, afford to continue to develop new medical technologies? Should developments such as organ transplantation and artificial heart implantation be allowed to proceed? As new therapies have become so costly that even middle-class families lack the resources to withstand the expense, society is forced to reevaluate the worth of the individual life as opposed to the cost to the society and to redefine the government's role in decisions related to the new technologies. There have been few values higher in priority in modern Western society than the importance of the individual life and the value of medical progress through science. Yet now questions are being raised about the cost of saving lives that could not be saved before. Should scientists be encouraged to develop expensive technologies that potentially can extend the lives of select groups of the fatally ill? The twentieth century has seen enormous progress in the conquest of disease and extension of the life-span; whether we can continue in this direction is at issue.

Current federal government policy continues to support greater medical progress and discovery despite controversy around the related issues.

Hundreds of millions of dollars have been allocated for cancer research; an amendment to the Social Security Act of 1972 legislates payment for almost all expenses of kidney transplant patients; and a government-financed comprehensive or catastrophic health insurance program may be inevitable. But serious scholars, radical medical groups, and others question the ethics and priorities involved.

In this volume we examine the consequences of one of the most dramatic of the new medical technologies—organ transplantation, particularly kidney transplantation, and the related technological advance of hemodialysis. Although unique in some important ways, the experience of organ transplantation parallels other less dramatic but almost equally expensive therapies and alerts us to possible effects of future medical advances. What have the consequences of this technology been for the norms and values within medicine and the larger culture, for the patient and his family, and for the society and health care delivery system? Are the gains for the patients and families sufficient to say that from their point of view this costly therapy is "worth it?"

The issues examined in this work are relevant to two audiences—general readers concerned with the impact of medical technology on patients, families, and the larger society; and behavioral scientists interested in the social psychology of the illness crisis and in the study of family altruism and decision-making under stress. Analyses presented here tell the story of kidney transplantation in particular and allow the general reader to evaluate the social and psychological consequences of this very expensive technological breakthrough from the point of view of costs and benefits. In addition, transplantation can be seen by the behavioral scientist as one example of a family and individual crisis, and its effects can be traced in this light. Because of the opportunity for family members to donate a kidney to their relative, an analysis of the consequences of family decision-making and of help-giving under stress become particularly relevant. Thus the data are applicable both to policy-relevant concerns and to issues of relevance to behavioral science theory.

The focus of this study is on *kidney* transplantation because the kidney was the first organ to be transplanted successfully in human beings. Kidney transplantation is also the only type of organ transplantation that has moved almost totally from the realm of experimentation to everyday practical therapeutics. Many of the stresses and problems that may be associated with large-scale heart, lung, and liver transplantation in the future can be foreseen by a study of kidney transplantation, as can the problems that may emerge from the development of an implantable artificial heart or an expensive cancer therapy.

THE TECHNOLOGY OF DIALYSIS AND TRANSPLANTATION

In end-stage kidney disease the kidney no longer can remove waste products from the blood; and without some help life cannot be maintained. Hemodialysis (the purification of a kidney patient's blood by means of an artificial kidney machine) was the first major advance in the treatment of end-stage kidney disease. It is used today on a short-term basis by patients awaiting transplantation and on a long-term relatively permanent basis by those patients who have no transplant operation in sight.

In a hospital, clinic, or even a home setting, the kidney patient is "hooked up" to the dialysis machine by means of needles and tubes connected to the blood vessels of his arm or leg. Various external or internal devices permit the patient's blood to flow through the machine, where it is purified, and then returned to his body. A period of 6 to 10 hours is required for this treatment, two or three times per week.

More than 10,000 patients are currently on dialysis, and approximately 77% survive two years or more (GAO, 1975). Dr. Fred Shapiro, Chief of Nephrology, Hennepin County Medical Center in Minneapolis, reports that 40% of his patients survive five years; however, when only those more recent patients who started dialysis since 1972 are considered, the survival rate is 15% higher.

Despite the life-saving nature of dialysis, as a therapy it has several disadvantages. The extent of time spent on the machine, the severe fluid and dietary restrictions necessary between treatments, and the fact that patients reported that they still did not feel well were incentives for the development of a more satisfactory technical solution.

Kidney transplantation attempts to remove the patient from the status of being "sick" altogether. In this operation a healthy kidney is transplanted into the ill patient. Because normal human beings have two functioning kidneys and only one is needed, a healthy individual can donate one of his kidneys to a dying patient or a healthy kidney from a newly dead cadaver can be utilized. The first successful series of kidney transplants with identical twin donor-recipient pairs took place in the early 1950s at the Peter Brent Brigham Hospital in Boston. However, because the body will immunologically reject and destroy tissue from all but identical twins, a new breakthrough was needed to allow the successful use of other types of donors. This advance was the development of immunosuppressive drugs (e.g., imuran and prednisone) which help to prevent this reaction. In 1959 the first successful transplant was performed between nonidentical twins, and the recipient is still alive and healthy 17 years later (Riteris, 1973).

According to the "Twelfth Report of the Human Renal Transplant Registery" (1975), more than 16,400 transplants have been done in the world (more than 9000 in the United States), and the current number of operations approximates 2500 annually. Approximately 74% of patients who received a kidney in 1972 from a living sibling and 43% of those who received kidneys from cadavers have survived two or more years with functioning kidneys. Kidneys from related donors survive better because the tissues are genetically more similar to those of the recipient and the body is less likely to reject the kidney immunologically.

At the University of Minnesota Transplant Center 60% of recipients with kidneys from siblings and 45% of those with cadaver kidneys currently survive at least five years with functioning kidneys. An additional 20% of patients in each group survive loss of the first transplant and are retransplanted or undergo chronic hemodialysis. Though even 5-year survivors will probably not have a completely normal life-span, the rate of patient loss after five years appears to be very low (Matas et al., 1976). These statistics indicate that kidney transplantation with related donors is more successful in providing a cure than are most standard operations designed to cure visceral cancer.

FUNDING FOR KIDNEY TRANSPLANTATION AND DIALYSIS

The history of scarcity of financial resources as a new technology develops is an interesting one in itself and is discussed in detail in Chapter 11. At this point, however, the costliness of the therapy must be documented. Kidney transplantation and dialysis, like other new medical technologies, require large numbers of highly specialized personnel as well as expensive equipment and laboratory facilities. The University of Minnesota Transplant Center, for example, utilizes a team of 15 physicians at various levels of training, 14 highly specialized nurses, and 53 other nurses and technicians as well as a variety of consultants and laboratory personnel. The cost for such large numbers of personnel and expensive facilities is considerable.

On the average, dialysis at a hospital center costs approximately $25,000 to $30,000 a year for outpatients; dialysis in the home setting costs $12,000 to $20,000 for the first year of training and an average of $7,000 a year thereafter. And the cost of a kidney transplantation averages between $12,800 and $20,000 plus $1000 in yearly follow-up. If a discharged patient later needs a second transplant or chronic hemodialysis, his bill is, of course, doubled, and sometimes charges for one patient can run as high as $50,000 to $100,000 with many complications

(Douglas, 1973; "The Kidney Care Issues," 1973; GAO, 1975; Metcalfe, 1976).

Until 1972, funding was inadequate, and many patients had to be rejected for treatment and, in effect, condemned to death. In 1972 a Chronic Kidney Disease Amendment to the Social Security Act was passed by Congress as the first foray into a type of catastrophic health insurance (see Chapter 11). According to this amendment, almost all kidney transplantation and dialysis expenses could be paid by the federal government starting in July 1973.* This law, PL92-603, is popularly known as the HR-1 amendment and is so referred to in this book. This revolutionary legislation meant that problems of access to treatment would radically change once adequate financial resources were available for the new technology. No longer would the ordinary patient have to be rejected for treatment.

The costliness of the therapy, however, has not been reduced. The burden has simply been transferred to the total society. Thus the question of whether the absorption of the cost is in the society's interest has become relevant. Many critics have indicated that the allocation of health resources should be directed mainly to primary and preventive care, not to the development of expensive new medical technologies (Somers, 1971; Thomas, 1973; Rettig, 1976). A set of *New York Times* editorials and articles criticized the kidney amendment as "medicarelessness," saying that the cost to save only a few patients would be too great at a time when government resources were needed for eradicating slums, improving education, or finding a cure for cancer ("Medicarelessness," 1973; Lyons, Jan. 11, 1973).

For this study we do not attempt to evaluate the consequences of allocating resources to technologies such as transplantation as opposed to assigning funds to competing needs. However, we try to ascertain the social-psychological costs and benefits of transplantation for families and patients involved. Are the problems for these persons, who are subject to the technological advance, great enough to give further support to the critics of this type of resource allocation?

THE ORGANIZATION OF THE STUDY

The bulk of this report is based on a set of quantitative and qualitative empirical studies. All kidney transplant recipients, donors, and families who were seen at the University of Minnesota Hospitals during a 3-year period were followed by a team of sociologists, both with quantitative

* No other catastrophic therapy was funded by this legislation (see Chapter 11).

questionnaires and in-depth interviewing. Based on these studies, Part II (Chapters 3 to 5) of the monograph is focused on the impact of kidney transplantation upon the recipients. Is their quality of life satisfactory enough to warrant the high level of energy and funds being devoted to this therapy? What are the psychological reactions of young children and patients with diabetes who are being rejected for transplantation by many centers but are accepted at Minnesota? The more general implications of these findings—that is, the nature of the psychological impact of the crisis of illness and of restoration to health upon different types of patients—are also examined. There is a particular emphasis on the consequences of the crisis for the self-image of the recipients.

Part III (Chapters 6 to 10) is concentrated on organ donors and their families. The effect of altruism of this extreme nature should be investigated. What are the long-term psychological consequences of sacrificing a body-part to save a relative's life? Do these consequences cast doubt on the policy of related donation or do they affirm it? We examine the stress for the family members as they attempt to decide who, if anyone, will give a kidney. Differences between family members who volunteer to donate a kidney and those who do not are explored.

In general, using the donor situation as an example, we also study how individuals and families make major decisions under stress. Family communication processes and emotional relationships between donor and recipient in this difficult situation are also analyzed. In addition, the impact of donation upon the family of the cadaver donor is explored.

Part IV is focused on larger health care delivery and funding issues.

Prior to presenting these analyses, however, Chapter 2 examines some of the overall unresolved ethical issues related to transplantation , namely the changing norms—medical, legal, and social—that have been affected by organ transplantation.

2

TRANSPLANTATION AND CHANGING NORMS: CULTURAL LAG AND ETHICAL AMBIGUITIES

Technological advances often exceed the resources and social organization necessary for their optimal use. Organ transplantation is clearly a prototype of this "cultural lag," as originally formulated by Ogburn (1922). In his classic analysis of social change, Ogburn's basic thesis is that various parts of modern culture change at different rates. Because there is a correlation and interdependence of parts, a change in one part of the culture requires readjustments in other correlated parts. However, subsequent to a new invention or discovery, there frequently is a delay in these latter readjustments during which ". . . there may be said to be a maladjustment." Typically, changes occur first in the "material culture"—that is, in technology—while appropriate modifications in social organization and public norms and attitudes fail to keep pace.

As a major new medical technology, organ transplantation may solve important health problems, but it has created unanticipated adjustment problems for the government, the general public, medical organization, and the patient and his family. In particular, transplantation has led to ethical and normative problems. New situations have arisen both within the medical world and in the larger society for which no clear norms or rules exist. There is a gap between the technological advance and the extant formal laws and informal norms governing its application. (See Simmons and Simmons, 1971.)

In some cases the existing regulations and customs inhibit the full development of transplantation potential. *Uncertainty* and *conflict* over the proper course of action (normative uncertainty) continue in many areas. The two major issues involved are the selection of patients for treatment and the use of organ donors.

PATIENT SELECTION

SELECTION WHEN RESOURCES WERE SCARCE

For many years the knowledge, personnel, and facilities for transplantation and hemodialysis were insufficient for the demand. Because medical centers normally accept all referred patients, the selection of only some patients for the new treatment became a major area of normative uncertainty. In many transplant centers the number of referred patients exceeded the limits of available care.* Before federal funding was available for transplantation, how was the crucial decision made as to who would live and who would die? The necessity for this type of decision is liable to reoccur in the future as other new technologies achieve therapeutic success prior to establishing adequate funding.

Physicians have had few established guidelines to help them decide how to reject patients for lifesaving treatment (Schreiner and Maher, 1965). As members of the transplant team from Duke University formulated the problem:

> Thus far, the available literature has contained little more than. . .general philosophical statements regarding problems and experiences surrounding the selection of donors and recipients for renal transplantation. . . .Although we believe that our own approach to the problem has been consistent with the general philosophy. . .we anticipate that some experienced physicians may not

* The University of Minnesota did not fall in this category. The transplant program was able to expand rapidly enough to handle the influx. However, before 1973 the financial resources of the hospital were threatened when many patients were unable to pay.

> agree with the manner in which such a philosophy was applied in each patient. Indeed, in a number of situations, we found that we were often uncertain ourselves as to the correctness of our decision (Hayes and Gunnells, 1969).

One attempt to create guidelines was the establishment of an anonymous lay board to select patients for the new dialysis procedures (Alexander, 1962). Such boards, designed in part to select persons whose lives have the most social value, would be expected to reject the unemployed, the worker whose job is "less important," the person who has few family ties or obligations, and the man with a history of deviance of any sort (see Duckeminier and Sanders, 1968; Fox and Swazey, 1974, Ch. 9; and Schreiner, 1966). However, almost all of these boards were discontinued, and the burden of selection fell onto the physicians themselves (Abram, 1969; Katz and Procter, 1969).

The situation remained unclear because physicians varied greatly in the criteria used for acceptance. Many centers set up "universalistic" medical criteria—that is, standards that apply to all, regardless of social background. In some of these centers the initial aim was to choose patients who were expected to have the least complicated medical course—that is, the relatively young patient with preterminal renal failure uncomplicated by other medical, surgical, or psychiatric disease. Arbitrary age limits were therefore established at most centers. In some centers selection was dictated by research protocols that emphasized the study of patients with specific medical problems such as diabetes or severe high blood pressure. In one center patients were chosen on a first-come, first-served basis for a period of time and then no more patients were considered for months until most of these transplants were completed.

Social and Psychological Criteria

Many programs, however, appeared to introduce less universalistic criteria into the selection process. Although their use is controversial, psychological and social variables were stressed in the past and continue to be emphasized, particularly in selection of patients for dialysis. Emphasizing the difficulty of the strict medical regimen, many clinicians believe that there must be careful screening for *willingness to cooperate with the treatment*.Scribner and associates (1965) advocated reserving dialysis for emotionally mature stable patients. Livingston (1970) reported that the psychological success of the dialysis program at Seattle was probably due largely to the selection of patients who were intelligent and stable enough to cooperate with the treatment. Moreover, based on a series of 28 dialysis patients, Dwarshius (n.d.) showed that more cooperative patients have a slightly higher IQ than their less cooperative peers ($p < .06$). In a survey of 87 dialysis centers Katz and Procter (1969) indicated that 97% of the centers believed willingness to cooperate with the treatment was an important criterion for selection, and 82% usually used *intelligence* as an indicator for such cooperation (Table 2-1).

There has been less agreement on the necessity for a full psychiatric evaluation of the patient or on the importance of the patient's "social worth" or his financial resources, although many centers have utilized such criteria (Table 2-1; Abram and Wadlington, 1968). In 1969 74% of the centers regarded likelihood of vocational rehabilitation to be important (Table 2-1).

Given the fact that psychiatric prediction is difficult and that uremia (kidney disease) itself can cause reversible intellectual impairment and even psychotic episodes, there has been discomfort among some centers in using psychological and sociological variables for selection (Abram, 1968, 1969). Although a series of articles from Sweden (Hagberg, 1974; Malmquist, 1973; Malmquist and Hagberg, 1974) indicated that patients who were better adjusted before dialysis were also better rehabilitated after 12 months on dialysis, the question remains whether psychiatrists can predict the reaction of a severely ill patient to medical therapy accurately enough to refuse him lifesaving treatment. One young man came to the Minnesota program after being rejected for kidney transplantation by another hospital because of several incidents of glue sniffing. The other center probably felt reticent to apply this extraordinarily expensive treatment to a man whose social rehabilitation appeared doubtful. After being transplanted successfully at this center, however, the patient's social behavior and personality functioning showed great improvement, and he obtained a full-time job.

Middle-Class Bias. Whatever the method of selection, lower-class patients probably have been at a disadvantage in the past—a situation that may continue. A key concern in medical sociology has been the availability and accessibility of medical treatment to the less-advantaged segments of the society. A lower-class person can be blocked from treatment at many points. First, a study by Rosenblatt and Suchman (1964) indicates that he is less likely to seek treatment. Second, if the lower-class person does not attend a major hospital clinic but visits a local physician, he may not be referred to a transplant center, either because of the physician's unconscious bias or fear that the costs will be too great. In the past the costs may actually have been too high for such a patient to afford (see Chapter 11).

In addition, once such a patient arrives at the transplant or dialysis

TABLE 2-1 *IMPORTANCE OF SELECTION CRITERIA USED BY 87 HEMODIALYSIS CENTERS*[a]

Patient Selection Criteria	Percent of Centers Believing the Criterion to Be Important and Using Such a Criterion Frequently
Medical suitability (good prognosis with dialysis)	97
Absence of disabling disease (other than that of renal origin)	95
Age	82
Sex	3
Willingness to cooperate in dialysis regimen	96
Intelligence (as related to understanding treatment)	82
Psychiatric evaluation	55
Social welfare evaluation of patient and his family	44
Patient judged congenial, likable by staff	22
Social welfare burden of patient's dependents if not selected	23
Patient's demonstrated "social worth"	32
Patient's future social contribution	42
Likelihood of vocational rehabilitation	74
Financial resources for patient's treatment	36
Research potential of patient for staff	15
Primacy of application for vacancy available in facility	54

[a] A. Katz and D. Procter, Social psychological characteristics of patients receiving hemodialysis treatment for chronic renal failure, Report of questionnaire survey of dialysis centers and patients during 1967, United States Government Printing Office Washington, D.C., July 1969.

center, his chance may be affected by the physician's unconscious bias toward more middle-class "respectable" patients, patients more like the doctor himself. This trend could be further reinforced by the frequent emphasis on more intelligent patients with greater "social worth," patients capable of vocational rehabilitation. Hollingshead and Redlich (1958) have indicated such a middle-class bias in the psychiatrist's treatment of mentally ill patients, as has Sudnow (1967) in the attention given by medical personnel to dying patients.

Katz and Procter's (1969) survey of dialysis centers showed that 91% of dialysis patients were white, 45% had at least one year of college education (in comparison to only 18% of the general U.S. adult population), and 60% of the patients had incomes (before dialysis) at or above the U.S. median family income. Crane's (1969) preliminary data on heart transplantation also indicate a slight bias in the direction of middle-class patients, but there is no systematic study of the social origins of kidney transplant patients or of the methods and norms used in selecting them (Hayes and Gunnells, 1969).

SELECTION OF PATIENTS WHEN RESOURCES ARE ADEQUATE

High-Risk Patients: Physiological Problems

With the passage of the HR-1 amendment, there should no longer be a shortage of facilities. Therefore, selection and rejection of patients will no longer assume the urgency it has in the past. Nevertheless, in specific cases difficult ethical decisions and normative ambiguities will persist. If a patient is at greater risk—that is, if the transplant is less likely to be successful—the question of acceptance for this therapy remains. Should older persons, diabetics, infants, and other high-risk patients be allowed this costly treatment? When the answer of the local center has been to refuse treatment to a particular type of patient, only the intelligent, wealthy, and aggressive in this category have been able to seek out a distant center that will accept the high-risk patients.

The following case reports are typical of the controversies surrounding this issue:

CASE 1 A 38-Year-Old Woman

The woman's medical history included a radical mastectomy for cancer of the breast. Two years later she developed end-stage renal disease. When her first kidney was removed, a cancer of the kidney was discovered, although this was not the primary cause of the kidney disease. A year later no other cancer had developed; the other kidney was removed and no further malignancy was found. The question of a kidney transplant was raised and became a controversial issue. A sister was quite eager to donate a kidney, but some staff members were uncertain whether it was ethical to risk a related donor.

Posttransplant the patient would have to receive medicines designed to suppress her immunological responses in order to reduce the likelihood of her destroying or rejecting the kidney. Statistics indicate that malignancies are more likely to develop in such immunologically suppressed transplant patients: 2–4% of such patients have been seen to develop cancers spontaneously (a rate in this age group 100,000 times higher than normal).

The physicians disagreed radically as to whether a patient who already showed a tendency to develop malignancies and thereby was a greater risk should be allowed this expensive treatment and what type of donation she should receive.

CASE 2 A 72-Year-Old Man

H.G. was admitted to the Renal Service complaining of progressive nausea, vomiting, weakness, and shortness of breath.

Physical examination and testing revealed an alert elderly male with end-stage kidney disease. In addition, the patient was found to have arterial-sclerotic heart disease and mitral insufficiency.

Dietary therapy for uremia was unsuccessful, and his condition deteriorated. Because of his heart failure and his age, the question was raised whether to attempt to save his life by placing him on dialysis. Hemodialysis was initiated one month after his initial examination. The dialyses were complicated by cardiac arrhythmias, suggesting that the dialysis-induced alterations of the extracellular fluid were detrimental to the diseased heart. Yet without the dialysis, life could not be sustained.

On 9/27/72 grand-mal convulsions occurred at home. Respiratory arrest occurred during the ambulance ride to the hospital. The patient was resuscitated. Once hospitalized, his heart disease continued to cause severe problems. Recurrent episodes of ventricular tachycardia* with transient loss of consciousness occurred. A temporary transvenous pacemaker was inserted into his heart. Despite this, episodes of ventricular tachycardia still occurred. Medical treatment had temporary success at best. Again the question was raised as to whether to continue dialysis.

Because the government is now paying for the therapy, many centers

* See glossary for definition of these terms.

have extended treatment to elderly and high-risk ill patients. Yet some physicians are concerned that such extensions will cause costs for this program to skyrocket so far above original government estimates that either the kidney program or other catastrophic disease programs may be jeopardized. These physicians feel caught between a concern for the societal ramifications of their actions and their obligation to particular patients who wish to take the gamble and try to extend their lives. The discomfort involved in turning away a patient when he has a small chance for success is very intense, because dialysis has been successful in maintaining the physical life of many elderly patients who otherwise would become bedridden, senile, and totally dependent. At least one dialyzer has attempted to solve the dilemma by accepting all patients for a trial of dialysis therapy with the understanding that if the "quality of life" of the elderly patient becomes sufficiently poor, treatment will be discontinued. The patient and family are informed that dialysis may be discontinued in case of severe medical complication, emotional maladjustment, or the requirement of permanent nursing home or other extended facility care. There is difficulty, however, in deciding when quality of life is too poor to warrant continuation, and conflicts among physicians, nurses, technicians and between the physician and family concerning this issue have sometimes been extreme.

Who Makes the Decision about High-Risk Patients? The point has been made by some that it is the patient's right to make such decisions. If the patient wishes to accept the added risk, however great and however costly, he should be allowed to do so; the physician does not have the right to adjudicate these issues. Whatever the merit of this viewpoint, the burden of such decisions probably will not be totally removed from the physicians. The implementation of the HR-1 amendment involves the certification of each individual patient for treatment (see Chapter 11). Regional peer review policy boards will perform this function with later approval by the Social Security Administration. Thus local groups of physicians will probably develop informal norms and policies regarding the types of patients suitable for such treatment.

If a kidney center wishes to extend treatment to groups at greater risk in terms of age or disease history, the extension may be defined a temporary experiment, as data with regard to the success rate are collected and evaluated. If the statistics indicate that the group has a low chance of a successful outcome, peer review boards, medical professional societies, and perhaps even the Social Security Administration may develop policies suggesting the exclusion of such patients. Currently no such policies bind the individual physician, and therefore government refusal to pay the costs for these patients would represent a major change of the health care delivery system. Physicians would probably be quite resistant to an attempt to "force" them to refuse care to any group of patients. Yet informal policies formulated by the physicians themselves at individual kidney centers may have the same effect. Undoubtedly the high cost of transplantation, especially in cases of failure, will always be a significant pressure against its widespread application to high-risk groups. Whether such pressures will inhibit research into improvement in care that could allow inclusion is a significant unanswered question.

A case in point is the transplantation of organs other than the kidney. Transplantation of the lung, heart, liver, and pancreas is successful in a minority of cases* and continues to be supported by NIH research funds. Yet no physicians are suggesting that all patients who wish to undergo these treatments be permitted to do so or that Social Security funds be extended to these groups. In fact, in the field of heart transplantation the original low rate of success has led to the controversial question of whether a moratorium should be declared and to a partially affirmative answer. Fox and Swazey (1974) note that this type of question is likely to emerge in the early stages of any new therapy. The initial results are likely to be bleak and discouraging and the choice of whether to continue will become acute for the physician involved. When the financial costs are great, as in cardiac transplants, the choice is even more difficult. The call for a moratorium has severely restricted clinical research in this area; only one center currently practices heart transplantation with a better than 35% long-term success rate.

Physicians organized in blue-ribbon panels and professional organizations have played the role of policymakers in these areas, although their policies have not been binding (Shelley, 1968). For example, the American Heart Association set up panels to deal with the issue of a moratorium on heart transplantation (Appel, 1968; Beecher, 1968; Stickel, 1966). These policymaking groups may have an informal influence on the allocation of federal research monies and on the availability of treatment to high-risk groups. Whether innovation will thereby be limited or whether treatment will be restricted to the best risks and costs cut accordingly

* According to world statistics from the Transplant Registry, in September 1975, 50 of 281 heart transplant patients were alive with functioning grafts (18%), 27 of 235 liver transplant patients (11%), none of 37 lung transplants, and 4 of 46 pancreas grafts (9%). The longest survival with a functioning graft has been 6.9 years for heart transplants, 6.1 years for liver, 10 months for lung, and 3.1 years for pancreas. Dr. Norman Shumway of Stanford University Medical School who currently performs most of the world's heart transplants also reports the highest heart transplant success rate. As of August 1975, he had performed 90 heart transplants. Of all of those who could have reached one year, 47% did so; the 2-year survival rate was 37%; the 3-year rate was 27%.

remains to be seen. How such panels and physician groups decide on the level of risk that is acceptable also remains a question. What are the factors that will enter into these decisions?

Professional Considerations Leading to Exclusion. Whatever policy is set by physician groups, individual centers may choose to exclude high-risk patients because of the attitudes of professional groups with whom the transplant and dialysis physicians expect to deal. The pressures on the physicians faced with selection decisions are not only those of limited facilities and resources, but also the more subtle influences of their peers and co-workers. For example, physicians are affected by the need to maintain reasonable morale among the nursing and paramedical staff who participate in patient care and who become discouraged by persistant or recurrent failure. When asked why he does not perform more cardiac transplants, one renowned pioneer in cardiac transplantation cited the morale of the nurses in the intensive care unit as the principal factor. Similar factors are operative in dialysis and kidney transplantation units in regard to high-risk patients.

A second factor discouraging physicians from taking risks is the threat that failure has for their local reputation within the medical institution. Critics within their own specialty are prone to look upon their worst results (frequently presented at complication or mortality rounds) as typical of the results of therapy. If only small risks are taken, few presentations at these conferences will be required, and the local reputation will grow.

Allied to this latter problem are possible impediments to the expansion of the therapeutic modality itself within the institution. A physician working in a highly experimental therapeutic area may not obtain referrals (i.e., patients with all types of renal failure) if his statistics largely reflect the poor results to be expected from treating high-risk patients. In fact, human experimentation committees, now required in all hospitals receiving federal (and sometimes private foundation) funds, may look unfavorably at results obtained only with the highest risk patient, and disapproval of the local program may follow. Such a fate probably befell many heart transplantation programs in small centers.

Finally, the physician fears for his national or international standing within his own reference group of clinical investigators. Most transplant programs, for example, compete with each other for favorable results. One can generally improve one's results by careful selection of recipients. Conversely, of course, one can explain away poor results as due to a high-risk group of patients.

A 10-Year-Old Girl

tient came from a family of nine children with a father who was a highly laborer earning $11,000 a year. The child had glomerulonephritis, and by e she was nine years old was suffering from end-stage renal disease. The olerated dialysis very poorly, screaming and crying during much of the s. She also tolerated the hospital regimen very badly in general and became ical, angry, and difficult. Family members were unwilling or unable to e kidney donors, and the child received a kidney from a cadaver source. discharged, she became much more active, began to grow, and side effects he necessary steroid medication appeared minimal. However, the kidney on was never completely normal; her blood tests indicated chronic rejec-

months after the transplant, kidney function seriously deteriorated to the where life could not be long maintained, and she was rehospitalized. The course of treatment at this point would be to remove the immunologically ed kidney, place the patient back on dialysis, and plan for a second trans- if the family desired. This was explained to the family, along with the fact he statistics for a second transplant were almost the same as those for a first plant, and that many second-transplanted children were doing very well.

use this case occurred prior to federal funding for transplantation and use the family's income was too high for Medicaid or welfare funds, the cost e treatment had been extreme in this large family. Half of the yearly income been spent for the child's bills, and some medical expenses were still unpaid.

parents felt cadaver donor statistics were not good enough and that the child ered too much on dialysis. They therefore decided to allow the child to die.

child, who was extremely ill, expressed a fear of death to one of the nurses. ne members of the medical staff were very angry and tried to convince the ily that their decision was an error. When the family insisted, some of the sicians raised the question of taking the family to court in order that dialysis ld be reinstituted to save the child's life. Yet because dialysis and transplanta- n were relatively new technologies and still called experimental by some, ether the courts would rule in their favor was unclear. The family was not en to court, and the child died within two weeks. Some staff members were set that the family had not been given more emotional support after making eir decision.

The issue of whether patient consent to withdraw treatment has been btained can be particularly difficult in cases where medical complica- ons have led to impaired communication. Such complications are more kely among high-risk diabetic patients. One diabetic woman had

High-Risk Patients: Psychological Problems

In the case of costly new therapies, then, it is likely that physicians will be confronted by difficult situations for which no clear norms have been established—particularly in relation to the selection of patients. A frequent reaction will be to set up national, regional, or local policymaking committees of peers to deal with these issues. However, some situations—particularly those involving the selection of patients at risk psychologically—will have to be handled by the physicians on an individual basis. For example, if liver transplants become more successful, "reformed" alcoholics may have to be evaluated individually for treatment (see Rybak, 1974). Psychiatrically vulnerable kidney patients currently present the staff with difficult decisions. In the following case, for instance, the physicians and staff were divided as to whether to recommend a second kidney transplant and whether to allow the patient to withdraw from dialysis (see Fox and Swazey, 1974, Ch. 10 for a similar case).

CASE 3 A 16-Year-Old Boy with End-Stage Renal Disease

A youngster with a history of delinquency tolerated the artificial kidney (dialysis machine) poorly and frequently failed to take the medicines designed to control his kidney disease. His family, which was from out of state, was unable to control this behavior and had given up attempting to do so. He particularly hated to be penned up in an institution and would run away from the hospital, although he never missed a dialysis treatment. His fear of death was great, and many staff members felt there was a direct relationship between his delinquent acts and events that to him appeared life-threatening.

The question in the minds of the medical staff was whether this youngster could show the discipline necessary to take the enormous battery of daily posttransplant pills necessary to prevent the kidney from being rejected, to have frequent blood-tests, and to show up at the hospital when called.

The transplant staff was reluctant to deny treatment on such social and psychological grounds and decided to accept him for transplantation. The next question was whether to risk a related kidney on him. Although his chances would not be so good with a cadaver organ, the staff decided against a related donor in his case. Within a few months he received a cadaver transplant which worked very well. However, posttransplant, perhaps in reaction to certain distressing aspects of his life, he continued delinquent behavior and twice stopped taking his medications for several days. Both times, he was readmitted to the hospital and treated for a rejection crisis. After the first occasion he was informed that if he destroyed his own kidney by failing to take the antirejection medicines, he would not be given a second transplant nor be allowed dialysis. This threat of death was an attempt to motivate him to follow directions; also the social work and psychiatric staff offered him much help. He was no longer living with his family at this point but had been placed in foster homes.

When he was readmitted the second time he said as he had previously, that he had learned his lesson and that he wished to live. His kidney lost all function and had to be removed.

The staff was in some conflict whether (1) the youngster should be put back on chronic dialysis treatment, which he tolerated poorly and which was very expensive, (2) a second scarce cadaver kidney should be allocated to him, or (3) he should be allowed to die.

The decision was made to remove the rejected kidney and place him back on dialysis for a considerable length of time before considering retransplantation.

After this procedure the youngster began to refuse treatment, although he was inconsistent in this refusal. The staff was not sure how to react to his refusal of treatment. Neither the psychiatrist nor the social worker appeared to be able to gain his trust at that time.

Withdrawal of Treatment

The original decision whether to accept a patient for treatment and the subsequent decision to withdraw treatment are inextricably intertwined. If in retrospect the original decision appears dubious, if the patient does not respond well to the treatment, one alternative is to terminate therapy, particularly if the patient is overtly suicidal himself. Yet the moral discomfort of allowing the life of a patient to end when the patient has been known intimately over a long time can be even greater than that involved in refusing treatment to a stranger (Fox and Swazey, 1974, Ch. 9, Epilogue). The issue of terminating therapy is definitely one of normative uncertainty and conflict for the physicians involved.

Insisting that the decision be the patient's alone would seem to remove the onus from the physician. If the patient wishes to continue treatment, the cost must be borne by government and staff. If he wishes to terminate after attempts at psychiatric therapy, he must have the "right to die." Yet there is much controversy among professionals as to the amount of intervention necessary when a patient expresses a desire to die. Professionals differ in the extent to which they believe a depressed patient is capable of making such a decision (Abram et al., 1971; Fox and Swazey, 1974, p. 62). There is a basic distinction between physicians who see the

depression as temporary and the individual as
life-stress if given extensive help and those w
life" for certain transplant and dialysis patien
continuation from any realistic standpoint.

The situation becomes more complex if the
seen as factors affecting the depression of the
transplant has failed and the patient is tolerat
causing great difficulty for the staff, feelings of ar
ness frequently emerge, according to social w
reports (Kaplan De-Nour and Czaczkes, 1974; Le
long-term interaction may result in the patient bei
A social worker from a busy transplant-dialysis se
ing case:

CASE 4 A 16-Year-Old Girl

The girl had rejected two transplants, each of which had
Due to very large doses of steroids, her face was extrem
giving her an abnormal appearance. Her growth had
shortness made her feel like an outsider. She commente
belong to the organized group of midgets and too shor
peers her own age. She had few friends and currently wa
with her parents.

When returned to dialysis after rejecting the second tr
depressed and suicidal. She was extremely uncooperative
ing and expressing hostility toward the nurses. The nur
others their belief that the girl had nothing to live for, and
that unconscious invitations to suicide were being made to
of an interesting aside, the girl was told by a nurse about th
death that sometimes results from ignoring dietary restric

The danger of accepting a suicidal wish at face value
also a strong feeling among many professionals that
have the right to terminate treatment and be supporte
termination period.

If the patient is an adult, his right to make his own de
as inviolable. The ethical problems for the staff when th
and the parents are the ones who wish to withdraw treat
even more difficult.

rejected two kidneys and had lost her eyesight and one foot due to diabetic vascular disease. She was too weak to walk. Then she became deafened as a rare side effect of some of her medications. After surviving dialysis for more than a year, she started to become intermittantly confused and would sometimes threaten her younger children. At that point the family and physicians agreed that the quality of her life was so poor and her suffering so great that dialysis should be discontinued. Although there had been a definite attempt to "discuss" this decision with the patient, the physician was unclear whether the deaf-blind woman comprehended until, as she was leaving the last dialysis, she turned her wheelchair around to face the staff and said, "Thank you for all you tried to do." One of the dialysis technicians, who was very attached to the patient, expressed anger that the patient's own feelings had not been the major basis of the decision.*

The National Kidney Foundation has recently recognized the severity of the problem of how to discontinue dialysis and has sent out a letter requesting information from all members as to their customs so that such information might be disseminated:

> A number of physicians have indicated increasing problems on how to discontinue dialysis. This situation seems to come about as the result of increasingly liberalized selection criteria and the fact that after many years of dialysis, patients can develop increasing signs of pulmonary, cardiac or cerebral disease. In the latter situation, patients may become very combative in the unit with physical abuse of personnel and equipment. It may lead to eventual confinement in a nursing home or state mental hospital. Despite intense psychiatric, psychological, and staff efforts over many months, a few patients never seem to adequately adjust to the treatment regimen. Some physicians have been threatened with law suits should they discontinue dialysis even under these somewhat adverse or even precarious situations.

ORGAN DONORS: SOCIETAL NORMS

Normative uncertainty related to patient selection and continuation of treatment is equalled by societal and medical uncertainties involving the selection of an organ donor. The patient's opportunity to receive a transplanted organ has been limited not only by the scarcity of personnel, hospital beds, financial support, and the need to meet selection criteria but also by the fact that transplantation requires the unique resource of healthy, transplantable human organs. As indicated earlier, transplant-

* See Crane (1975) for other discussions of discontinuation of lifesaving therapy.

able organs may be obtained from one of three potential donor sources: (1) living donors related to the potential recipient; (2) living donors unrelated to the recipient; and (3) cadaver organ donors. At present the demand for organs exceeds the supply. Because the prognosis is so favorable, a certain proportion of donated organs will be provided by relatives. However, kidney patients who have no related donors may wait on dialysis for years for a suitable organ because of the shortage of cadaver organs (Gallagher and Morelock, 1974). With the increase in patients being accepted for treatment due to the HR-1 government support, the shortage appears to be increasing. In New York City one transplanter reports that there are more than 1500 patients waiting for cadaver kidneys.

The unprecedented demand for this type of resource has created a situation in which appropriate medical and social norms have been lacking and laws have been absent.

CADAVER DONORS: MEDICAL NORMS

Three basic issues should be considered regarding the ethical problems and normative uncertainty surrounding the use of cadaver organs: When can a potential donor be defined as dead? How can the powerless cadaver donor be protected? Should family or individual consent for the donation of cadaver organs be eliminated?

Definition of Death: Medical-Legal Norms

With the need for cadaver donors has come a redefinition of death itself. As will become evident below, this area has clearly been one of cultural lag; laws have not kept pace with the new technological potential. The attempt to create new medical norms has been impeded by lags in the legal system in this and other societies and by uncertainties as to proper action.

Within the medical world itself there has been a widespread ethical concern about the determination of death for the cadaver donor, and most medical centers have formulated careful guidelines to redefine death in accord with new medical standards. In the past conventional definitions of death had depended on cessation of heart action, but such a definition has threatened to encumber transplant technology by "unnecessarily" ruining the relevant organ (Stickel, 1966). When the heart and the circulation of blood stop, the kidney or other organs can be badly damaged. Under the leadership of Beecher at Harvard Medical School a new concept of brain death has been carefully defined. Utilizing specific signs and tests, physicians can declare death before the heart has stopped beating, and the circulatory system can be maintained until the time the organ is removed from the body (Moore et al., 1968; "New Dimensions in Legal and Ethical Concepts for Human Research," 1969).

In line with this new concept of brain death, currently in the United States most prospective donors are declared dead when the physicians are certain there is no brain activity and that life cannot be continued without artificial support. The patient's respiration and heartbeat are then maintained by the artificial respirator until the healthy organs to be transplanted can be removed. Only at that point is artificial support of the circulation and heartbeat abandoned.

While the brain death criterion has been widely used by individual physicians in the United States, ethical debate has been rampant. In many other countries, such as Sweden, the utilization of brain death was not originally considered legal—such a concept was not thought to afford adequate protection for the patient-cadaver ("Kidney Grafting in Sweden," 1973). In the United States the lag in the legal system has taken another form. The issue is not that brain death is definitely thought illegal, but that the absence of a law about the issue has caused considerable difficulty. Nine states have laws recognizing the legitimacy of brain death and several others are considering such legislation ("Bar Assn. Urges," 1975; "Dearth of Donor Organs," 1974). In most states, however, the patient is defined as dead when a physician has declared him so and signed a death certificate.

Because of this lack of any law, lawyers have warned that the physician exceeds the law whenever he takes a patient off a respirator (McFadden, 1972; Arnet, 1973). In fact, brain death has been challenged through the courts. In a Virginia court case in 1972 a donor's family claimed that the transplant surgeons who removed the heart had been responsible for the death.* The jury ruled against the donor's family, declaring the donor had been legally dead because of the prior irreversible death of his brain. This was considered a landmark case, the first instance of the court's acceptance of the concept of brain death (Schmeck, 1972; "Virginia Jury Rules," 1972).

Yet even by 1974 the issue had not been settled. In two cases in California that year brain death was again legally challenged by lawyers

* Tucker's Administrator vs. Lower. Case #2831. Court of Law and Equity, Richmond, Virginia, May 25, 1972. Similarly, in Buenos Aires a heart transplanter was tried for the murder of two cadaver donors ("Transplant Pioneer Faces Murder Charge," 1968), and in England a murderer claimed it was the transplanter who killed the donor (Leavell, 1973) because the heart had been beating in the brain-dead patient before it was removed for transplantation.

for two men accused of murder and manslaughter. In these cases the murder victims had been hospitalized and placed on the machinery that artificially maintained their heartbeat and respiration, and physicians later declared them "brain dead" before removing their hearts for transplantation. The defence lawyers in the cases claimed their clients could not be found guilty of murder, because the heart was beating at the time it was removed for transplantation, and therefore the donor was alive. The concept of brain death would no longer have been a viable one if the two alleged murderers were released on the grounds that their victims were not legally dead until later when their hearts were removed by transplant surgeons. The California court, however, ruled against the defendants and in favor of the criterion of brain death.

Many transplanters are in favor of resolving these legal ambiguities through clear-cut laws that would not only provide legal protection for the transplant surgeon but would help to persuade certain "gatekeepers" to aid transplantation efforts. For a transplant surgeon to utilize a cadaver donor, another physician has to approach the family and refer the patient; frequently that physician (or another physician or a committee) has to declare the patient brain dead without disconnecting the respirator. If there is a question of homicide or suicide, the medical examiner or coroner has to give authorization for use of the organs. All of these "gatekeepers" may be dissuaded by the threat of legal complications or suit. In fact, major conflicts have occurred between transplant surgeons and state examiners who were unwilling for homicide victims to be used (Connally, 1968; Graham, 1973; "Kidney Grafting in Sweden," 1973). In New York transplanters deliberately made use of the organs of a homicide victim despite this official opposition in order to force a court test of brain death (Prial, 1975).

Laws recognizing brain death could resolve this conflict in favor of transplantation. The House of Delegates of the American Bar Association recently voted in favor of the passage of such laws at the state level "Bar Assn. Urges," 1975). Lawyers point to the danger of operating through the courts (Capron and Kass, 1972) and particularly of allowing the definition of death to depend on the vagaries of the jury system. While one jury, as in Virginia, may rule in favor of brain death, another jury in a different case could make a very different decision.*

The American Medical Association (AMA), however, is worried that any specific legal definition of death will be inappropriate for certain situations and will be rapidly outdated by scientific advances. In addition,

* In fact, in earlier cases when the issue was not transplantation, but which spouse died first and which spouse's will took precedence, the courts ruled against brain death and insisted upon cessation of heartbeat (Arnet, 1973).

insofar as such laws remove the determination of death from individual physician judgment, they are regarded by the AMA as a threat to professional autonomy and as a political roadblock to future technological progress. Thus the House of Delegates of the American Medical Association adopted a resolution that "the present statutory definition of death is not desirable or necessary. . . .Death should be determined by the clinical judgment of the physician using. . .currently accepted criteria" (Masland, 1975). Other nonmedical persons, however, emphasize the necessity for nonphysicians to be involved in this ultimate question of the definition of death (Capron and Kass, 1972).

State laws like those of Kansas, California, and Georgia* that simply recognize the legitimacy of brain death are more acceptable to organized medicine than laws that attempt to define it specifically ("Dearth of Donor Organs," 1974; Frederick, 1972). Yet several law review articles press for explicit definitions to protect the cadaver donor and the transplant physician; indeed, some lawyers appear to want a list of definite signs and tests such as that advanced by the Harvard group (Arnet, 1973; Frederick, 1972).

The fact that at present brain death is not a clearly defined clinical entity makes matters more complex and uncertain. There is a wide difference of opinion between doctors as to what precautions are justified and important in identifying the death of the brain (Arnet, 1973; Black, 1975; Hamburger and Crosnier, 1968; Masland, 1975; Van Till-d'Aulnis de Bourouill, 1975; Vaux, 1969; Visscher, 1970). Although there usually seems to be little problem in identifying a particular patient as having irreversible loss of brain function, the tests currently considered necessary to confirm this judgment differ from center to center. Some feel the Harvard criteria are too strict; others feel that they are not strict enough; and some will not accept responsibility for brain death at all. In some centers the heart and lung machine must be turned off after death is declared to be certain the patient is incapable of breathing on his own; in others the machine is discontinued only after the organ is removed ("New Dimensions in Legal and Ethical Concepts," 1969; Silverman et al., 1969). Some physicians do not use the electroencephalogram (EEG) routinely; some physicians believe that the EEG should be flat for three to four hours; while others insist on 24 to 48 hours (Savage, 1969; Silverman et al., 1969).

Still other physicians claim the EEGs are inadequate indicators because a few patients have recovered after registering lack of brain activity for somewhat longer periods (Durdin, 1968). The American Electroencephalographic Society reports that such cases exist but are very few in

* The passage of the law in Georgia resulted almost immediately in an increase of cadaver donors, apparently because referring physicians felt "safer."

number: Out of 1665 cases of flat EEGs surveyed, only three recovered some cerebral function. Based on a study of its members, this society reports that most members accepted the Harvard criteria of brain death but felt no absolute indicators could be established—the physician must decide in each case (Silverman et al., 1969).

Whatever the rational acceptance of this new criterion of brain death, family and medical staff have reported emotional difficulties and uncertainty when they have seen potential cadaver donors apparently still breathing (see Chapter 10 and Munster, 1974). As the wife of one cadaver donor put it:

> But when I walked in and saw Sam, there he was breathing, his chest moving up and down. I felt he was alive, even though he couldn't recognize me, even though the machines were breathing for him. Dear God, Sam seemed alive. But all the time, even before they pronounced it—he was dead. It was strange (Graham, 1973).

From a 1970 survey of doctors and nurses in two general hospitals in Great Britain, Crosby and Waters (1972) report that approximately half agree that they have misgivings about cadaver donation because of "difficulties regarding the decision on when a patient has actually died." British physicians have been reluctant to recognize brain death and still rely on a circulatory criterion of death.

The end of life has become ambiguous. Largely due to the requirements of transplant technology, a new fundamental distinction has been made between the death of the body and the death of the person. However, this change appears minor in comparison to the "grotesque" science fiction-type outcome envisioned by Gaylin (1974). If technology improves enough to maintain the brain-dead in respirators for several years, he feels that there is the possibility of institutions full of "neo-morts," full of "warm, respirating, pulsating, evacuating, and excreting bodies requiring nursing, dietary, and general grooming attention." Such living dead would be incapable of pain or perception and could be utilized as sources of organs, blood, and bone marrow. They could also be used as experimental animals and as training vehicles for neophyte physicians and surgeons. Gaylin questions whether the revulsion engendered by this picture is simply the conservative reaction to any major change or represents a valid reaction to a fundamental loss of human dignity. Aside from the medical and economic problems of this fantasy, one might ask whether individuals can separate personal identity from the body sharply enough to allow such an institution?

Of course, alternate technological advances may obviate the need for cadaver donation altogether. Immunological breakthroughs allowing the use of animal organs in humans could eliminate the entire problem. Although animal-to-human heart transplants have been attempted, success will require major innovations. The possibility of an artificial man-made heart also could reduce the need for cadaver donation.

In the interim the uncertainties surrounding the determination of the moment of death remain, and the potential cadaver donor requires protection.

Protection of the Potential Cadaver Donor

In addition to the question of how to define death, standards concerning who should declare death have had to be established. To avoid conflict of interest, the agreement has generally been made that the prospective donor should be cared for by a group other than transplant surgeons and that the transplant team cannot be involved in the declaration of death (Merrill, 1968b).

The situation is more complex than is often recognized. No one questions the fact that a donor's own chance for life must be protected and that the transplant team should not be allowed to hasten the process of death. But the question arises whether the neurologist and the transplant team should consult each other before the donor's death concerning treatment that will benefit the *organ* to be donated. If insufficient attention is paid to the fluid balance of the patient, as occurs sometimes with hopeless patients, the patient will die with a useless kidney. Should the transplant team be allowed to question this type of inadequate therapy? Fortunately what is good for the kidney will usually be good for the patient (Stickel, 1966). At the University of Minnesota and elsewhere, several patients who were expected to die, recovered, partially because of the advice of the transplant team (Crosbie, 1970). Whatever the benefits that might accrue to the dying donor himself, some discomfort and uncertainty has been expressed concerning the institution of any therapy designed *primarily* to benefit the needed organ (Stickel, 1966).

In much of the discussion of this problem in the literature, the larger context has been ignored (Wasmuth, 1969). The question is not simply when a prospective donor should be declared dead, but how long any apparently hopeless patient should be treated by extraordinary means. Transplantation has alerted the society to an already existing problem, and this may be the reason physicians seem to be less disturbed by the issue than are outsiders who are less aware of existing practices. Patients whose brains are destroyed have routinely died in the past, not because their bodies could not be kept alive for a longer period but because extraordinary care either was not instituted or was purposefully discontinued (see Leavell, 1973).

In fact, the unconscious brain-damaged donor is frequently kept alive longer because of transplantation. If the hopeless patient had not been selected as a donor, some of the extraordinary treatment would have been discontinued: The respirator machine would have been turned off; corrective fluids and blood transfusions would not have been used; and cardiac massage would not be utilized if the heart stopped. For the cadaver donor all of these extraordinary measures persist until brain death can be definitely declared, sometimes prolonging the agony for relatives. The relatives are told that although all brain activity has not yet ceased, their comatose relative is essentially dead. Yet during the waiting period, unrealistic feelings of hope can alternate with grief and anxiety over the correctness of the decision to donate. Usually this extension of life amounts at the most to two or three days. However, in one case an unconscious patient with extensive brain damage stayed alive without the artificial respirator for six months after donation had been suggested because the brain in fact was not yet dead.

Changes in any laws that specify brain-death criteria should have an impact on all terminal patients requiring artificial respiration, not simply cadaver donors. In this era in which emphasis is being placed on the right to die with dignity and without unnecessary, expensive, and extraordinary care, such laws may force physicians in the opposite direction. The widely publicized Karen Quinlan Case ("In the Matter of Karen Quinlan," 1976) led lawyers to envision a lawsuit similar to the Virginia case in which a physician who removes a hopeless patient from a respirator is accused of homicide, although cadaver donation was not an issue. As one physician comments in regard to the brain-death criteria:

> (These) criteria. . .have their usefulness primarily in relation to. . .organ transplantation. . . .It would be a *reductio ad absurdum* that every terminal patient must be placed in a respirator and kept there until he has a flat EEG before being declared dead (Masland, 1975, p. 52).

Cadaver Organs and the Ethics of Consent

Currently in the United States cadaver donation can be made only if the individual has willed his organs earlier or his family gives consent when brain death becomes apparent. The disadvantage of this system is the severe shortage of cadaver organs. A more rapid way to tap the potential source of cadaver organs would be a widespread change in the law to permit the state to remove organs without family permission unless the individual had expressed opposition to donation during his lifetime (Castel, 1968, 1972; Duckeminier and Sanders, 1968; Louisell and Kilbrandon, 1966). Countries such as Israel, France, Sweden, Hungary, and Austria have had similar laws (Herbich, 1972; Wright, 1969), and one has been proposed recently in Great Britain ("Transplant of Human Organs," 1974). Even in the United States there are four states (Virginia, Maryland, California, and Hawaii) that have passed laws permitting medical examiners to give permission for the use of organs for transplantation without the consent of family or prior consent of the individual if there is not enough time to notify the family and if they have no known objection ("The Sale of Human Body Parts," 1974). Unclaimed bodies could be considered appropriate under this law. For example, according to California's Diligent Search Act, organs can be used for transplantation if no relatives are found after an extensive 24-hour investigation that includes searching missing-person files, the patient's belongings, questioning all visitors, and so on (Chatterjee et al., 1975).

However, the question of whether consent is ethically necessary for cadaver donation is far from settled. One widely publicized court case arose as a result of the law in Virginia. Family members sued the hospital and the transplant physician for failing to exert enough effort in reaching them before allegedly terminating the life of the patient by removing the heart. The family of Bruce Tucker, a 54-year-old black laborer, claimed that they had been unsuccessfully calling the hospital for information; while the defendants said they had been unable to find a family member (Schmeck, 1972; "Virginia Jury Rules," 1972). Similarly, in South Africa where there is a comparable law, a widow of a transplant donor claimed that Dr. Barnard and authorities neither asked her permission for the donation nor informed her of her husband's impending death. She allegedly was under the impression her husband was improving only hours before his heart was removed. The authorities who gave permission claimed they did not know the donor was married ("Racism Is Charged," 1971; "Widow," 1971).

In both cases racism was an issue because the donor was black and the recipient white. The publicity attached to these cases and to two recent court cases in California threatened to erode the sympathy many lay persons, referring doctors, and coroners had toward organ donation (Capron, 1974; Graham, 1973).

Whether a law allowing the removal of organs without family permission could pass in most states is problematic. Organized resistance to such a law might develop in many regions (Frye, 1969), but the generally positive attitudes toward organ donation might permit passage in some states. A Gallup poll taken in January 1968 indicated that 70% of the adult

American population claims to be willing to donate an organ upon their death.

Mechanisms to Obtain Voluntary Consent

Without laws obviating the necessity for explicit signed consent, cadaver donation is dependent upon favorable attitudes in the population at large. In the future attitudes may become favorable enough for organ donation to become the custom. Over time norms could emerge such that the family and the physician of a dying patient would consider donation a social obligation thereby increasing the cadaver organ supply. Currently, however, while a favorable attitude exists in some population segments, there are still significant ethical concerns and uncertainties about cadaver donation that have been expressed in the popular literature.

Many popular articles have detailed the *ethical dangers* of transplantation. One major concern has been that the poor and powerless will be exploited as donors for more advantaged citizens (Kass, 1968). Fear of undue pressure to donate organs and of inferior medical care of the dying patient has also been expressed. The fear that physicians will hasten one's threatened death rather than provide vigorous treatment has even been dealt with humorously in the popular culture. At one point a lapel button was manufactured that read "Drive Carefully, Dr. Barnard is waiting." Underlying ambivalence toward organ donation undoubtedly exists, despite the generally positive attitudes of 70% of the population.

Whether the lower classes are particularly fearful of exploitation in this regard is unknown. However, according to the Gallup poll and several other studies, the less-educated segment of the population is less positive toward organ donation (see Cleveland and Johnson, 1970; Fellner and Schwartz, 1971; Simmons et al., 1974).

The more negative attitudes of the less educated correspond with other research on the attitudes of blue-collar and white-collar persons toward medicine. Blue-collar subjects in New York City were less knowledgeable about illness; less likely to take preventative medical precautions; less acceptant of the sick role; and most important, more skeptical about the efficacy of medical care (Rosenblatt and Suchman, 1964).

Favorable attitudes toward cadaver donation are thus not distributed evenly throughout the population. In addition to the less educated, older individuals are also less positive, perhaps reflecting a more traditional view of death. In fact there is evidence that persons more favorable toward organ donation demonstrate a different configuration of life attitudes than do others. Simmons et al. (1974) showed that persons willing to sign donor cards that legally bequest their organs for transplantation after death held less traditional more secular attitudes toward religion, death, and funeral practices than a control group of neighbors, even when age and education were controlled. They were more likely to relate to religion in a less conventional manner; they attended church less frequently; they were more likely to believe that religious values were congruent with modern science; and they seemed more favorable to science in general. They were less sure of the existence of an afterlife, less likely to see the body as sacred after death, more positive toward cremation, and less committed to having the body present at the funeral.

Thus while favorable attitudes toward cadaver donation are widespread, uncertainties exist in certain categories of the population. Still, Gallup has projected the 70% of persons favorable into 80 million individuals, a vast source of potential donors. There are legal mechanisms to facilitate donation for those who wish to do so.

All legal limitation to donating one's own body has been rapidly erased because of a vigorous well-organized campaign by physicians and lawyers. All 50 states have passed the Uniform Anatomical Gift Act, which allows persons to will their organs for transplantation simply by signing a wallet-sized card with two witnesses (Castel, 1972; Leavell, 1973; Sadler et al., 1970; Schmeck, 1970). That opposition to the bill was minimal is remarkable in the face of concern about the ethical issues.

There is a great difference, however, in the motivation necessary to sign the donor card and that required to express a simple positive attitude on a poll. We cannot assume that the 70% of American adults who answered the Gallup Poll question favorably have actually signed the cards or will sign them, although there has been considerable interest in the program (see Moores et al., 1976; Sadler et al., 1969a).*

Even if a number of persons carry these cards, there are still great logistical problems in identifying such donors and in contacting a transplant center rapidly enough (Louisell and Kilbrandon, 1966). In most cases the next of kin still has to inform the local physicians of the dying patient's wishes, and the local physicians and hospital have to be motivated to expend effort in setting the process in motion. The emotional character of the death intensifies the difficulties. Because the organs of elderly patients are not so useful, the best donor is a relatively young person whose death is usually a sudden tragedy for the family—as in the case of an automobile accident. During this highly emotional time the

* In Minnesota more than 3000 individuals responded to a TV and newspaper donor campaign and requested a card to sign that would volunteer their organs in the event of their death. *Modern Medicine*, a magazine that is sent to 210,000 physicians, received requests for 32,000 donor cards from physicians and medical societies after an issue publicized the uniform donor card and included a sheet of six cards.

cadaver donation issue may not occur to the family, and the physician who has "failed" to save the brain-dead patient may experience emotional difficulty in reminding the grieving family of the possibility of donation (see Chatterjee et al., 1975).

Therefore, it is unlikely that a great number of those who sign donor cards will ever actually contribute organs; the supply of organs will probably not be increased directly by this means. In the six years since the donor-card program was instituted in Minnesota, only three or four donor-card signees have actually been used. However, the campaign and publicity about donor cards may have important *indirect* effects. The local physicians and the population in general may become more alert to the possibility and the need for donation; some may find it easier to consider donating the body parts of a dying relative or patient. Although customs related to religious and emotionally significant events are notoriously slow to change, in the long run the campaign may help to produce some change.

In summary, there are many normative and ethical uncertainties regarding the use of cadaver donors. Problems of the definition of death, of protection of the potential donor, and of the necessity for explicit consent have received much attention. Currently in the United States mobilization of the scarce cadaver donor resource has depended upon voluntary consent of individuals and families. While favorable attitudes appear widespread in the population, certain subgroups appear to be more ambivalent. Laws removing the necessity for explicit consent on the part of the potential donor or his family and laws recognizing the validity of brain death would appear to facilitate the efficient use of cadaver donation, at the same time as they raise ethical concerns. Different countries and even different states within the United States vary in their acceptance of such laws. As Titmuss (1971) and Fox and Swazey (1974) have noted, society can encourage or discourage the altruistic tendency in man, and in this case the existing laws have not always been encouraging.

LIVING UNRELATED DONORS: MEDICAL NORMS

Should They Be Used?

One method of alleviating the kidney shortage and avoiding many of the cadaver problems would be to utilize living volunteers unrelated to the organ recipient. However, the lack of clear norms governing such a situation has discouraged many centers from tapping this source.

At one time at one center penal volunteers were used as unrelated kidney donors (Crosbie, 1970). The practice was discontinued on the grounds that "the use of penal volunteers, however equitably handled in a local situation, would inevitably lead to abuse if accepted as a reasonable precedent and applied broadly" (Starzl, 1966a).

Most other centers have refrained from using unrelated living donors due to ethical considerations of this type and to the failure of such kidneys to function any better than cadaver kidneys. However, the University of California Hospitals in San Franciso at one point did use living unrelated volunteers. Sadler (1970) and associates studied the psychiatric aspects. In one year three public appeals for volunteer donors generated calls from 200 persons; 22 became serious volunteers. Careful screening indicated that 17 of these were without psychological problems and that most were middle-class stable citizens, married, with children. No social and psychological complications were noted in the donors.

Seventeen additional donors a year is not an inconsiderable number for a transplant program. Fellner and Schwartz (1971) surveyed a random sampling of adults in one midwestern city and reported that a considerable number of people were willing to consider donating an organ to a stranger. In a survey in Detroit, Gade (1972) found 41% so willing. However, most transplant surgeons are unsure of the ethics of subjecting an unrelated person to a nephrectomy and the small risk to his life and health without a significant advantage to the recipient over cadaver donation. Fellner and Schwartz (1971) criticize the medical profession for an undue distrust of the motives of such potential donors (also see Katz and Capron, 1975 and Chapter 6 for more discussion of the donor issue).

In addition to strangers, several other types of living "unrelated" donors are not generally used. The most willing family member, the patient's spouse, is genetically unrelated to the recipient. Close friends are also not allowed to donate. Yet in informal discussions some transplant surgeons have raised the possibility of screening spouses or close friends for particularly good tissue matches. At the moment the existing norms seem to have prevented such a course at most centers.

Should Donors Be Paid?

The issue of whether both living and cadaver donors are to be paid has been extensively discussed. J. Hamburger, President of the Transplantation Society, in 1970 sent a letter to the French Ministry of Health urging an international convention that would forbid the purchase and sale of organs. Hamburger noted the dangers of blackmail, of unfair advantage over the poor and the captive and of coercion in nations where personal liberties are not protected. However, the reaction to this letter at the First International Symposium on the Socio-Medical Aspects of Organ Transplantation at Houston, Texas, March 1970, indicates that this area also has been one of normative uncertainty. One physician reported that a wealthy patient at his center had advertised internationally for a kidney. He asked how the hospital should react if the patient arrived at the center with a matched and willing donor. Strong opinions were voiced on both sides of the question. One clergyman, who believed no stance should be taken on this issue, noted that in the American culture, "He who pays, gets." He suggested that the area of organ donation need not be an exception (Savage, 1969). Others did not wish to pass premature laws at this time that might restrict transplantation at a later date.

In contrast, other members of the symposium noted that most transplant facilities had been heavily supported with public funds. This discussion took place prior to the passage of the HR-1 amendment to fund kidney transplantation, and some members thought that if scarce places in these programs were filled by persons who could afford to purchase an organ, there would be even less opportunity for the poor to secure treatment, even though they had contributed to the taxes that supported the program.

The prices for organs are likely to involve thousands of dollars. In July 1971 *Newsweek Magazine* published a story of a suffering dialysis patient who was offering $3000 for a cadaver kidney with appropriate match and suitable for transplantation ("I Can't Take It Anymore," 1971, p. 51) (Figure 2-1). The patient received several offers, and the next week *Newsweek* reported that he had received a kidney ("A Kidney in Time," 1971). In fact the hospital had refused to accept a "bought" kidney, but

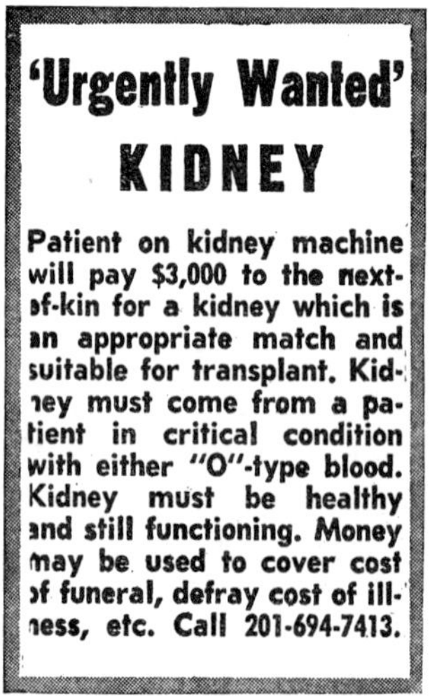

'Urgently Wanted'

KIDNEY

Patient on kidney machine will pay $3,000 to the next-of-kin for a kidney which is an appropriate match and suitable for transplant. Kidney must come from a patient in critical condition with either "O"-type blood. Kidney must be healthy and still functioning. Money may be used to cover cost of funeral, defray cost of illness, etc. Call 201-694-7413.

Figure 2-1.

this refusal was not made clear in the national magazine. If advertisement were to become general and there was an opportunity to secure such high prices, voluntary donation of organs both from relatives and cadaver families might be decreased.

In September 1970, prior to the *Newsweek* articles, the International Transplantation Society meeting in the Hague issued a policy designed to discourage such practices. But more recently an article in the *Michigan Law Review* ("The Sale of Human Body Parts," 1974) recommended a reversal of this policy to increase the supply of cadaver organs.

The issue would be completely different if the model of blood donation were imitated and if the government, hospital, or insurance company paid for the organ. Because the recipients would not have to pay out of their own resources, all recipients would still have an equal chance to obtain the scarce cadaver organ (see Etzioni, 1974). But the cost of transplantation would rise significantly. Interim guidelines of the government dealing with the implementation of the HR-1 amendment state clearly that for any kidney patient whose treatment is federally supported, no program reimbursement may be made for the kidney itself—that is, if the donor sells his kidney, the purchase price may not be reflected in any program payment. Thus the government will not pay for cadaver kidneys, though the costs involved in removing and transporting the organ are covered by Medicare. The patient himself is not prevented from paying the donor's family for a kidney. The ethical problem is still left unsettled. No normative consensus exists on this issue or on most issues involving organ donation (Hamburger and Crosnier, 1968).

MEDICAL NORMS CONCERNING RELATED DONORS

Should They Be Used?

Physicians are also uncertain regarding the controversial issue of related donors. The attitude of the staff toward the ethics of donation and the physician's own role in this area seem to vary from institution to institution. In several institutions the policy has been to discourage living donors. In Australia only 2% of the transplants have utilized living donors and in Europe only 15%; in contrast, in the United States as a whole 35% have utilized living donors (Salaman, 1974), and 66% have been used at the University of Minnesota. The sacrifice of a normal organ and the jeopardy to a normal life is considered unethical in many places (McGeown, 1968; "Kidneys from Living Donors," 1974). In the words of one Swiss surgeon:

> The question whether in fact this [related organ donation] should be done is still unanswered; we ourselves believe. . .only material from cadavers should be used and that removing kidneys from living donors. . .is now out-of-date and should cease. . . .It is true that the success rate. . .of cadaver material is somewhat lower, but rejected grafts can be replaced, and it is better to operate twice on a recipient than to operate once on him and once on a healthy donor (Largiadèr, 1971).

Opponents to related donation have also emphasized the danger of family blackmail and involuntary consent on the part of the donor (Brewer, 1970; Katz and Capron, 1975).

On the other hand, some centers try to restrict their patients to those with living related donors because they wish to devote the limited resources of equipment, money, and personnel to the cases that have the best prognosis. Such centers are aware of the Human Renal Transplant Registry statistics showing that 74% of patients with sibling donors survive two years posttransplant with functioning kidneys, in comparison to only 43% of the patients with cadaver kidneys ("Twelfth Report of the Human Renal Transplant Registry," 1975). Viewed from a different perspective, the chance for failure is 30% for sibling kidneys and nearly double that figure for cadaver kidneys. Furthermore, the advocates of related donors point out the fact that rejected grafts often cannot be successfully replaced and that the death rate following cadaver transplantation is much higher than for related transplantation. To the personnel in these programs the tremendous added benefit to the recipient seems to outweigh the slim risks to the donor (Hamburger and Crosnier, 1968) and the chance that a few donors will conceal their reluctance (Stickel, 1966). (However, there is evidence that improved tissue typing for cadavers may in the future lead to better survival of cadaver grafts. Whether the discrepancy between cadavers and related will ever be effectively erased remains an open question.)

Still other institutions accept patients regardless of their donor source and expend either more or less effort in obtaining a family donor. If no related donor can be found, a cadaver is used. The Minnesota Kidney Transplant Program is in this category, and great emphasis is placed on securing related donors if possible. To these surgeons not only is the success rate better, but the patients who must obtain a cadaver kidney are benefited because the waiting list is shortened when those who can secure family donors are removed.

In programs where related donors are used, the transplant surgeon may find himself in a difficult position—asking a relative to donate a kidney is stressful for the doctor and virtually unparalleled in his experience. In a fundamental sense the situation is contrary to medical norms and role expectations. *Primum non nocere* ("First of all, do no harm") is a traditional medical norm. The doctor's task is to help cure patients. Yet in this situation he must ask a person to assume a surgical risk and to undergo a major operation, with no physical benefit for himself as the donor. The risk of the operation to the patient's life has been calculated to be 0.05%, and the long-term risk is 0.07% (Hamburger and Crosnier, 1968; also see Chapter 6).

Approaching and Selecting Related Donors: The Issue of Consent

While attempting to influence a potential donor, the doctor is placed in an ethical role conflict between his obligation to the donor and his commitment to save the life of his kidney patient. Although the dilemma has been widely discussed (Hamburger and Crosnier, 1968; Stickel, 1966; Wolstenholme and O'Connor, 1966), no clear norms have emerged to guide the doctor, except for the necessity of "informed consent." There is agreement that the prospective donor must be informed about the degree of risk and the inconveniences that will occur. There is no consensus, however, concerning the degree of effort a doctor should exert to secure a family donor, nor about the method he should use (Hamburger and Crosnier, 1968).

Some centers have routinized the selection procedure and instituted psychiatric review boards to reject any prospective donor whose ambivalence and anxiety appear too great and whose volunteering is considered more the result of family pressure than individual desire (Hamburger and Crosnier, 1968; Stickel, 1966). In some programs the policy has been to make volunteering difficult for the donor, and a member of the team tries to talk him out of donation (Pierce, 1970), or the donor is not accepted until he has offered many times (Korsch, 1970). Renee Fox and Judith Swazey (1974) report a case in which the "gatekeeping" physicians refused to allow a willing donor to proceed because his wife was opposed; the donor was told that he was ineligible, although this was not the fact. The Minnesota service does not force family members to beg to donate, nor does it refuse to allow donation if there is some family opposition. In addition, the onus of intervention has not been given to the psychiatrists but remains with the physicians and surgeons responsible for patient care. They are the ones who must advance the idea of family donation and explain both the need and the risks.

At a center, such as Minnesota, where a large number of both cadaver and related kidneys are transplanted, there appear to be strong structural pressures on the physician to resolve the conflict in favor of the recipient and to press hard for a family donor. The surgeons and nephrologists are likely to have had much more contact with the patient than with the donor before any decision is made, and they expect this differential contact to persist. Because of their greater exposure to the patient, they are likely to be extremely motivated to save his life. In addition, the doctor is constantly reminded by his own experience that the recipient will do considerably better with a related kidney than with a cadaver kidney. Almost all of his patients with related kidneys do well, but many of the cadaver recipients return sooner or later with irreversible kidney rejection. The small risk to the donor appears less real to the physician, especially if there have been no problems with donors on his own service.

Despite any strong bias in favor of the recipient, direct solicitation of a prospective donor can be extremely uncomfortable. The physician is conscious of the norm against exerting undue pressure, but he has no clear normative guidelines. What *is* undue pressure in a specific case? If the potential donor expresses doubts, at what point should the physician respond by informing him he should not donate?

Merton (1957) suggests that a mechanism for resolving role conflict is to abridge the role set, to cut off relations with one of the conflicting parties. Such a mechanism has developed at the Minnesota center. The relationship between the doctor and the potential donor has not been eliminated, but contact is kept to a minimum during the early decision-making period. This pattern allows the physician to urge donation by family members but enables him to avoid direct confrontation with ambivalent potential donors. A number of physicians participate in this process, but the pattern for all is similar. The physicians inform the potential adult recipient (and perhaps the spouse) of the great need to secure a biologically related donor to increase the chances of functional survival. In this way the doctors communicate the statistical urgency of the problem without applying direct pressure on the donor. This task is left to the recipient himself. This tactic appears to alleviate some of the physician's discomfort about his ethical role. However, it may place the patient in an uncomfortable position, because he has to request his family to save his life. Whatever the degree of stress on the patient in this situation (see Chapter 9), the device appears effective in recruiting family donors. For example, several patients referred to the Minnesota service as potential recipients of cadaver kidneys have been convinced of the urgency of family donation and have later obtained volunteer family donors for themselves.

However, this emergent pattern has not been formally institutionalized. Therefore, the physician's role differs somewhat from case to case, partially due to his own uncertainty about the correct course and to situational differences. The physician may come into contact with a prospective donor who is visiting the patient, or a family may request a consultation. In some cases the patient may be reluctant to approach the extended family himself and may request the doctor's intervention.

If a family member consents to be a donor, the procedure followed by most centers appears to be more uniform. Blood and tissue typing will be carried out to determine compatibility with the recipient. The donor will also receive a thorough medical work-up to assure that his kidneys are normal and that his general health is adequate for donation. He will also be informed about the nature of the operative risk and discomforts. If at this time he decides he does not wish to donate, the doctors at most centers will give him a medical excuse to avoid embarrassment in facing the recipient (Hamburger and Crosnier, 1968). However, centers and physicians seem to have no clear-cut rule specifying when and if the possibility of a medical excuse is mentioned. Should all potential donors be told about the possibility of a medical excuse or only those who express significant ambivalence? Should a physician respond to donor ambivalence by giving him the choice of a medical excuse or should a medical excuse be applied without even the donor's knowledge that it is untrue?

Which physician should care for the related donor? At the University of Minnesota a separate donor service has been established with a donor physician who is not responsible for recipient care. The donor's physician assumes responsibility for the potential donor at the time of the work-up and throughout the transplant period. The organizational mechanism has been used to resolve some of the ethical problems. It is based on the feeling that a physician less committed to the individual recipient will be more likely to protect the ambivalent donor and that he would have more time to listen to the donor than the physicians whose major efforts were devoted to the crisis-prone recipients. In fact in one case a donor became extremely agitated and frightened the night before the transplant, alternating between stating that he wanted to withdraw and that he was willing to proceed to donate to his sister. The signals he was emitting were unclear, and it became evident that the donor's doctor and the recipient's physician would have interpreted these signals differently. The recipient's physician emphasized the donor's willingness to proceed and predicted the donor would feel great guilt if he withdrew. The donor's doctor, however, had the final responsibility and refused to allow the donation to proceed, even though the donor kept repeating that he wished to donate despite his extreme fear. The donor was given a medical excuse.

In other cases, where the ambivalence is less strong, even the donor's physician can be unclear as to how to proceed. For example, in Case 6, the donor doctor was unsure of how seriously to interpret the donor's remarks.

CASE 6

A donor, who had expressed some ambivalence about donation early but who had decided to donate, seemed quite positive upon admission to the hospital and signed the operative consent. However, as the preanesthesia medication was being administered, the donor said to the nurse: "I'm not sure I want to go through with this." The recipient was already anesthetized and in the operating room. The nurse ran to notify the donor's doctor, concerned that the donor would be asleep from the medication in a few minutes. The doctor was unsure of what action to take in the few minutes left. Was the donor simply expressing the fear that everyone feels just before an operation, or was she withdrawing consent. The physician immediately returned to the donor so that if she were serious she could repeat her remark. However, he chose not to confront her with the problem but rather to ask her in general how she was doing. The donor did not repeat the remark; the transplant proceeded; and the donor expressed positive feelings posttransplant. She never mentioned the preanesthesia incident to the staff nor in the confidential posttransplant interviews with the sociologists.

There are other unsettled questions in addition to the central problem of whether family members should be used and what the physician's role in recruiting these donors should be. Should minors in the family be used? Should relatives institutionalized due to retardation or mental illness be allowed to donate? Hospitals have been unwilling to make this decision themselves, and in several instances have referred the matter to the courts (Kane, 1973; "The Sale of Human Body Parts," 1974; Savage, 1969; Wasmuth, 1969). In some cases such persons have been approved as donors after the court concluded that the death of the recipient would be psychologically disadvantageous for the potential donor. However, these decisions are controversial, and how a general precedent will be established is unclear. At the University of Minnesota no donor under 16 is considered, and all those between 16 and the age of majority must go to court for consent. This consent has been easy to obtain. However, the use of younger donors is a more difficult issue. In one Connecticut case the court approved donation by a 7-year-old identical twin on the grounds that the parents were unable to donate and the loss of her twin would be a severe emotional problem for the potential donor (Kane, 1973; Lewis, 1974).

ORGANIZATIONAL RESPONSES TO AMBIGUITY

The ethical and normative uncertainties raised by transplantation have generated an unusual amount of organizational activity (Page, 1969). On the national level hearings on the issues have been held in Congress (Schmeck, 1969), and national and international professional organizations have also been involved. The Sadler brothers, who were largely responsible for the origination and success of the Uniform Anatomical Gift Act and the uniform donor card, worked through highly prestigious and influential organizations. They helped set up an *ad hoc* committee of the National Research Council of the National Academy of Sciences consisting of 51 representatives of medical and other concerned groups (Sadler et al., 1969a, b, 1970). The uniform laws and donor cards were drafted by the National Conference of Commissioners in Uniform State Laws and approved by the American Bar Association, a committee of the American Medical Association, and the *ad hoc* committee of the American Heart Association.

Within the medical world, international and national symposia on transplantation have been held (Sadler et al., 1969a; Silverman et al., 1969; Wolstenholme and O'Conner, 1966), and blue-ribbon panels have been set up to establish ethical guidelines for physicians within organizations such as the American Heart Association, the Judicial Council of the American Medical Association (Shelley, 1968), the World Medical Association, the Council for International Organization of Medical Sciences (Corday, 1970; Wright, 1969), the International Federation of Societies for Electroencephalographic and Clinical Neurophysiology (Silverman et al., 1969) and others (Frye, 1969). Editorials have been written in influential medical journals, and experts have been polled (Allgower and Gruber, 1970; Silverman, et al., 1969). In all of these meetings, committees, and editorials, the basic ethical issues have been examined: How should recipients be selected? How can a potential cadaver donor be protected against premature termination of his life? Is family or individual consent necessary for cadaver donation? What is the acceptable definition of death? Should living unrelated donors be used? Should living donors be paid? Should heart transplantation be continued (Appel, 1968; Beecher, 1968; Stickel, 1966)?

The most publicized of these blue-ribbon groups may be the Harvard Medical School Committee headed by Beecher, which set up guidelines for determining brain death in a cadaver donor. These guidelines were approved by the American Heart Association's *Ad Hoc* Committee and were widely published (Beecher, 1968; "New Dimensions in Legal and Ethical Concepts", 1969). The effect and efficacy of such guidelines are unknown. The extent to which they inhibit inadvisable procedures or technological advance remains to be investigated. Whether they will be institutionalized is also an open question. In general, despite all the groups that have met, most of the difficult ethical problems related to organ transplantation remain unsettled. Wide differences in practice among institutions persist.

II

REHABILITATION AND SOCIAL-PSYCHOLOGICAL ADJUSTMENT OF THE POSTTRANSPLANT PATIENT

Transplantation has given rise to a host of ethical ambiguities and unsolved problems in the delivery of health care. For many the momentum of the technological battle against death necessitates the toleration of all such difficulties. The physical success of kidney transplantation makes every other issue pale into insignificance.

Yet several investigators have claimed that while transplantation extends the physical life of the patient, his psychological and social life may be untenable.

> Almost all transplant patients live a life of nervous uncertainty (Dempsey, 1974, p. 59).

> Other problems include. . .creation of psychological problems in recipients; and. . .unrealistic expectations of the populace. At present the great com-

mitment of skills, efforts, and funds often results in failure [or] the salvage of a partially functioning individual. . . .It is suggested that the cost of one organ transplant, if allocated instead to education, or to case-finding and preventative services, would produce a markedly better cost benefit ratio ("Should We Transplant Organs or Efforts?" 1969, p. 1567).

While maintenance hemodialysis failed to vouchsafe a satisfactory life, renal transplantation was found to be no more likely to guarantee an acceptable existence, at least not immediately (Beard, 1969, p. 30).

Kidney transplantation as a therapy is an attempt to remove the patient from the role of social invalid. There would be little sense in making such a large expenditure in funds and energy to rehabilitate the patient physically if he were to remain a social-psychological cripple.

In this section of the book we ask whether transplantation is "worth it" from the point of view of the patient and his family. Is the quality of life high enough to warrant the full enthusiasm of the society's support? Renal transplantation for many subcategories of patients, such as diabetics and children, has elicited particular controversy. Many transplant centers have refused to accept such patients. The effect of transplantation in such groups is important to investigate.

Chapter 3 is focused on our studies of the rehabilitation and life-enjoyment of the adult posttransplant patient. In Chapters 4 and 5 we discuss children ill with kidney disease and those undergoing transplantation.

The impact of stress upon mental health is of great theoretical and practical interest. The stress of a dangerous and chronic long-term illness followed by major surgical intervention and a massive attempt to restore health would appear to place the individual psyche at significant risk. In fact when the sources of potential stress are detailed, the ability of *any* patient to withstand the pressure appears amazing. The focus here is on the patient's self-image in the face of severe challenge.

Although the prediction that the self-image and mental health of these patients would be adversely affected appears reasonable, much of the current literature on individuals at risk points to the surprising resiliency of the human animal (Anthony and Koupernik, 1974; Bleuler, 1974; Garmezy, 1974 a, b). Among children growing up in households with one schizophrenic parent, only 10% themselves become schizophrenic; where there are two schizophrenic parents only 35% of the children succumb (Rosenthal, 1972). According to recent quantitative studies, black children subject to extreme poverty, societal prejudice, and a higher rate of broken families emerge with self-esteem and levels of happiness as high as their white counterparts (Rosenberg and Simmons, 1972). The majority of families split by war adapt and emerge from the crisis basically healthy (Hill, 1949). In disaster situations most individuals are able to regain enough self-control quickly to aid themselves and others (Fritz, 1957). Studies of crisis point to a bifurcation of reaction: Some individuals emerge from the experience strenghened and matured, while others are weakened and experience long-term suffering and permanently impaired mental health.

The question at issue here is what proportion of patients are able to withstand the crisis of life-threatening illness and transplantation. What dimensions of adjustment are particularly vulnerable, and under what conditions is the reaction to stress more severe?

3

SOCIAL AND PSYCHOLOGICAL REHABILITATION OF THE ADULT TRANSPLANT PATIENT

The purpose of kidney transplantation as a therapy is to produce dramatic improvement in the patient's health and thereby to increase his productivity, enhance his self-image, strengthen his general adjustment level, and reduce tension in the family. Before turning to the question of whether this goal is achieved, we outline the aspects of disease and therapy that challenge the adult patient's adjustment. The potential sources of stress confronting him are extreme.

SOURCES OF STRESS

PHYSICAL STRESSES PRETRANSPLANT

Perhaps the most significant stress for the dialysis patient with end-stage kidney disease is the constant physical sensation of illness. Despite dialysis, the patient still feels ill most of the time. One woman who had adjusted fairly well stated that she was fatigued the day before and the day after dialysis. With two treatments per week requiring 7 to 15 hours each, this woman's disease severely restricted her activities for the better part of 6 out of every 7 days. (Some patients are dialyzed in the evening and thereby lose less time.) Another patient in the same series said, "You have to remember that you never really feel well with this condition. You have to keep working at it to keep going" (Brand and Komorita, 1966). Symptoms of uremia—nausea, dizziness, fatigue, and weakness—return as the time for the next treatment approaches. In our series of 139 non-diabetic pretransplant patients, 82%–89% experience weakness or tiredness "sometimes" or "very often"; 53% are bothered by nausea, 50% by swelling of body parts, and 41% by headaches. Insomnia, itching, neuropathy, or numbness in the extremities are also prevalent.

In addition, there appear to be psychophysical effects of severe uremia that are partly chemical in origin and that are improved but not eliminated by dialysis.* Among these are apathy, drowziness, inability to concentrate, restlessness, tolerance for only short bursts of activity, irritability, depression, and cognitive impairment revealed in slow speech, erratic memory, confusion, and lower performance on IQ and other tests. Kaplan De-Nour and associates (1968) and Blatt and Tsushima (1966) report on impaired cognitive functioning among dialysis patients. In severe uremia a psychosis with paranoid hallucinations can develop. The final stages of dialysis itself can aggravate some of these symptoms. One British patient says:

> I become increasingly restless, tense and irritable and start to feel sick and usually vomit. By then I'm screaming to get off the machine. My whole inside is brimming over. I'm tense but I can't keep still. I'm sure it's doing my kidneys a lot of good, but it is not doing me much good (Menzies and Stewart, 1968).

In addition to the chemical changes and distressing symptoms in the body itself, the medical regimen, with its severe dietary and fluid restrictions, can intensify physical sources of stress. Patients frequently are forbidden salt and are kept extraordinarily thirsty. Many patients are unable to conform to these rules.† Suicidal binges are reported in which patients defy the food and fluid restrictions.‡

* See Baker and Knutson (1946); Kemph (1966); Menzies and Stewart (1968); Salisbury (1968); Schreiner (1959); Tyler (1965).

† See Cutter (1970); Gombos et al., (1964); Katz and Procter (1969); MacDonald (1967); Salisbury (1968); Shea et al., (1965).

‡ See Abram (1968); Retan and Lewis (1966).

SOCIAL-PSYCHOLOGICAL STRESSES PRETRANSPLANT

To physical sources of distress must be added equally severe psychological onslaughts (Levy, 1974). The constant threat of death and uncertainty of life-prognosis are the most fundamental challenges (Christopherson, 1973). Ten percent of dialysis patients under 60 die each year; 35% of diabetic dialysis patients die the first year, and 25% per year thereafter (Shapiro, 1974). Even if the patient remains healthy, he is likely to be aware of complications and death among other patients at the dialysis and transplant center.

The alteration of one's life-patterns and self-image to fit the role of invalid also appear to be stressful (Cramond, et al., 1967). In some cases renal failure, with its accompanying symptoms, appears rapidly, and the diagnosis of end-stage disease is sudden and unexpected. In these situations the family and patient may have to cope with a grief-like reaction to the sudden loss of the healthy self. For most other patients the disease is insidious and gradual. For example, diabetics may have a long history of the sick-role. In all of these cases, assuming the role of a chronically ill patient can be difficult for an adult who has internalized societal values of achievement, independence, and self-reliance.

Although any illness imposes dependency, the reliance on the artificial kidney is seen as extreme (Kaplan De-Nour et al., 1968; Leopold, 1968). To survive, the patient must lie in the hospital for 6 to 10 hours two or three times a week, dependent on a machine through which his blood flows. Mechanical difficulties are real and fearsome possibilities; when dialysis is a long-term therapy, no end to this process is in sight. Loss of control over the environment is great. Many investigators posit that the feelings of dependency can be reduced in a home dialysis situation in which the patient (with a relative) is encouraged to assume the major responsibility for his own care (Merrill, 1968a; Rae et al., 1968). At home, however, without the security of medical staff at hand, the fear of fatal hemorrhage, mechanical difficulty, and chemical imbalances may become more severe.

As the new role of a chronically ill person can be difficult to assume, the old roles become severely impaired. The attempt to maintain family and social relationships can be difficult, and family tensions may be quite high (MacNamara, 1969). Parsons and Fox (1969) have pointed out that the modern nuclear family is ill-equipped to absorb the stress of a sick member. Role demands are already high and must be fulfilled by a small number of persons. Sickness can augment these demands to an unbearable degree, and the entire equilibrium of the family can be disrupted. The mother of a severely ill child will find fulfilling her obligations to all family members especially difficult (MacNamara, 1967). If the mother is the patient, such problems will be magnified.

Shambaugh et al. (1967) studied spouses of 18 patients on home dialysis. These spouses were frequently responsible for the patients while they were on dialysis, a time at which hemorrhaging or other life-threatening emergencies could occur. Fifteen of these spouses were found to have significant adjustment problems, 12 of which were severe. They were subject to depression, grief, and fear of the patient's death. In addition, several felt hostility toward the patient because of his dependency, his irritable childlike behavior, the financial sacrifices involved and the deprivation of recreation and sex. The fact that kidney patients frequently become impotent or lose interest in sex is a great strain on a marriage. In another study of spouses who are trained to be responsible for the patient's medical care during home dialysis, Bailey (1972) showed that 12 out of 106 became embroiled in malignant dependency relationships in which either the spouse became the destructive "parent" or the patient, the overdemanding "master."

Participation in the outside world can also be difficult. Although many patients continue full-time employment, others cannot (Sullivan, 1973). Financial problems arise from reduced income and can result in a loss of status for the family as job, home, and possessions are given up (MacNamara, 1967; Meldrum et al., 1968; Wright, 1969).

Plans for the future and even leisure-time activities become difficult to make, partly because of financial difficulties but also because of the inability to predict when the patient will be feeling well.* This inability of the patient to maintain customary roles within and without the family would appear to challenge his self-esteem.

If the decision is made to attempt a transplant, the stresses of a donor search impinge upon the patient. With a shortage of cadaver donors, the wait for a kidney is often long and frustrating. The alternative is to ask a family member to make the sacrifice and donate one of his kidneys; the discovery of which family members are willing and which unwilling to donate may be painful (see Part III).

PHYSICAL STRESS POSTTRANSPLANT

Although the transplant operation is a relatively minor physiologic trauma with a 30-day postoperative death rate less than 1%, a number of significant medical problems can be encountered. Postoperative com-

* See Goodey and Kelly (1967); Katz and Procter (1969); Short and Alexander (1969); Wright et al., (1966).

plications such as bleeding, infection, or the development of a urinary leak requiring reoperation are not infrequent and are more dangerous to these patients, whose immune systems are suppressed. Bleeding tendencies are more likely in this group because they receive anticoagulants as part of their preoperative dialysis regime. Healing of the incision may be difficult for the diabetic patient, and the immunosuppressive drugs make control of his diabetes much more difficult.

Because of immunosuppression, susceptibility to infection increases, and certain infections can be life-threatening and may require the physicians to abandon the kidney to save the patient's life—a battle that is not always successful. Even after the patient is discharged from the hospital, viral and bacterial infections, which healthy individuals ignore, can be life-threatening.

In addition, rejection episodes occur frequently in the first three to six months. At this time the body's immune systems are liable to attack the kidney severely enough to require rehospitalization where more vigorous antirejection therapy can be instituted. In some cases the rejection process is irreversible, and the kidney must be removed and dialysis reinstituted. However well the patient feels, he is always aware of the threat of rejection and the potential return to dialysis.

For some patients the kidney never works at full capacity, but shows gradual chronic rejection, with the patient experiencing some symptoms of uremia and being forced to take very high doses of steroid medication. Within a few years at best, these chronically rejected kidneys must be removed.

Even when kidney function is excellent and the patient is discharged from the hospital in a few weeks, the posttransplant medical regimen can be stressful. Although energy and cognitive clarity return, the patient's life is dependent upon immunosuppressive drugs and he must adjust to taking a minimum of three or four and as many as a dozen different varieties of medication. Some of the medications have distressing side effects. The high doses of steroids may cause muscle-wasting and a redistribution of body and facial fat so that an unattractive fat "moon face" and rotund figure result ("Cushingoid" appearance). Acne may develop in teenagers, and impotence sometimes occurs or persists among male adults. Other frequent problems are neuropathy (a numbness in the extremities which is particularly common in diabetics), bone damage, hair loss, cataracts on the eyes, and mood disturbances.

Yet as the patient improves, the steroid doses are reduced along with many, but not all, of these side effects. The initial need for thrice-weekly blood tests and weekly hospital visits is also gradually reduced.

For the diabetic patient, the problems of diabetes and its management remain. Transplantation relieves some of these problems: The loss of strength and sensation in the legs (neuropathy) is *somewhat* reduced, and the progressive loss of eyesight characteristic of these patients is often arrested (Kjellstrand et al., 1973). But a functioning kidney does nothing to reduce the progress of vascular disease, which leads to heart attacks, and to foot gangrene with resultant amputations. Many of the post-transplant diabetics, then, are semiblind persons who have difficulty in walking. The combination of blindness and neuropathy is a difficult one because sensation in the feet helps the blind person to compensate for defects in sight, and the lack of this sensation intensifies the difficulty of the blind person in manoeuvering. Currently, transplantation of diabetics is undertaken earlier, before the kidney function has completely disappeared, in order to save the eyesight and reduce neuropathy.

SOCIAL-PSYCHOLOGICAL STRESSES POSTTRANSPLANT

The constant threat of rejection, the uncertainty of the long-term prognosis, the psychological acceptance of a body-part from another individual are potential sources of stress (see Part III). Whenever the patient is hospitalized, either at the time of the operation or subsequently, he is probably surrounded by other transplant patients who are in grave difficulty. Although most patients do well, those who do not are concentrated on one small hospital ward. The variety of ways that the transplant and patient can fail are salient to both patient and staff. In fact, because of continual interaction with the problem cases, dialysis and transplant staff members who have little contact with the large number of successful posttransplant patients can easily become pessimistic about transplantation as a therapeutic modality.

Several studies have indicated that an identification develops between the two patients who receive kidneys from the same cadaver—they become "surgical twins" (Abram, 1972; Schowalter, 1970) and carefully watch each other's progress. Because 40% or more of transplants using cadaver kidneys are unsuccessful, depending on the center, one of these surgical twins is liable to discover that the other patient has lost his kidney or has become seriously ill.

After years of assuming the dependent role of invalid, some kidney transplant patients may have difficulty resuming an independent role. Idelson et al., (1974 a, b) describes the stages of adjustment through which heart attack patients pass as they return to normal life. Stress is induced by the uncertainty of prognosis and the impossibility of knowing whether one should define oneself as healthy or ill, whether one should indulge in a full range of normal activities or be prudently restrictive, whether one need notice each slight body symptom or whether these can be safely ignored. Families in this situation may be overprotective.* The benefits of the sick role in terms of extra attention, fewer responsibilities, and disability allowances may be difficult to surrender (Dansak, 1972; Reichsman and Levy, 1974).

In addition, there are societal barriers to the vocational rehabilitation of the well patient who is defined as ill. Former jobs may not be available, or employers may hesitate to hire a transplant patient, especially the diabetic, because of the fear he will be rehospitalized or because he has been receiving Social Security disability assistance. In some cases employment may be impossible because the patient cannot be insured as part of a union or employee group health insurance plan. In other cases the unskilled laborer may be afraid of returning to heavy labor (Hickey, 1968).

REACTION TO STRESSES

Our experiences and those of most other investigators indicate that the early posttransplant period can be difficult for many patients, because this is the time when threatened rejection is most liable to occur and steroid doses are at their highest level. If the transplant fails or threatens to fail due to rejection, infection, or serious complication, the distress of the patient and his family is likely to be extreme. If the transplant is not followed by a subsequent successful organ graft, transplantation obviously has not been "worth it." In these cases the distress engendered by the destruction of hope, the physical suffering involved, and the increased chance of death render the transplant less satisfactory than the more conservative therapy of dialysis, despite all of dialysis' problems (Eady, 1973).

In evaluating transplantation as a therapy, however, we should focus on the long-term medically *successful* patient. If transplantation fails, the outcome is certainly not worth the cost. But is it worth it if the kidney functions as planned?

Our own research had as its object the examination of the quality of life of the patients who have reached a year posttransplant with functioning kidneys (see Simmons and Schilling, 1974). How does their level of adjustment compare to that of pretransplant patients?

There has been little quantitative data available dealing with the kidney transplant patient's level of rehabilitation (Banik et al., 1974; Blagg et al.,

* See Bois et al., (1968); Cramond (1967); Hertel and Kemph (1969); Hickey (1969).

1973; Burns, in preparation; Sampson, in preparation). For this reason in our own research we have used quantitative scales and indicators to measure the patient's adjustment level in three major areas: (1) the patient's preceived level of physical rehabilitation—his feelings of health and physical well-being; (2) his general social-psychological adjustment including his satisfaction with major role-relationships, his changes in self-image, his feelings of happiness or depression and his anxiety level; and (3) his ability to perform in occupational or school roles. In addition, we have attempted to document the extent of gross psychosis or suicidal behavior that his presented itself to the medical staff.

One aspect of the patient's social-psychological adjustment that has been of particular concern is his self-image. Several subdimensions of the self-image have been measured including the patient's self-esteem, the stability of his self-picture, his preoccupation with himself, his feelings of control over his destiny, and his feelings of independence-dependency.

METHODS

Our data were collected by interviewing all adult patients over 16 years of age who received renal transplants or were placed on the list to await a cadaver donor at the University of Minnesota Hospitals between October 1970 and June 1973. The population totals 208 male and female patients: 200 were transplanted here; five never received a graft; three were transplanted elsewhere. Questionnaires were administered to 178 patients pretransplant; 177 again at their first posttransplant clinic visit, usually three weeks posttransplant; and 156 at a year after the transplant. The discrepancy in numbers is due to the fact that our study began prior to the development of the questionnaire so that some patients who received a year posttransplant questionnaire were not measured pretransplant. In addition, we do not have year posttransplant questionnaires for the patients not transplanted here, nor for the 40 patients who died or rejected their kidney before the year had passed (20% of all those transplanted here). The refasal rate is very low: Only three patients refused the questionnaire at any point and only five altogether.

As part of this population, 41 patients had diabetes, 33 of whom had reached a year posttransplant with functioning kidneys. It should be noted that 99% of all patients were being maintained on hemodialysis while waiting for transplantation. The length of time they were on dialysis varies from two weeks to five years, with 27% on dialysis for longer than six months.

For patients receiving kidneys from related donors, questionnaires were administered five days prior to the scheduled transplant. For patients who were to receive cadaver kidneys, the questionnaire was given as soon as possible after their names were added to the waiting list. Year posttransplant questionnaires were administered within one month of the first transplant anniversary. These questionnaires contained both multiple-choice questions and open-ended material.

Scales to measure social-psychological variables were taken from Rosenberg (1965), Rosenberg and Simmons (1972), Kohn (1969), and Coleman (1966). These scales were designed to measure dimensions of the self-image, level of happiness, and level of anxiety. They were constructed from several multiple-choice questions and were tested for reliability and, where possible, validity—that is, they were tested first to make certain the scale items had internal consistency and were tapping the same dimension and second to assure that the scales were validly measuring the concept claimed. All scales show satisfactory reliability; the self-esteem scale in particular is the most extensively and satisfactorily validated. The exact scale items along with reliability and validity information are presented in Appendix A.*

As a further validity check on our findings, Minnesota Multiphasic Personality Inventories (MMPIs) were given to a subpopulation of patients pre- and posttransplant. The goal was to administer MMPIs to all eligible patients three days prior to removal of their own diseased kidneys between February 1971 and May 1972 and again to the same patients *after a year* posttransplant. Patients whose kidneys were not removed at our hospital, those who were scheduled at the last minute, and those who were blind could not be given the MMPIs. Only patients who survived with functioning kidneys were given the year-post transplant tests. Failure to complete the MMPI occurred in seven patients pretransplant and four patients at a year posttransplant. Fifty usable MMPIs were secured pretransplant and 27 at a year posttransplant. Thus, the MMPI results are not so clearly representative as the questionnaire results. As a validity check, however, they should still be useful.

All instruments were administered by the sociological research staff. All patients were informed of the independence of this staff from the medical personnel and were assured that no information communicated

* Scores on social-psychological scales do not have absolute meaning. However, by comparing individuals and groups to one another, it is possible to determine in a relative sense which groups are more likely to score high in "happiness" or "self-esteem," and it is also possible to identify individuals whose scores are located in extreme categories relative to the normal distribution of scores in the group. Similar measures exist in many fields—for example, certain chemicals with biological activity are measured in "units" of activity relative to an arbitrary standard. Such measures may have great utility in medicine or engineering.

by them would be transmitted to the medical staff or to family members. While general policy recommendations would be made on the basis of patient opinions, no individual patient would be identified in this process. This confidentiality was never violated.*

FINDINGS

Because the University of Minnesota Hospital is unusual in its large number of diabetic patients and because this group is particularly controversial, findings throughout are presented for both diabetic and nondiabetic cases (see Simmons and Schilling, 1974).

Level of Adjustment

In general there is no doubt that for the vast majority of patients (both diabetic and nondiabetic) who have a functioning kidney at the end of a year, the therapy is regarded in a positive light. In answer to multiple-choice questions, 90% of the patients "agree a lot" with the statement "Now that the transplant operation is over, everything seems better"; 98% believe that all the money and effort going into kidney transplantation is "worth it"; 99% feel transplantation is a more satisfactory treatment for them than dialysis; and 99% respond that they would still have had the transplant if they knew before what they know now.

To what extent does this positive attitude derive from a significant improvement in health and quality of life? To what extent is it reflected in a more positive self-image?

1. *Physical Well-Being*. To measure the extent to which patients perceived their health as interfering with their lives, the following three questions were asked both before and after transplantation (Table 3-1):

> I'd like to ask you now about your health, about how you feel, and about how the (disease/transplant) has affected your life. Which of these statements best describes your life during the past month? I am
>
> (1) well and doing most things I did before my illness
> (2) well but not performing many customary activities
> (3) up most of the day but quite restricted in activity
> (4) confined to a wheelchair when out of bed

* In case histories reported throughout this volume we have changed key identifying material that is irrelevant to the points being made to further protect the subjects. Other than details that would identify the patient, however, all material is accurate.

(5) confined to bed but feeling well
(6) confined to bed and not feeling well

How much of a problem has the disease been for you? Has it been

(1) a very great problem
(2) somewhat of a problem
(3) a small problem
(4) no problem at all

How do you feel now? Do you feel

(1) very sick
(2) moderately sick
(3) not very sick
(4) not at all sick

TABLE 3-1 HEALTH OF DIABETIC AND NONDIABETIC PATIENTS BEFORE AND 1 YEAR AFTER TRANSPLANTATION

	Diabetic patients		Nondiabetic patients	
	1	2	3	4
Multiple-choice questions	Before transplant (38 patients)	1 year after transplant (32 patients)	Before transplant (139 patients)	1 year after transplant (124 patients)
Percentage classifying themselves as "I am well and doing most things I did before my illness."[a]	8	63	20	85
How do you feel now? Percentage "not at all sick"[a]	14	81	28	77
How much of a problem has your health been for you recently? Percentage "no problem at all"[a]	0	34	3	64

[a] According to a chi-square test of the differences between pre- and post-transplant patients, $p < .001$ both for diabetics and for nondiabetics.

In addition, patients were asked at both points in time how often they experienced problems with the usual symptoms of uremia (i.e., kidney disease) (Table 3-2), and whether they had any difficulty with a series of ordinary life activities due to their health (Table 3-3).

Tables 3-1 through 3-3 show dramatic improvements for all of the one-year posttransplant patients including those with diabetes. For example, before transplantation only 20% of the nondiabetic patients classified themselves as well and doing most things they did before their illness, in comparison to 85% at a year after transplantation. Before transplantation only 28% of the nondiabetic patients could say they do not feel at all sick, in contrast to 77% after transplantation. With the exception of problems with eyesight and confusion, all uremic symptoms related to kidney disease had been considerably reduced for diabetics as

TABLE 3-2 PERCENTAGE OF DIABETIC AND NONDIABETIC PATIENTS REPORTING SYMPTOMS OF UREMIA "VERY OFTEN" OR "SOMETIMES"[a]

	Diabetic patients (%)		Nondiabetic patients (%)	
	1	2	3	4
Symptoms	Before trans-plant (38 patients)	1 year after trans-plant (32 patients)	Before trans-plant (139 patients)	1 year after trans-plant (124 patients)
Nausea	65	0*	54	1*
Weakness	92	45*	82	25*
Headaches	46	16†	41	20*
Tiredness	97	52*	89	44*
Pain	43	16	30	13*
Swelling of body parts	68	32‡	50	31†
Eyesight	78	79	37	38
Confusion	23	33	40	18

[a] According to a chi-square test of the difference between pre- and posttransplant patients:
 * $p < .001$.
 † $p < .01$.
 ‡ $p < .05$.

TABLE 3-3 PERCENTAGE OF DIABETIC AND NONDIABETIC PATIENTS HAVING DIFFICULTIES WITH DAILY ACTIVITIES[a]

	Diabetic patients		Nondiabetic patients	
	1	2	3	4
Activities	Before trans- plant (38 patients)	1 year after trans- plant (32 patients)	Before trans- plant (139 patients)	1 year after trans- plant (124 patients)
Getting out of bed	44	6*	16	7‡
Walking	86	52†	41	28‡
Dressing	56	10*	12	5‡
Bathing	67	6*	36	4*
Eating	47	10*	25	11†
Housework (women)	100	31*	70	27*
Preparing meals (women)	71	6*	42	4*
Care of children (women)	67	25	40	4*
Climbing stairs	89	68‡	67	37*
Lifting things	89	81	73	44*
Eyesight	83	87	36	41
Reading	80	64	34	27
Shopping	82	52‡	48	12*

[a] According to a chi-square test of the differences between pre- and post-transplant patients:
* $p < .001$.
† $p < .01$.
‡ $p < .05$.

well as nondiabetics (Table 3-2). Patients were having considerably less difficulty with most life activities (Table 3-3).*

In addition, 95% of the patients said they were "more healthy" and felt "better" than they did when they were sick with kidney disease.

* All differences reported in this chapter remain if we remove from the comparison those pretransplant patients whose kidneys were not to survive to a year after transplantation. In fact if we compare the *exact same* patients at the two periods in time, in almost all cases the percentages are virtually identical to those reported above; and where they are not, differences tend toward making our initial results even stronger. Since there is no distortion in findings, the data presented throughout the paper have been based on all of the cases, in order to increase sample size.

Yet, with all this improvement, both pretransplant and posttransplant diabetic patients have more physical problems than nondiabetic patients. (In Tables 3-1 through 3-3, compare column 1 to column 3 and column 2 to column 4.) At a year after transplantation only 34% of the diabetic patients could say their health was no problem, in comparison to 64% of the nondiabetic patients (Table 3-1).

Table 3-3 indicates that the major difficulties for the patients with diabetes at a year after transplantation involve blindness and problems with walking. With the termination of uremic neuropathy (numbness in the limbs) and the greater level of energy, walking improves for many patients after transplantation. In fact, prior to the transplant, 24% of the diabetic patients were confined to bed or to a wheelchair, whereas a year after transplantation only one patient was so limited. However, at a year after transplantation, 27% of our diabetic patients had very little remaining vision; almost 20% of the diabetic patients were hardly able to walk. Twelve out of 33 (36%) had major problems in one or both areas. Eleven (33%) seemed to have either no problems or only minor difficulties.

Thus, although their level of health appears to have improved substantially after transplantation, diabetics are left with significant health difficulties. It should also be noted that a minority of nondiabetics still have difficulty with some daily life activities.

2. *Social-Psychological Adjustment*

(a) Happiness and Anxiety. Scales designed to measure the patient's level of happiness* (Rosenberg, 1965) and anxiety (Kohn, 1969) show substantial increases in perceived happiness at a year after transplantation and a reduction in anxiety level for both diabetic and nondiabetic patients (Table 3-4). The correlation between the patient's level of happiness and his transplant status—that is, whether he is pre- or posttransplant—is sizeable: $r = .46$ ($p < .001$). Perhaps most revealing is the fact that when

* For example, the items making up this scale are as follows:

Do you agree or disagree with the following statement? I get a lot of fun out of life. Do you (agree/disagree)?

On the whole I think I am quite a happy person. Do you (agree/disagree)?

Right now, on the whole, how happy would you say you are? Are you (very happy/fairly happy/not very happy/not at all happy)?

How often do you feel downcast and dejected? Do you feel that way (very often/fairly often/occasionally/rarely/never)?

In general, how would you say you feel most of the time—in good or low spirits? Are you in (very good spirits/fairly good spirits/neither good nor low spirits/fairly low spirits/very low spirits)?

Do you agree or disagree with this statement? I wish I could be as happy as others seem to be. At this point in your life do you (agree/disagree)?

TABLE 3-4 PERCENTAGE OF DIABETIC AND NONDIABETIC PATIENTS SCORING MOST FAVORABLY ON SCALES OF PSYCHOLOGICAL ADJUSTMENT

	Diabetic patients (%)		Nondiabetic patients (%)		All patients
Psychological scales	Before trans-plant (38 patients)	1 year after trans-plant (32 patients)	Before trans-plant (139 patients)	1 year after trans-plant (124 patients)	Pearson's correlation between pre- and post-transplant status and scale for all patients
High in happiness	9	72	37	81	$r = .46$*
High in self-esteem	27	48	28	50	$r = .30$*
High in self-image, stability, feelings of a firm identity	24	63	32	61	$r = .08$*
High in independence	24	50	46	80	$r = .58$*
High in feeling of control over one's destiny	28	46	48	68	$r = .38$*
Low in anxiety	32	57	36	58	$r = -.22$*
Low in preoccupation with oneself and one's illness	24	47	22	59	$r = -.37$*
					Canonical[a] correlation 67*

[a] The canonical correlation measures the association between pre- and posttransplant status and all of the psychological scales together. A correlation of .67 indicates that as much as 45% of the common variance in these measures is attributable to whether the patient is pre- or posttransplant.

* $p < .001$.

asked whether their lives were "completely satisfying," "pretty satisfying," or "not very satisfying," 57% of the *pretransplant* patients chose "not very satisfying" in comparison to only 13% at a year after transplantation. At both points in time, however, diabetic patients describe themselves as less happy than do nondiabetic patients.

The dramatic quality of the change becomes even more evident when we compare the recipients to normal control groups. Table 3-5 shows the distribution of these patients' responses to a question that has been widely used to measure happiness. In comparison to national control

TABLE 3-5 HAPPINESS OF TRANSPLANT PATIENTS AND CONTROL GROUPS

Taken all together, how would you say things are these days—would you say you are very happy, pretty happy, or not too happy?

	Very happy	Pretty happy	Not too happy	Total
Nationwide samples [a]				
1957	35%	54%	11%	100% (2460) [d]
1963	36	55	9	100 (2062)
1963	32	51	16	100 (1501)
1965	30	53	17	100 (1469)
Minneapolis–St. Paul samples [b]				
Signers of donor cards (1969)	37	54	9	100 (75)
Control group of neighbors	37	56	6	100 (78)
Samples from transplant Study [c]				
Related donors pretransplant	34	58	8	100 (134)
Related nondonors posttransplant	26	68	5	100 (174)
Recipients pretransplant	18	58	25	100 (171)
Recipients year posttransplant	57	36	7	100 (150)

[a] Bradburn, 1969, p. 40.

[b] The entire study is reported in Simmons et al., 1974.

[c] A chi-square analysis indicates significant differences. Among the last six groups in the table: $p < .001$. Between recipients pretransplant and the Twin City and related controls: $p < .001$. Between recipients posttransplant and these four controls: $p < .001$.

[d] Numbers in parentheses indicate total number of individuals in sample.

groups, to local control groups from Minneapolis and St. Paul, and to relatives from the recipient's own family, the desperately ill *pretransplant* patient is by far the least likely to say he is "very happy" and the most likely to rate himself as "not too happy." While 30–40% of all unrelated control individuals report themselves as "very happy," only 18% of the pretransplant patients so classify themselves. Many investigators have noted the high level of denial among dialysis patients and have therefore questioned the ability of some multiple-choice questions to tap the patient's underlying depression (Glassman and Siegel, 1970). Yet whatever denial is operating among these patients, it has not rendered this particular question insensitive or invalid as a measure. These patients demonstrate significantly more unhappiness than normal controls.

At a year posttransplant the reverse is true. The recipients become the most likely to report themselves "very happy"—more likely than all of the control groups:* 57% of the recipients then rate themselves as very happy.

For many patients restored health and physical well-being bring a great exhilaration. In the words of one typical patient:

> I'm much more active than I was before. I'm happier. I probably have even a greater appreciation of life than I had before. . . .I expected to be sick and I haven't been. Every day I wake up and—My God, I (am not sick). Jubilation!

The theme of rebirth is frequently voiced in our research and that of others.

> Having been given a second chance to live has given me a much greater appreciation of the true meaning of life (Mock, 1973, p. 41).

> I now wake up each morning feeling that I can move mountains. I can run instead of walking slowly. When my hematocrit was as low as ten to twelve [during dialysis], this was not possible. I can care for my three children and husband; housework is a pleasure to do! . . .I recently, in six weeks time, prepared for a private art show. . .my coloring is clear and rosy, instead of muddy and grey; moist, soft skin has replaced the dry, itchy skin of dialysis days (West, 1973, p. 12).

Whatever the strains of the posttransplant regime, these difficulties are considerably less overwhelming to many patients than the problems of end-stage kidney disease or treatment on the dialysis machine.

(*b*) *Self-image*. Does restored health also affect the self-esteem of these patients? Several writers (Parets, 1967; Wright, 1960) have suggested that the self-image of the chronically ill patient is adversely affected by his illness. Yet there are few data to verify this contention and some theoretical reasons to suspect it. How highly one rates oneself as a person is of central importance to the individual's sense of well-being and mental health. Indeed, many theorists have postulated that the need to maintain a high self-esteem is one of the most important, if not the most important, motivational components of the personality. Murphy (1947), Allport (1943), Rosenberg (1965), and Rosenberg and Simmons (1972) have shown that the individual resists challenges to his self-esteem through

* See Chapter 6 for discussion of changes among donors.

various defense mechanisms. Several such defense mechanisms are available to the person sick with kidney disease. If he has been healthy for a good proportion of his life, he can define his illness and the limitations caused by his illness as temporary, atypical, and not reflective of his true abilities and potentialities. Such a defense mechanism would be less suitable for patients with diabetes, who have been chronically ill for the larger part of their lives, however. A second defense mechanism—the reduction of aspirations for the self—is available for both diabetic and nondiabetic patients. As William James noted in 1890, satisfaction with the self is a function of the relationship between aspirations and attainments. If one reduces one's goals, one can protect his self-esteem against the pain of failure. As one patient noted after transplantation, "I'd been sick for five years. . . .You get used to dragging around at half-speed. You think it's normal—you think everyone feels like this. Now I know." Accustomed to the lack of energy, she had no longer expected very much of herself and did not devalue herself because of her inability to sustain activity. Denial aids this process.

Therefore, one must test whether kidney disease is a powerful enough stimulus in reality to overcome these defense mechanisms and damage the self-esteem, and, consequently, whether kidney transplantation can benefit the self-picture.

Table 3-4 indicates that the self-esteem is, indeed, responsive to changes in health. At a year after transplantation, both diabetic and nondiabetic patients reveal markedly higher self-esteem. In fact, if we compare the patient's self-esteem scores to those of the same Minneapolis–St. Paul controls and to the same members of his own family used in Table 3–5, we find that the ill patients prior to the transplant score considerably lower in self-esteem than all control groups. In contrast, the patients with *successful transplants* score higher than the members of their own family who did not volunteer to donate an organ (nondonors) and almost as high as the Twin City controls. (Only 38% of the pretransplant patients score high in an abbreviated self-esteem scale,* compared to 59% of the nondonors, 80% of the Twin City control group, and 70% of the year posttransplant patients.)

Restoration to health, then, apparently leads to dramatic improvements in the individual's self-esteem.

Other dimensions of the self-image also appear to benefit markedly from the transplant therapy. A five-item scale† was included before and

* See Appendix. See Chapter 6 for a discussion of donor's self-esteem.

† The items from the scale were as follows:

> Do you think the experience of being sick has caused your opinions of yourself to change a good deal, or do your opinions of yourself always continue to remain the

after the transplant to measure the stability of a patient's self-picture, the firmness of his identity (see Erikson, 1956; Lecky, 1945). One could predict that the major changes brought about by illness might challenge the core of a person's identity; he might be less certain of the type of individual he is. After a successful transplant, his identity might be reintegrated and his self-image stabilized. Our data show that both diabetic and nondiabetic posttransplant patients indicated significantly greater stability—that is, they were less likely than before to say they felt "mixed up" about themselves and what they were like; they were less likely to say that their "opinions about themselves" changed a good deal.

In addition to a higher self-esteem and a more stable self-picture, our results in Table 3-4 indicate that the posttransplant patient is less preoccupied with himself. Lederer (1960) and King (1963) describe the chronically ill person as intensely self-preoccupied with a severely constricted interest in the outside world. For example, 45% of the pretransplant patients say they think about themselves "almost always" or "often," in contrast to only 19% of the recipients at a year posttransplant.

Finally, in terms of the self-image, the posttransplant patients show marked improvement in their view of themselves as independent beings, in control over their own destiny (see Table 3-4). For example, when asked how much help they needed to get things done, 45% of the diabetic and 78% of the nondiabetic patients said they needed "no extra help" at a year after transplantation. Before transplantation no diabetic and only 10% of the nondiabetic patients reported they could get along with "no extra help."

Table 3-4 indicates that along some, but not all, of these psychological and self-image dimensions, the diabetic begins or ends less well-off than the nondiabetic patient. This disadvantage is particularly noticeable for feelings of independence and control over one's destiny.

The marked improvement in psychological well-being that we have shown is evident almost immediately after the transplant along most

same? Would you say your opinions of yourself (change a great deal/change somewhat/change very little/do not change at all)?

How sure are you that you know what kind of a person you really are these days? Are you (very sure/pretty sure/not very sure/not at all sure) about what kind of a person you are?

Since you have been sick, how often do you feel mixed up about yourself, about what you are really like? Does it happen (often/sometimes/never)?

Do you agree with this? Since I have been sick I have found that my ideas of who I am and what I am like seem to change quickly. Do you (agree/disagree)?

Someone told me: "Some days I am happy with the kind of person I am, other days I am not happy with the kind of person I am." Since you have been sick, do your feelings change like this (yes/no)?

dimensions. On our questionnaires at the first clinic visit (usually three weeks posttransplant), elation is as high as at a year posttransplant. Feelings of physical well-being and great hope occur quite rapidly. And for the patient who retains his graft, such emotions are still evident at the first anniversary of the transplant.

(c) *The Donated Organ and the Self-image*. In Chapter 6 we discuss the stress associated with donation. However, at this point we should note that many investigators have described cases in which the recipient had difficulty incorporating the donor organ into his body-image (Abram, 1972; Cramond, 1967; Kemph, 1966). Abram (1972) reports a case in which a white Ku Klux Klan member became active in the NAACP after receiving a kidney from a black cadaver; Viederman (1974) tells of a black man who fantasized that his kidney from a white donor was attacking him. A heart transplant patient was reportedly haunted by a hallucination in which the cadaver donor returned for her heart (Castelnuovo–Tedesco, 1973; Lunde, 1969). Some males have felt feminized by organs from female donors (Castelnuovo–Tedesco, 1973; Viederman, 1974). A brother acted as if his masculinity was threatened when he discovered that his donor brother was a homosexual (Lefebvre, 1973). Viederman (1974) concludes that if the related donor is not liked, the kidney becomes a hostile "introject" and chances for rejection are enhanced.

These psychoanalysts see the fantasies attached to the new organ as similar to

> . . .the phallic-oedipal struggle in young men, involving castration and the fantasied acquisition of the penis (Muslin, 1972, p. SS-6).

> The object image of the new kidney is seen to merge with the object of a mother, life, a phallus, a baby. . .(Muslin, 1972, p. SS-7).

However, Biörck, and Magnusson (1968) and Banik et al. (1974) report little difficulty in this regard for their series of patients (see Basch, 1973).

In any case, as Abram notes (1975), the evidence is difficult to evaluate. Although the cases are each well-documented, there is little data indicating the frequency of such problems. The applicability of psychoanalytic theories must remain tentative. In our own data few adults indicate severe problems of this sort (see Chapter 5 for a discussion of children's fantasies). In only one case were we aware of difficulty. A mother who received a cadaver kidney from an 11-year-old boy became depressed because her own son was the same age. However, our adult patients were not interviewed routinely by a psychiatrist unless clinical problems arose. Their fantasies and dreams were not regularly probed. We did ask both the related donor and recipient whether either ever referred to the kidney as the donor's at a year posttransplant. Two-thirds of the recipients of related kidneys and their donors reported that this identification of the kidney occurred at times, and approximately 60% agreed that the donor sometimes said, "Take good care of my kidney." We also asked whether anything else either joking or serious was ever said about the kidney. Twenty-three percent of the related donors at a year posttransplant reported jokes that referred to some merging of identities:

DONOR (sister to the recipient). We've kidded back and forth because she seems to have more ambition than I do. I said "You must have got the ambitious kidney."

RECIPIENT (brother is the donor). We joke about becoming the same person. Being myself more active than he is, he says I got the better kidney. All kinds of jokes—basically, he says that I'm younger than he is, though I'm older, that I got the better kidney. I look younger, I'm more active.

DONOR (sister three years older than the recipient). She and her husband always say I gave her a new life and we are twins.

DONOR (sister who donated to a brother). Oh, one time I said something to him like: "If you get turned on when you walk past a man, blame it on me."

Certainly humor may function to release real tensions, but our impression is that few of these instances reflected serious psychiatric problems. We have no evidence to contraindicate the use of cross-sex kidneys (see Cramond 1967 for a suggestion that men with blurred sexual concepts of themselves be given male kidneys). Whether the sex and age of the cadaver donor ought to be withheld from the patient as has been recommended (Castelnuovo-Tedesco, 1973) remains an open question. There is no particular benefit in revealing this information to the patient, although the logistics of secrecy may be difficult in practice. At the University of Minnesota there is no policy to withhold any knowledge other than the name of the cadaver, and most patients seem to know something about the donor.

(d) MMPI Results. Results from the Minnesota Multiphasic Personality Inventory further verify our picture of a significantly improved emotional adjustment posttransplant. Sampson (in preparation) reports that both short-term and long-term transplant patients ($N = 29$) showed better adjustment than dialysis patients ($N = 18$) in the MMPI and the Bell Adjustment Inventory (also see Pierce et al., 1973b; Banik et al., 1974). While dialysis patients in his series demonstrated poorer adjustment the

longer they remained on dialysis, the reverse was true for transplant patients. He compared two groups of successful posttransplant patients: those who were between one and two years posttransplant and those who had retained their grafts for more than two years. The latter group showed less anxiety, fearfulness, pessimism, desperation, and depressive symptomatology than those for whom the experience was more recent.

Our study compares a small group of pretransplant patients to themselves at a year after transplant. Of the 27 patients, four were diabetics; all had been on dialysis for varying lengths of time. In Figure 3-1 the scores of the recipients pretransplant are compared to their own posttransplant scores as well as to a control group of living related donors and a "normal" Twin City group* of 50 middle-class men and 50 women.† The higher scores on Scales 1–10 indicate more maladjustment in a variety of areas. On all but one of the 10 scales (Masculinity–Femininity), the pretransplant recipients are the most likely to demonstrate maladjustment, and in all cases these differences are statistically significant. Furthermore, at a year after the transplant, the patients show improvement on all but two scales (5 and 9), although in many areas the posttransplant patients still indicate more problems than do the normal controls. Pretransplant patients are particularly liable to demonstrate concern with their bodily functions, depression, denial and repression, anxiety, and bizarre thinking patterns. Although the posttransplant patients indicate greater mental health in all of these areas, they remain significantly lower in morale than normal and higher in scales measuring anxiety, alienation, and euphoria.

The transplant patients can also be compared to other persons with medical problems. In comparison to a sample of 50,000 medical outpatients seen at the Mayo Clinic in Rochester, Minnesota (Swenson et al., 1973), the pretransplant patients exhibited higher mean scores on all but Scale 5. The year posttransplant patients, however, were neither consistently more or less maladjusted.

There are some limitations in using the MMPI with patients who have physical symptoms, because physical complaints are included among the indicators of Scales 1, 2, 3, and 8—that is, among the measures of somatic concern, depression, denial, and alienation. In our population such items

* We wish to express gratitude to Professor James Butcher for making these data available to us.

† In all groups there are a few high L, F, or K scores. Whereas one might not wish to use these MMPIs for clinical decisions, it is customary to include them in research presentation. In terms of T-scores above 80, there is one recipient posttransplant with an F-score this high, one donor and one "normal" control who have L-scores elevated to this extent.

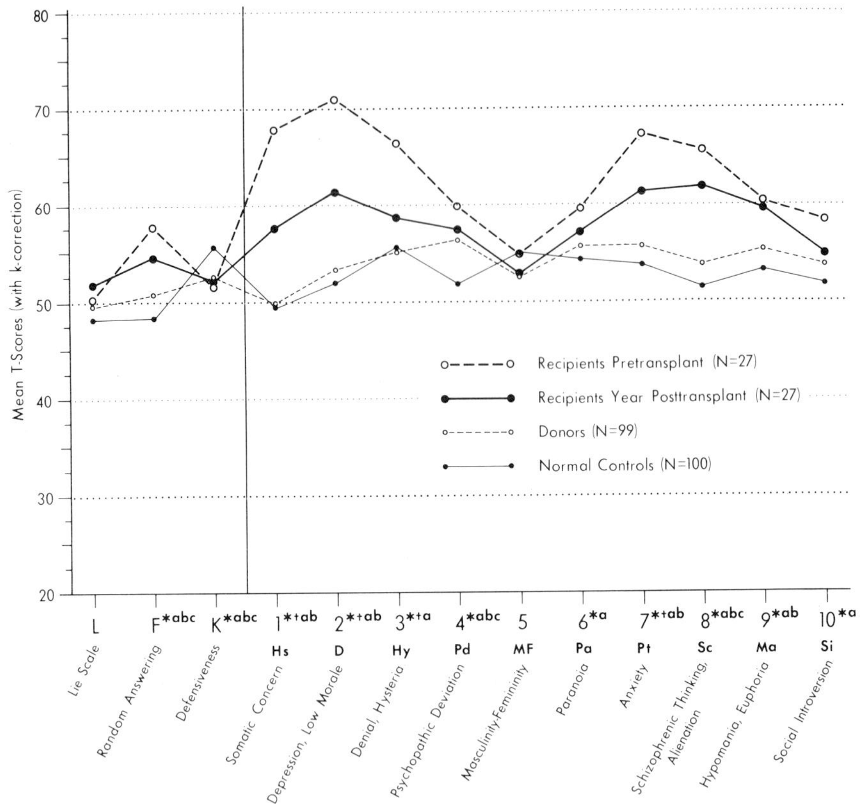

Statistical Significance

* Differences among the four groups are statistically significant p ≤ .05 (analyses of variance)
+ Differences between recipients pre and post are also statistically significant p ≤ .05
a Difference between recipients pre and either donors or normal controls is also significant p ≤ .05
b Difference between recipients post and either donors or normal controls is also significant p ≤ .05
c Difference between donors and normal controls is also significant p ≤ .05

Figure 3-1 MMPIs of recipients pretransplant and posttransplant and controls.

may be accurate reflectors of the disease process—kidney disease, diabetes—rather than valid measures of psychological distress. However, many other items are also used in these scales, and our purpose in this analysis of a small sample of MMPIs is a modest one. We are attempting to validate the general picture that is emerging from an examination of our other measures of the larger transplant group. Indeed, both analyses point to psychological improvement after a successful transplant.

We now turn back to the *entire* population of transplant patients and to the questionnaire data.

(e) *Satisfaction with Major Role-relationships*. Not only do posttransplant patients demonstrate a greater level of happiness, a lower degree of anxiety, and a more satisfactory self-image than they did prior to the operation, but dissatisfaction with the occupational, recreational, and social areas of their lives decreases and they appear to be socializing more with people outside the family (Table 3-6). Again, patients with diabetes are less satisfied than others in all of these areas before transplantation, although almost all of these differences disappear in the posttransplant period (compare Column 1 to Column 3, and Column 2 to Column 4).

Perhaps most important, the transplant appears to have positive benefits for the *marital relationship*. Although there is no reported difference in marital happiness, both diabetic and nondiabetic patients report less dissatisfaction with their role as a spouse at one year after transplantation than before transplantation. This attitude change may be because they are no longer so much of a burden to their spouses and families economically, emotionally, or physically. In fact, 85% of the patients at a year after transplantation report that their health "hardly

TABLE 3-6 PERCENTAGE OF DIABETIC AND NONDIABETIC PATIENTS DISSATISFIED WITH LIFE ROLES[a]

	Diabetic patients		Nondiabetic patients	
	1	2	3	4
Role relationships	Before transplant (38 patients)	1 year after transplant (32 patients)	Before transplant (139 patients)	1 year after transplant (124 patients)
Job situation	57	33	43	30‡
Recreation	68	29†	51	18*
Social life	63	19*	38	14*
Relationships with friends	32	6†	20	8‡
With role as a (husband, wife)	37	8‡	24	8†
With role as a parent	38	16	9	7

[a] According to a chi-square test of the differences between pre- and posttransplant patients:
* $p < .001$.
† $p < .01$.
‡ $p < .05$.

ever" or "never" interferes with family routine, compared to only 24% before transplantation. Further, at a year after transplantation fewer patients (12% compared to 24%) characterize their families as "somewhat" or "very tense and nervous." Families of both diabetic and nondiabetic patients show these improvements, although the nondiabetics are better in these regards both before and after transplantation.

One of the major problems before transplantation for male patients is sexual impotence. Patients with uremia experience a great deterioration in sexual functioning (Levy, 1973). Based on a sample of the membership of the National Association of Patients on Hemodialysis and Transplantation, Levy indicated that 56% of all male hemodialysis patients and 43% of all male transplant patients considered themselves partially or totally impotent (also see Foster et al., 1973). Our data indicate that 86% of all married men before transplantation experienced at least some difficulty with sexual performance, and 43% experienced "a lot of difficulty." At a year after transplantation fewer men were having problems—52% had at least "some difficulty" and 22% "a lot of difficulty." Impotence is substantially reduced but remains a very significant problem for both diabetics and nondiabetics.

For all married patients, both men and women, 81% report before transplantation that their sexual activity had decreased since their illness, and 74% reported that their sexual desire had decreased. Nondiabetic patients were only a little less likely than diabetics to report these decreases in activity and desire. At a year after transplantation 35–40% of the patients reported increases in activity while 20–22% reported further decreases. Although marital relationships appear significantly improved after the transplant, sexual problems persist in a sizeable minority of the cases for both diabetic and nondiabetic patients and for both sexes.

We have been discussing the patients who remain married after the transplant. The question arises whether the incidence of divorce is particularly high in the first year after a successful transplant. One might predict that the stress level would be too extreme for some couples. In other cases the spouse might feel free to leave once the patient is "restored" to health and is no longer in active crisis, dependent on the dialysis machine to live. Or the newly independent patient may now feel capable of taking such a step. The findings, however, indicate that the vast majority of patients maintain their marriages. Only six married patients out of 108 (6%) were separated or divorced in the year following the transplant. Three of these were diabetics. The data show that 12% of all married diabetics and 4% of nondiabetics were divorced or separated during the year after the transplant.

3. *Vocational Rehabilitation*. In terms of vocational rehabilitation, 88% of

the nondiabetic males and 44% of the nondiabetic females were working or going to school at a year after transplantation, and the large majority of women (73%) had no difficulty with their housework (see Blagg et al., 1973). Five of the seven nondiabetic males who were not working at a year posttransplant had significant health problems: One was in need of hip surgery due to side effects of the steroids; one had developed Parkinson's disease; another had a minimally functioning kidney and had been put back on the list to await a cadaver donor; a fourth had severe neuropathy and difficulty in walking; and the fifth was suffering from a heart condition.

Diabetic patients are less likely to be able to work because of diabetic blindness and neuropathy. Only 44% of the diabetic males and 27% of the diabetic females were working at a year after transplantation. As can be seen in Table 3-7, fewer diabetic patients were working at a year after

TABLE 3-7 PERCENTAGE OF DIABETIC AND NONDIABETIC PATIENTS WORKING OR IN SCHOOL[a]

	Male patients (%)		Female patients (%)	
	Diabetics	Nondiabetics	Diabetics	Nondiabetics
Before the disease became serious	100 (21)	99 (71)	76 (17)	74 (66)
In the year previous to the transplant	67 (21)	83 (71)	47 (17)	49 (63)
One year after transplant	44 (18)	88 (56)	27 (15)	44 (64)

[a] Numbers in parentheses indicate total number of individuals in category.

transplantation than had held jobs at some time in the year prior to the transplant. However, of the 10 diabetic men who were not working at a year after transplantation, only two had still been working three months prior to the pretransplant nephrectomy. All the others had stopped work at least four months before the transplant.

Of the ten diabetic men, who were not working, four probably were healthy enough to work after the transplant, although only one was without either some eyesight or walking difficulty. The other six had very little vision, and three had major difficulty in walking. Rehabilitating the diabetic patient vocationally has involved many of the same problems as rehabilitating the blind. However, if early transplantation preserves the diabetic's eyesight, one would expect dramatic improvements in vocational rehabilitation.

On the other hand it is important to note the role of Social Security disability regulations in encouraging diabetic patients to stay unemployed. The same factors would also be expected to affect individuals with other chronic illnesses. If a person is unable to work and is on Social Security disability allowance for more than two years, he qualifies for full immediate Medicare coverage in case of hospitalization. The patient who has had diabetes since childhood cannot secure private insurance, and coverage through other means, such as Medicaid and county welfare assistance, is possible only if his assets and income are low enough to meet poverty standards (see Chapter 11). Because hospitalization for a diabetic-related problem is probable, prudence would seem to dictate remaining on his disability allowance. A long-term hospitalization could pauperize his family if he returned to work and dropped the disability allowance and Medicare coverage. One of the blind diabetic males at two years posttransplant was doing volunteer work for a fund-raising agency 40 hours a week; he was not interested in earning a salary and withdrawing from his disability allowance.

The nondiabetic patient is not in this bind, for he does not expect to be extensively hospitalized for other than transplant-related problems, problems which usually will be covered financially by the new "kidney amendment." He is also more likely to have secured insurance prior to his kidney disease.

Ideally, in evaluating any treatment, one would wish to compare it to alternate therapies. In this case the alternative to the massive surgical intervention of transplantation with its attendant difficulties for organ donors is the dialysis machine. However, the question of whether vocational rehabilitation is greater for transplant patients or long-term dialysis patients is a difficult one to answer because of the lack of comparative data. Dr. Christopher Blagg from the Northwest Kidney Center in Seattle has provided us with data on the rehabilitation of 98 patients (aged 15–60) on home dialysis for one year or more. Comparing our nondiabetic* one-year posttransplant subjects to those patients, we find a somewhat

* Because none of the dialyzed patients were diabetic, we use nondiabetics in all these comparisons. Comty and associates (1974) indicate 21% of their diabetic males on dialysis for a year were employed full or part time, in comparison to 44% of our diabetic transplant patients. However, the number of cases in our series is too small for such a difference to be statistically significant.

higher percentage of transplanted males either employed or in school (88% vs. 61%).* Regardless of age, the transplant patients are more likely to demonstrate vocational rehabilitation. For men 40 years old or less, 94% of the transplant patients, compared to 74% of those dialyzed one year or more, are working or in school. For male dialysis patients over 40 the picture is particularly unfavorable, with only 44% of them at work or in school, compared to 78% of the transplant patients of the same age. In other words, the difference between the two groups is particularly evident among the older patients. The vast majority of men under 40 are performing quite well regardless of therapy (see Kramer et al., 1975, for similar results).

The transplanted nondiabetic females, regardless of age, are much more likely than those on dialysis to be employed or in school instead of, or in addition to, being housewives (44% vs. 10%).

Yet without more careful prospective studies, there is no way to be certain that these dialysis and transplant patients were comparable prior to selecting dialysis or transplantation as a therapy. Possibly the less-good surgical risks are assigned to dialysis, or persons who feel more strongly about a vocation choose transplantation. Regional economic differences could also be responsible for these results.†

Transplantation appears to be accompanied by a definite increase in income. Blagg and associates (1973) report that transplant patients are much more likely than home dialysis patients to report personal income increase. Recomputing data from Levy (1973), we again find that transplant patients are better off then are patients who have been on dialysis a year or more. Compared to before their disease became serious, 36% of the transplant patients in his study, but only 23% of the long-term dialysis patients, showed an increase of family income of $1000 or more.

Our data also indicate that transplanted males tend to show an improvement in mean and median income over the year pretransplant when most of them were on dialysis. However, at neither time does their mean or median income equal their incomes before they became sick with kidney disease. Among males who were working at all three points in time, the *mean* incomes began at $11,815 prior to illness, were reduced to

* Somewhat fewer of both groups are employed or in school full time: 70% of the male transplant patients, 54% of those being dialyzed.

† However, Blagg's data appears quite similar to that reported by Gottschalk (1967) based on 79 patients dialyzed at 12 centers around the country. Gottschalk combined men and women and showed that 71% were either fully employed or engaged in normal housekeeping duties, although there were some discrepancies among centers. Approximately the same proportion of Blagg's patients (67%) fall in this category. Seventy-eight percent of our nondiabetic transplant patients are also this well rehabilitated (also see Abram, 1972; Burns, 1976; Burns et al., in preparation; Hughson et al., 1974).

$10,425 during the pretransplant year, and partially restored to $11,017 at a year posttransplant.* In at least 20% of the cases, the increase in income is quite substantial, and well above inflation rates.

In summary, the vocational and income rehabilitation of the nondiabetic transplated patient appears to be excellent. The diabetic and the dialysis patient do not appear to do so well, although measurement problems frustrate dialysis-transplantation comparisons. We have been quite careful to distinguish various dimensions of the patients' quality of life; and vocational rehabilitation is only one such dimension. Sullivan (1973) and others (Abram, 1974) have suggested that the evaluators of these therapies should not become obsessed with traditional vocational rehabilitation. Several patients who are unable to find suitable jobs lead active and functional lives. As is clear in Table 3-3, for example, the vast majority of diabetic posttransplant women report no difficulty with housework. Similarly, Blagg's (1973) data and Burn's and associates results (in preparation) indicate that a majority of women on dialysis are functioning housewives, even though few are employed outside the home.

4. *Psychosis and Suicide*. Although the mental health of patients in terms of happiness, anxiety, and self-image appears to be generally improved after transplantation, the stress level of this situation is expected to be too extreme for certain individuals. Gross psychiatric episodes and suicidal attempts (Abram, et al., 1971; McKegney and Lange, 1971; Penn et al., 1971) occur in a small number of the transplant patients at some time during their course. Out of the 208 patients studied, one patient committed suicide after transplantation, 10 patients made threats or suicidal attempts that became known to the staff (five of which occurred in relatively healthy posttransplant patients with functioning kidneys), and eight patients (two of whom were diabetic) experienced psychotic episodes. The suicide rate is 0.5% and the rate of psychotic episodes is 3.8%.

The psychotic episodes were all self-limited, and after transplantation they occurred primarily among patients who were physically ill or seriously rejecting their kidneys (also see Penn et al., 1971). In only one case did such an episode occur in a physically healthy posttransplant patient. This patient was a diabetic who, at two years after transplantation, exhibited some borderline psychotic behavior.

Abram and associates (1971) have shown that the rate of suicidal

* In terms of measuring the true income level *at a year* posttransplant, we did not wish to include the first two or three months of the prior year when the patient was likely to be out of work recuperating from the operation. Therefore we asked the year posttransplant patients for their income during the past month and multiplied that by 12.

behavior among dialysis patients is higher than the suicide rate of one out of 10,000 in the normal population;* similarly, the suicide rate appears much higher than normal among transplant patients (see Goldstein and Reznikoff, 1971). Both groups not only experience greater than average stress, but they also are confronted with more opportunities for self-destructive behavior. Refusing to keep to their diet, refusing dialysis treatment, or withdrawing from the antirejection drugs posttransplant can place the patient in a life-threatening situation. The one clear suicide case involved a delinquent teenager who tried several of these methods which are unavailable to the ordinary person. First, after the transplant he withdrew from the steroid treatment, although this behavior was in part an impulsive test rather than a suicidal act. The kidney was then rejected; and subsequently he became severely depressed, intermittently refused dialysis, and finally pulled out his arteriovenous shunt† and hemorrhaged to death.

It is interesting to note that all but two of the suicidal patients in our series were either teenagers or diabetics: Five were teenagers and four were diabetics—that is, 10% of all diabetic patients and 22% of all adolescents were suicidal either pre- or posttransplant. Of the five persons who were suicidal after transplantation despite organic health and functioning kidneys, three were teenagers and two had diabetes (see Chapters 5 and 6 for more discussion of adolescent suicidal behavior).

We may be underestimating the extent of suicide and suicidal gestures in our population. As we noted, only one patient clearly committed suicide by pulling out his shunt. For other patients, the extent to which their own acts led to their death or to the rejection of their kidney must remain ambiguous. In most cases we cannot determine whether a patient has withdrawn from his medications against medical advice. We were able to identify potential suicides only among patients who made suicidal threats or took suicidal action that became known to the staff.

Although suicidal behavior appears to occur more frequently than normal among posttransplant patients, as far as we can tell it is a problem affecting only a small minority of all such patients, few of whom have been transplanted successfully. The incidence of these severe psychiatric disturbances in our transplant population is not so significant as to cast doubt upon transplantation as a valid therapy for diabetic or nondiabetic patients. Yet with an illness such as this one, extra psychiatric help for

* See Chu (1971) for criticism of Abram's statistical calculations.

† The shunt is the site where connections are made so that blood can flow through the artificial kidney machine. It is a connection of the vein and artery made outside the skin. Currently the connection is usually made under the skin and is called a fistula. Fistulas do not lend themselves as easily as shunts to suicide attempts.

patients at risk, particularly diabetics and adolescents, would appear warranted.

Other studies indicate that somewhat higher proportions of transplant patients are subject to severe psychiatric problems at some time in their course of treatment (see Table 3-8, derived from Abram, 1972). However, most of these investigators do not report the percentage of *long-term successful* patients with such psychiatric problems. Because approximately 30% of related kidneys and 60% of cadaver kidneys are rejected in the first two to three years posttransplant, the proportion showing psychiatric difficulty might be directly reflective of the medical failure rate. Penn and associates (1971), for example, note that the bulk of the difficulties in their series were attributable to an associated medical problem such as the threatened rejection of the kidney. If the complication resolved satisfactorily, depression usually cleared.

Which Patients Do Better

Aside from the diabetic–nondiabetic distinction, can we predict which patients will adjust more fully and which will need more psychiatric and social work support? There are four types of characteristics to examine: the patient's general background statuses, his level of health during the year posttransplant, his relationships with his family and the donor, and his psychological adjustment pretransplant. The relationship between each of these factors and the depression, anxiety, and self-image scores at a year posttransplant has been analyzed (see Table 3-4 for a list of the scales).*

1. *Background Statuses*. Levy and Wynbrandt (1975) report that female dialysis patients have resumed more of their usual life activities than the men, and we also find some tendency for females to be better adjusted. At a year they score lower in anxiety (66% vs. 50%), lower in depression (85% vs. 72%), higher in self–image stability (85% vs. 70%), and indicate feelings of greater control over their own destiny (74% vs. 53%).† These findings are particularly interesting, given contrasting evidence from studies of "normal" adults. A nationwide survey showed that women score higher in anxiety than men (Bradburn and Caplovitz, 1965), and other research indicates that adult females are more likely to become mentally ill than men (Bamber, 1973; Gove and Tudor, 1973; Silverman, 1968). Yet when faced with transplantation females apparently fare better

* Scales not mentioned throughout this section show no differences among comparative groups with the exception of "preoccupation with self" which varies somewhat unpredictably.

† $p \leq .05$ in this section.

TABLE 3-8 PSYCHIATRIC COMPLICATIONS OF TRANSPLANTATION REPORTED IN THE LITERATURE[a]

Author	Proportion showing psychiatric problems		
		%	
Abram and Buchanan (1975)	(7/30)	23	Moderate psychiatric complications and psychosocial upheaval
	(2/30)	7	Psychoses
Blazer et al. (ms.)	(9/215)	4	Psychoses
Colomb and Hamburger (1967)	(9/44)	20	Depression or anxiety
Ferris (Abram, 1972)			
One transplant	(23/47)	49	Psychotic or emotional decompensation
Multiple transplants	(7/7)	100	Emotional disorder
Penn (1971)	(94/292)	32	Significant psychopathology
	(32/294)	11	Psychoses
	(7/292)	2	Attempted suicide
	(1/292)	1	Actual suicide
Perez de Francisco (1971)	(6/6)	100	Psychiatric problems
Short and Harris (1969)	(2/19)	10	Psychotic depression

[a] Derived from Abram (1972).

psychologically, at least according to the measures used in this study. In fact, the MMPI data also indicate greater adjustment for females both before and after the transplant.

The burden on the ill and recuperating female in our society may be less. Traditionally greater passivity is sanctioned for the woman, and she is not expected to be so active occupationally and financially. The financial responsibility for the family is not so likely to be defined as hers. Thus, full acceptance of the housewife role will be interpreted by herself and others as full rehabilitation. For the man to be rated as successful, he must secure a job and maintain a high quality of occupational performance. Whereas the housewife role is readily available to the married woman, the vocational one is more problematic and more dependent upon the will of others. In addition, the fact that the role of the wife-mother is *so important* for the functioning of the family may be important in motivating her to resume normal activities (Deutsch and Goldston, 1960). As Litman (1974) says:

> . . .she [the mother] may exhibit a great deal of reluctance to accept the sick role. Mechanic, for instance, observed that mothers were more likely to seek medical care and advice for their children than for themselves and appeared much more willing to accord their children the right to the sick role than themselves. . . .Mothers apparently are considered to be less vulnerable and their activities too important to be disrupted by illness.
>
> In contrast to her husband, her own illness or prolonged incapacitation may be viewed as a serious threat to the family functioning. . . .Hollingshead and Rogers found that while chaos tended to accompany the mental illness of the wife, this was not the case for mentally ill husbands. . . .The same was true in our own study, where unlike her husband, the illness or prolonged incapacitation of the wife was regarded as a potentially serious blow to family functioning (pp. 505–506).

Age might also be expected to make a difference. Older patients may be more accepting of health problems as an expected part of their stage of the life-cycle. Young adults may very well find all restrictions more difficult. In fact, Bailey (1972) reports that geriatric patients adjust better than young adults to dialysis. Our data, however, show no consistent age differences among the adults at a year posttransplant.

Although religious background has little effect on adjustment, higher education and income are associated with higher self-esteem (r = .14* and .15). In fact, higher income of oneself if male and one's husband if female is associated with favorable scores on five out of the seven scales including scales of happiness and anxiety. Bradburn and Caplovitz (1965) show that in the normal population also, education and income relate positively to high happiness and low anxiety. Money and education are apparently resources that help to protect one against the full impact of life-stresses, including that of a major health problem. Those patients in our population who are still worried about finances at a year after the transplant are also among those most anxious and least happy in general.

Since our population is primarily white, we are unable to test for racial differences in rehabilitation. There is some tentative evidence from other centers suggesting less good vocational rehabilitation among non-whites. (H.H. Sadler, private communication.)

2. *Health Status*. One would certainly predict that those patients who had fewer health problems at a year after the transplant would demonstrate higher levels of adjustment. The fact that the diabetics frequently indicate less favorable scores supports this reasoning. We asked the patients how much of a problem their health has been for them recently and whether they have had any medical difficulties with rejection

* $p \leq .10$.

episodes posttransplant. Nondiabetic patients who currently define their health as a problem show significantly more maladjustment than healthier patients on six out of the seven psychological scales.*

The impact of body-image upon mental health is also of interest, especially because patients who threatened to reject their kidneys were given higher steroid doses and therefore were more likely to develop the unattractive, full moon-face characteristic of the Cushingoid appearance.

The interviewers were asked to rate the appearance of each patient as to whether he or she was

Very Cushingoid—would look abnormal to anyone
A little Cushingoid—would look normal to a stranger
Not Cushingoid

High doses of steroids had made 18% of the patients look grossly abnormal, with Cushingoid moon-faces; and 50% of them a little full-faced, but within normal limits. Thirty-two percent had a perfectly normal appearance, according to the interviewer. The less Cushingoid the patient, the lower his anxiety (58% vs. 35%), the higher his level of reported happiness (80% vs. 73%), and the higher his level of stability (78% vs. 64%).

3. *Family Relationships*. A close family would be expected to help soften and mediate the stresses of illness and recuperation. First, the immediate family with whom the patient lives should assume an important role. While marital status itself makes little difference, rejection by the spouse appears to be associated with long-term maladjustment. *Prior* to the transplant the patients were asked the following question:

Some people say that when they're sick they feel rejected by their (husbands, wives). Would you say you feel this way
Often
Sometimes, or
Never

Only 14 patients admitted to any feelings of rejection. With so few cases, our conclusions must be quite tentative, but this group appears to be very vulnerable. At a year posttransplant they score more unfavorably than others on six out of the seven scales, and on five of these the differences reach statistical significance levels of $p < .07$ despite the small number of cases. (The only exception involves preoccupation with the self, where there are no differences.) Anxiety† and low self-esteem‡ are particularly

* $p \leq .01$ on 4 scales; $p \leq .10$ on 2 scales.
† $p \leq .05$. ‡ $p \leq .10$.

characteristic of this group. The causal sequence here must remain hypothetical. Rather than family rejection leading to a low self-picture, patients with low self-esteem before illness may be the ones who perceive family rejection once illness occurs. In either case, individuals pre-transplant who can be identified as feeling rejected by spouses are at particular risk in terms of their long-term adjustment after transplantation.

In addition, patients were asked both pre- and posttransplant how close their immediate family was as a whole. The ratings pretransplant had little predictive power, but those who rate their families as closer at a year demonstrate lower anxiety,* higher esteem,† greater stability,* and more feelings of control over their own destiny.

Adult transplant patients frequently have two families of moment—their immediate family, which may be an important source of comfort, and their family of origin from which a related donor is sought. One might predict that patients who receive kidneys from a relative would fare better psychologically, because they have received concrete proof of familial love and their posttransplant medical course is less risky and more likely to be smooth. Yet in reviewing the literature Abram and Buchanan (1975) point tentatively to a pattern of higher adjustment in recipients of cadaver kidneys. Such recipients do not have the problems of indebtedness to a living donor. Our data, however, show no overall difference in the adjustment of recipients of cadaver or related kidneys on any of the seven scales.

However, patients who see themselves as well-liked by the members of their family of origin before transplant and who rate these families as more helpful than average during their illness, seem to be among those with higher self-esteem,† greater happiness, and lower anxiety* at a year posttransplant. (Again, without a measure prior to the illness it is difficult to determine causal sequence—to determine whether perceiving one's family as supportive produces a high self-picture or whether a long-term high level of self-esteem enables individuals to perceive their families as supportive during an illness. In either case, by determining those individuals who regard themselves as rejected by their families pre-transplant, we can identify a particularly vulnerable group in terms of long-term adjustment to the transplant.)

Difficulty with the donor relationship at a year posttransplant also appears to be associated with a lower level of adjustment. Which is the cause and which the effect is difficult to determine. Whereas the majority of recipients report few problems in this regard (see Chapter 6), the few

* $p \leq .05$. † $p \leq .10$.

who do are more likely to be anxious, less likely to be happy at a year posttransplant, and less likely to feel in control of their own destiny than those who perceive no problems with their donor. The difficulties of concern here involve recipient guilt and donor overprotection (see Chapter 6 for further discussion).

4. *Prior Psychological Adjustment*. Malmquist (1973) has indicated that one of the best predictors of adjustment to long-term dialysis therapy is prior adjustment to crisis in general and to the kidney disease in particular. Similarly, patients with a more favorable self-picture and higher level of happiness pretransplant are more likely to remain better adjusted at a year posttransplant. The correlation between self-esteem measured pretransplant and a year posttransplant is .47 ($p < .001$), between anxiety at the two points is .37 ($p < .001$), and between the two depression measures is .33 ($p < .001$). These correlations, however, are far from perfect and indicate the power of many other variables upon adjustment during this momentous time in the patient's life.

5. *Staff Optimism*. Although we have no data, we have noticed that there are differing levels of optimism about patient prognosis at various centers. While some centers perceive transplantation to be a way of extending a patient's life a few years, others such as the University of Minnesota regard a long-term lengthening of life to be quite possible. We would predict that both patients and donors would react more positively psychologically where the staff is more optimistic, provided their success rate does not belie this positive attitude.

SUMMARY AND DISCUSSION

"Quality of life" is a general and imprecisely defined concept. Yet the attempt to measure the quality of life of patients undergoing innovative expensive new therapies is vital. With this end in mind, we have specified several dimensions of life quality: the patients' feelings of *physical* well-being; their *psychological* well-being including their level of happiness and anxiety, the quality of their self-picture, and the tendency to psychiatric symptomatology; their *social* or interpersonal adjustment—that is their satisfaction with various life-roles including marital and sexual relationships; and their *vocational* rehabilitation.

On almost all of the dimensions, the 156 patients at a year after a successful kidney transplant show dramatic improvement compared to the period pretransplant when they were ill with kidney disease or on the dialysis machine. Overall happiness and a favorable self-picture seem extraordinarily affected by the return to health. In fact there is some evidence that their rescue from ill-health and imminent death has produced an exhilaration greater than that in the normal population. While their psychological state prior to the transplant was considerably less favorable than that seen in normal control groups, posttransplant they are even happier than ordinary individuals. The successful emergence from a severe crisis appears to produce a greater appreciation of the life they almost lost.

Not all categories of individuals responded equally well to this crisis experience. A small minority of patients in our population and a larger minority in other studies demonstrated psychotic behavior or suicidal tendencies. Gross psychopathology in our own and other studies appears directly responsive to health difficulties—episodes of kidney rejection, actual rejection, severe infection, or other complications. Rejection or failure of the kidney is a stress even more difficult for the individual and the family than adapting to chronic disease and certainly more difficult than adjusting to long-term dialysis. Health difficulties in general are associated with a less high level of psychological well-being.

For example, in many spheres diabetic patients start out before transplantation and end up at a year after transplantation in a less advantageous position than nondiabetic patients. Blindness and severe problems with walking make vocational rehabilitation difficult. Suicidal gestures also appear more frequently during the course of treatment, although only one long-term successful diabetic patient revealed such tendencies to the staff. Although these problems may be more difficult than those of nondiabetic patients, the data suggest that a large proportion of diabetics responds well to transplantation. The improvement as they perceive it is very real. The ethical problem of whether they should be accepted for treatment should perhaps take second place to an increased effort to rehabilitate them after transplantation.

Another vulnerable group in need of extra psychiatric support, in this and probably other diseases, appears to be adolescents, who demonstrate a greater suicidal propensity than do adults. The adjustment of the child and adolescent to illness and transplantation is more extensively discussed in Chapters 4 and 5.

In addition, there is evidence indicating that the following groups are more likely to be at risk: men in contrast to women, persons of lower income and education, individuals who show less favorable adjustment pretransplant, patients whose appearance has been very negatively affected by the steroid medication, individuals with less apparent emotional support from the family with which they live and less closeness to the family from which a donor must be sought, married patients who prior to the transplant feel rejected by their spouses, and the relatively few patients who report difficulties with their donor at a year posttransplant.

Alternative Explanations

We have been assuming in this discussion that the restoration to health and the successful resolution of a crisis is responsible for the generally favorable results. However, several alternate hypotheses should be considered. First, these posttransplant patients are ingesting high doses of steroid medications, and such medications are known to affect mood in some cases. Could the exhilaration observed here be simply a steroid "high?" Although we cannot isolate the exact effects of the medication, we do know that at a year posttransplant the dosage is much lower than earlier and yet the increased happiness is still evident. In addition, patients who are on the highest doses of steroids are those who are threatening to reject their kidneys, and the depression of these patients is palpable. The patients who report more rejection episodes and other complications score least favorably in our scales. The reality of their threatened situation overrides any possible mood-elevating effects of the steroids.

Another alternative explanation for these findings is that they are produced by denial—since denial is a major defense mechanism used by the ill (Hagberg, 1974). Yet the motivation to repress reality is certainly as great for the pretransplant as the posttransplant patient, and in fact it is among dialysis patients that denial has been stressed (Kaplan De-Nour, 1968). The MMPI results show that general denial and defensiveness (the 3 and K scales) are as or more prevalent for the pretransplant patients than for the posttransplant subjects. Whatever denial is operating, the pretransplant patients still score less favorably on our questionnaire measures than do "normal" controls, while the posttransplant patients frequently score higher.

It is also possible that posttransplant patients might exaggerate their pleasure with the transplant procedure, because to fail to do so would be to admit that all the pain and sacrifice they experienced was in vain. Theories of cognitive dissonance would lead to this conclusion. However, it seems unlikely that *such dramatic differences* would be produced by cognitive dissonance alone, that posttransplant patients could remember where they had rated themselves a year previously in enough multiple-choice questions to demonstrate the improvement we have shown, or that the differences between diabetics and nondiabetics or between those more and less close to their families would occur if motivated distortion were all that was operating. Would not diabetics and persons less close to their families be motivated to exaggerate as much as the other respondents?

We have attempted to use a variety of indicators—constructed scales, MMPI results, gross psychopathology, vocational and income statistics—to minimize validity problems in any one measure. On all indicators, transplant patients who have functioning kidneys do very well. And whatever the complex psychodynamics involved, from their point of view transplantation has clearly been "worth it," and is a much superior therapy to dialysis.

Different Treatment Modalities

In attempting to compare the quality of life of long-term dialysis patients to that of successful transplant patients, we are frustrated by measurement problems. Blagg et al. (1973), Levy, and Sampson present some evidence that long-term transplant patients function at a higher level in terms of vocational performance, income, and MMPI results. Our subjects are more likely to be employed than are Blagg's home dialysis patients. Comty (1974) indicates a high degree of psychosocial difficulty among dialyzed diabetic patients. Dialysis centers differ widely in their reports of patient rehabilitation with some reporting that 70–80% of those on dialysis live "really good lives" (Scribner, 1974) and others indicating that fewer than 25% are engaged in full-time activity (see Abram, 1968; Gottschalk, 1967).*

Few studies use the same measures in comparing patients undergoing transplantation, home, or center dialysis (Burns et al., in preparation; Freyberger, 1973). Initial selection differences among patients compound the problem. Our patients, for example, have chosen transplantation frequently because dialysis is intolerable for them, although many long-term dialysis patients react more favorably to the experience (Berman, 1973).

Among clinicians there appears to be general agreement that when the transplant is successful, the patients feel better and function more satisfactorily. The decision to place a patient on dialysis or transplantation is based not only on life-quality considerations but also on survival chances. Although the mortality loss appears the same for dialysis as a related

* Also see Brown et al., (1962); Foster et al., (1973); Goldstein and Reznikoff, (1971); Gonzalez et al., (1963); Johnson et al., (1966); Kolff et al., (1962); Levy and Wynbrandt, (1975); Norton, (1967); Rubini and Goldman, (1968); Sand et al., (1966); Schreiner and Maher, (1965); Scribner et al., (1965); Shapiro et al., (1974); Shea et al., (1965); Short and Alexander, (1969).

transplant, cadaver transplantation is significantly more risky (Eady, 1973; Lowrie et al., 1973). The stress of rejection and threatened loss of life appears to be greater than that of adapting to dialysis. How one weighs a safer lower-quality existence on dialysis against the gamble of cadaver transplantation is a problem confronting all physicians and surgeons in the field as well as all patients. In our series the vast majority of patients who survived the rejection of a first kidney chose to have a second transplant rather than stay on long-term dialysis (i.e., 16 out of 19 of all such patients and 12 out of 14 of those who would have to use the riskier cadaver donor the second time).

Nephrologists and transplant surgeons tend to see more of each other's failures than successes and thereby often become even more committed to their own therapy over time. The nephrologist must treat the patients who have returned to dialysis after a rejected transplant, and the transplant surgeon is in contact with many patients who find dialysis intolerable and therefore have elected transplantation. This cleavage often seen between the two groups of physicians, as they criticize the therapy offered by the other, may intensify the difficulties for the undecided patient (see Calland, 1972).

In the view of other critics resources should be allocated more heavily to research into the prevention of disease rather than to either of these expensive technologies that treat end-stage kidney disease once it has developed. At the present moment, although some research funds have been allocated to prevention of kidney disease, no breakthrough has occurred that will halt the progression of most of the kidney diseases that lead to total kidney failure. Due to the lack of progress in this area, end-stage kidney disease and the problem of its treatment will be with us for some time. The object of this chapter, however, is not to speculate on the potential costs and benefits of a larger disease-prevention program as opposed to the current allocation of resources to kidney transplantation. It is, rather, to examine the social-psychological costs and benefits of kidney transplantation for the patients concerned.

Resiliency

Throughout this chapter the distinction has been made between potential *sources* of stress and patients' reaction, in terms of their actual level of *distress*. Not all succumb psychologically, even though the pressure may be great. Distress and damage to the self-image in response to chronic illness pretransplant do appear to be considerable. However, the crises and stresses of a successful transplant are ones with which the majority copes very well. In fact, this crisis appears to have positive consequences for many subjects. Individuals who have successfully emerged from this extreme situation report a greater maturity, a clearer sense of values, and a deeper appreciation of life.

Reichsman and Levy (1974) report a similar elation among dialysis patients who are new to the therapy. Dialysis makes them feel considerably better than they did at the last stages of kidney failure. Yet this period of exhilaration is short-lived, lasting from six weeks to six months, and is followed by a period of disenchantment and discouragement. For the transplant patients, this marked emotional improvement has persisted to a year posttransplant, and Sampson (ms.) indicates that the MMPI results improve even more after two years. Yet the question remains as to how long the positive benefits of such a crisis can persist. Will the heightened sense of pleasure in life and the more fundamental values erode to usual levels as the patients define themselves more and more as physically normal persons, as the period of crisis recedes more into the background. Or will a disenchantment with the limitations of a posttransplant existence and steroid side effects eventually lead to active discouragement? The final psychological outcome for these adults is, of course, also dependent on the long-term physical success of transplantation.

* * *

Because there has been substantial controversy over the suitability of *children* for transplantation, the next task is to evaluate children's quality of life after a successful transplant to learn if they react as favorably as do the adults. However, prior to addressing this question of whether transplantation is also a worthwhile therapy for children (Chapter 5), we shall take a brief detour. Both as a backdrop against which the impact of pediatric transplantation can be understood and to pursue some of the theoretical issues raised above, in Chapter 4 we explore the sociopsychological reaction of children and their families to *chronic kidney disease*. At issue first is the question of whether children, like adults, react to *chronic disease* with reduced levels of happiness and lower self-pictures, and then whether *transplantation* has positive effects for youngsters' emotional adjustment as it does for adults. The positive consequences of stress and crisis for children and their level of vulnerability and invulnerability is of major concern, as it has been in the above chapter* (Garmezy, 1974a, b, c; Anthony and Koupernik, 1974).

* For readers less interested in the details of the adjustment of children and more interested in the family issues of kidney donation, the conclusions of Part II are summarized on p. 146 and Chapters 6 to 10 deal with the donation problem.

4

THE PSYCHOSOCIAL IMPACT OF CHRONIC KIDNEY DISEASE ON CHILDREN

SUSAN D. KLEIN, Ph.D.
and ROBERTA G. SIMMONS, Ph.D.

Chronic illness in childhood might be expected to challenge the coping mechanisms of both the child and his family. Pain, fatigue and other symptoms, the trauma of prognosis, and changes in the child's treatment by family and peers all appear to provide sources of stress for the child (Mattsson, 1972). Some have suggested that disease poses more of a problem to the child than the adult. "In a child, physical illness and emotional disturbance threaten to, or actually do, interfere with the process of growth itself, and are expressed in distortions or blocks in development" (Murphy, 1961, p. 218).

Although there is a sizeable literature on the chronically ill child, most of it is based on case-study material and small samples and lacks standardized quantitative measurement and normal controls (Litman, 1974; Richardson, 1961). Our major task in this chapter is to examine and measure quantitatively the effects of *chronic kidney disease* on the child's psychosocial development. The adjustment of chronically ill children is compared to the adjustment of control groups of "normal" children.

Children with kidney transplants who have been "restored to health" are discussed in Chapter 5 in comparison to chronically ill youngsters. Our focus in Chapter 3 was primarily on *transplanted* adults; in this chapter we concentrate on children chronically ill with kidney disease.

Chapter 3 showed negative psychological reactions on the part of adult kidney patients prior to transplantation, especially in comparison to healthy control groups and to their adjustment after transplantation. One purpose of this chapter is to investigate whether the psychosocial consequences of chronic illness in children are also highly negative, even though many of the children with chronic kidney disease are not so ill as the pretransplant adults and will never require transplantation. In particular, what dimensions of "adjustment" or quality of life are likely to suffer? What is the specific impact on the self-image? Which types of children are particularly vulnerable?

A number of variables might be expected to affect the vulnerability of the child—for example, disease severity (Pless and Roghmann, 1971), visibility or invisibility of the condition (Goldberg, 1974; McAnarney et al., 1974), the actual symptomatology of being sick (Eichhorn and Andersen, 1962), and the patient's perception and definition of the illness (Eichhorn and Andersen, 1962; Offord and Aponte, 1967). The effects of these and other characteristics of the child and of the disease are explored.

Because of the interdependence of the child and his family, we have also sought to analyze the impact of the child's disease upon the family. Different aspects of the crisis and factors associated with the family's vulnerability in the face of crisis are differentiated. Patterns for coping with the disease are explored, including strategies for managing the sick child and their consequences for his or her adjustment.

The general picture of the adjustment of the chronically ill child is unclear in the literature. Although many case studies detail the disruptive impact on the child of long-term illness, the few quantitative studies are contradictory in their findings. Some research shows little difference in adjustment between ill children and normal controls (Collier, 1969; Crain et al., 1966; Gates, 1946). Yet behavioral and academic problems were reported by Pless and Roghmann (1971) and by Sultz and associates (1972). High rates of hospitalization and school-related problems are frequent difficulties, according to the parents of chronically ill children ($N = 390$) in Sultz's research (1972). The Rochester Child Health Survey is one of the most methodologically rigorous studies, consisting of a probability sample of 1700 children of whom 350 were chronically ill (Pless and Roghmann, 1971). In reviewing the results from this survey and two similar British studies, Pless concludes that about one-third of all chronically ill children develop secondary social and psychological problems. Neither of these studies, however, explores the impact of chronic disease on self-esteem and other aspects of the self-image (also see Haggerty et al., 1975).

Pless and Roghmann, (1971) estimate that about one out of every 10 children will have at least one chronic illness by the age of 15. An understanding of the effects upon self-image and upon other dimensions of adjustment is important. The chronic kidney diseases studied here are similar to other noncrippling nonvisible diseases like asthma and diabetes. Like these diseases, the symptomatology, severity, and prognosis of chronic kidney diseases may vary greatly. In many cases the child is unlikely to have severe problems, but in other instances the outcome is uncertain. Because of new medications and other medical innovations, most of these conditions are no longer fatal and will not result in complete kidney failure. In some cases, however, the disease is almost certain to progress to a terminal stage requiring dialysis or transplantation. Although the incidence of kidney failure resulting from chronic kidney disease is difficult to determine, it has been estimated at 1 to 3.5 per 1.5 million population a year for children between 1 and 14 years of age (Meadow et al., 1970; Scharer, 1971). Only a small and very sick subgroup goes on to transplantation.

To provide relevant empirical data and to explore the impact of different severities of kidney disease upon children, three different approaches have been used: Chronically ill patients and their families have been interviewed with survey questionnaires, a group of children with long-term successful transplants have been similarly interviewed, and all transplant children have been evaluated psychiatrically before and after surgery. The first aspects of the research effort are discussed in this chapter, the other two in Chapter 5.

METHOD

Population

Chronically Ill Children. A population of 72 chronically ill patients from 8 to 20 years old was selected from the University of Minnesota Pediatric Renal Clinic. Because many of the children attending this clinic have acute and nonserious conditions and we wished to study only those whose disease was serious and chronic, a duration criterion of at least one year from time of diagnosis was used to help ensure that the disease was chronic, and to enable us to concentrate on children and families whose coping mechanisms were likely to have achieved some stability. The physicians were asked to classify every patient who had an appointment at the Renal Clinic within the designated time period. Their identification of seriously ill children was largely based on the existence of the following major diseases: chronic pyelonephritis, chronic glomerulonephritis, polycystic kidney disease, congenital interstitial nephritis, diabetic glomerulosclerosis, chronic end-stage renal disease (undetermined etiology), hypoplasia, or lupus erythematosis.

The mothers of all children who were designated by the physicians as meeting the criteria were contacted by telephone to confirm that the child was of proper age (over 8 and still in the home) and that the child had been under treatment for a year. All children who met these criteria between May 1972 and October 1973 were interviewed, except one whose parents refused to cooperate. Hence, we interviewed the entire population rather than a sample of the more seriously ill patients attending this clinic. Only nine of these patients had reached the stage at which they required hemodialysis or transplantation; 10 others had the very serious systematic disease of lupus erythematosis, three of whom classified themselves as severely ill at present.

In addition to the chronically ill patients, 44 "normal" siblings closest in age to the sick child were interviewed and serve as a control group. Sixty-five mothers were interviewed as well, thus providing three separate perspectives on the meaning of the disease to the child and his family. Although there were no actual refusals to be interviewed by the mothers whose children were studied, one out-of-town mother was unable to travel the long distance to the clinic, one family had no mother, and five mothers of children who would soon be transplanted were already being extensively studied as part of the larger research project (see Part III); we did not feel we could ask them to complete these questionnaires as well. In 16 families there were no siblings at home of eligible age to be interviewed, seven out-of-town families could not arrange to have the normal sibling travel the long distance to the clinic, and three siblings of pretransplant children were being intensively studied as part of the larger study and were not asked to participate in this aspect of the study. Only two in-town eligible siblings could be counted as refusals because they did not seem able to arrange the time for the interview.

Because normal siblings may be affected socially and psychologically by the disease in the home, an additional control group was also used from a prior study by Rosenberg and Simmons (1972). In a two-stage random-sample study of Baltimore school children, 25 schools had been sampled and 1918 children from grades 3 to 12 had been interviewed, using many of the same measures used here. Because the Baltimore sample was 63% black, we attempted to make the sample more comparable by using only the 621 white children, aged 10 to 18.

Measures

The research instruments included both closed and open-ended items. The questionnaires for the chronically ill children and their siblings were in two parts. Section 1 contained mainly closed-ended questions to measure multiple aspects of the self-image. Section 2 dealt more specifically with the child's illness, how he feels when he is sick, and what kinds of limitations he has experienced. Other questions probed his role in the family as well as his school adjustment and other activities. The mothers of the chronically ill children completed a written questionnaire as well as an interview that provided further background data and information on the impact of the disease on the child and his family.

An important focus of this research was to assess the effects of chronic disease on the adjustment of individual family members. The measures of psychosocial adjustment were adopted from previous research where they had been tested for reliability and validity, and reliability was satisfactorily established for this population (Klein, 1975; Rosenberg and Simmons, 1972). Most of the same dimensions of the self-picture that were investigated for the transplanted adults were also measured (see Chapter 3 and Figure 4-1), although the indicators have been modified to make them suitable for children ages 8 and over (Simmons et al., 1973) and the order of presentation is slightly different. The relevant scales measure level of happiness (or at the other extreme, the level of depressive affect) as well as the degree of anxiety and the disturbance along various dimensions of the self-image: self-esteem, stability of the self-concept, self-consciousness, estimate of popularity, and satisfaction with looks (see Appendix B for discussion of reliability of these measures; for more detail see Klein, 1975 and Simmons et al., 1973b).

FINDINGS

To measure adjustment or quality of life of the chronically ill child, we must specify the dimensions of quality of life. Basically the same dimensions are used here as for the adults with an overall focus on (1) physical well-being and ability to perform daily activities, (2) emotional well-being, and (3) social or interpersonal adjustment (see Figure 4-1).

Physical well-being
- Global feelings of well-being and symptomatology
- Ability to perform daily activities

Emotional well-being
- Happiness level
- Self-image level
  - Self-esteem
  - Self-consciousness
  - Stability of the self-picture
  - Sense of distinctiveness
  - Satisfaction with body-image
  - Perceived opinion of significant others (perceived popularity)
- Anxiety level
- Gross psychopathology and suicidal behavior

Social well-being: In major life roles
- *Social life*
  - Satisfaction
  - Participation
- *Vocation or school adjustment*
  - Satisfaction
  - Participation

Adjustment of other family members
- Family disruption
- Individual adjustment

Figure 4-1 Dimensions of adjustment for adults and children.

Physical Well-Being and Daily Activities

The child's sense of physical well-being is a most basic indicator of the effects of his disease and whether he defines himself as ill. In response to a general closed-ended question about how healthy they feel, only 21% of the children with chronic kidney disease, as compared to 57% of their siblings, describe themselves as "very healthy." The chronically ill child, his sibling, and mother all agree that this child is sick more often than other children (see Table 4-1).*

* Although data concerning the transplanted children are presented in these tables, they are discussed in Chapter 5.

TABLE 4-1 PERCEPTION OF ILLNESS BY FAMILY MEMBERS[a]

Compared to other kids, do you think you (your child, your sister) are sick more often than other kids, sick about the same, or sick less often?

	Chronically ill child regarding self	*Sibling regarding chronically ill child*	*Mother regarding chronically ill child*	*Normal control sibling regarding self*	*Transplanted child regarding self*
	%	%	%	%	%
More often	29	32	22	0	11
About the same	49	39	44	32	49
Less often	22	29	34	68	40
	(N = 72)	(N = 44)	(N = 64)	(N = 44)	(N = 37)

[a] $p < .001$.

In addition, these patients report they tire more easily ($p < .001$). They are also more likely than their siblings to worry about their health and to report that their mothers worry about how they feel. In comparing the child to his peers, the mother feels he is less active and at a disadvantage when *physically* competing with other children. More than half of the children were reported by their mothers to have experienced limitations in their school activities. Only 68% of the children reported that they go to gym classes; of those, only about two-thirds engage in all the regular activities.

School is an important focus of much of the child's activity, and other researchers have found academic difficulties associated with chronic illness (Pless and Roghmann, 1971; Sultz, 1972). In terms of absenteeism, a global measure of interference with academic life, these chronically ill children are at a disadvantage. Thirty-seven percent of the mothers answered that absenteeism had been a problem. Mothers were asked separately about days of school missed on the average by the sick and normal child. The sick children missed more days, with 18% missing more than five days a month whereas none of the siblings missed so many days.

In terms of quality of academic performance, 25% of the children were reported to have stayed back at least one year in school, and one-fourth of those repeats were specifically attributed by the mother to sickness. In addition, 52% of these children have needed a tutor. Although rates for normal children are unavailable, the levels of absenteeism and below-grade performance for this group seems high.

Other information was gathered about outside-school activities. Open-ended questions were asked of all three family members regarding clubs, hobbies, interests, and what the child did after school. Because of the qualitative nature of these data, differences were considered significant only if they were verified by more than one source and if they persisted when sex of the child was controlled. A variety of evidence suggests that the normal sibling is more physically active; he more often reports working outside, a significant fact for rural families. The most important differentiation in activities seems to be between team sports and social interaction groups (e.g., Girl Scouts). Consistently, according to all three groups of respondents, the normal siblings are more often *physically active* by participating in team sports, and the sick child is more involved in *social* activities. The difference in physical activity was expected; the latter difference was not. Are these sick children really more socially competent?

Social or Interpersonal Well-Being

These chronically ill children seem to have some obvious social liabilities—for example, a lack of energy. In addition, 42% of the mothers admit they make a special effort to keep the child away from others who are sick. Despite these obstacles, however, a series of questions about numbers of friends and frequency and type of social contacts revealed virtually no difference between the sick and normal children. There is limited evidence, in fact, that the sick girls may be more socially competent: The mothers report that these girls get along somewhat better with other children than do their female siblings (83% vs. 62%), although there is little difference between the sick boys and their brothers.

Thus, in terms of physical and academic performance but not social activity, these children with chronic disease seem to be at somewhat of a disadvantage in comparison to their siblings.

Disease and Emotional Well-Being

One of the major focuses in this research has been to explore the impact of chronic illness and transplantation on several dimensions of the child's psychological or emotional well-being, particularly on multiple aspects of the developing self-image. As a general indicator of mental health and adjustment, there are probably few factors as important to the individual as his picture of himself (see Rosenberg, 1965; Wylie, 1961).

In a large study of 1918 normal school children in Baltimore, Simmons and associates (1973b) showed that several dimensions of the self-image were particularly vulnerable to the stress of adolescence. We already know that adults seriously ill with kidney disease demonstrate more self-image problems than when they are later "returned to health" with a transplant (see Chapter 3). Thus, we hypothesized that the combination of illness and adolescence would be particularly stressful. We predicted that preadolescent and adolescent children who were chronically ill would indicate even greater disturbance in self-image than their healthier age-peers.

First of all, *global self-esteem*—the child's overall positive or negative evaluation of himself—might be adversely affected by being physically impaired and different. Second, an increase in *self-consciousness* may accompany illness as it does normal adolescence. The self, which is different because of illness, may become so salient in interaction with others that the interaction becomes embarrassing for the individual. Third, the question arises whether the *stability of the self-picture*—the sense of identity—is shaken with the uncertainties related to changed health status, as it is with the changes of early adolescence (see Erikson, 1956; Lecky, 1945). Fourth, because chronic kidney disease often retards growth, the *body-image*—the child's satisfaction with his looks—may also be affected. Finally, the *accorded self*—the opinions he believes others hold of him, his estimates of his own *popularity*—which take a negative turn in normal adolescence, might also be unfavorable because of the stress of being ill and different from one's peers.

Other dimensions of the self-image—including the extent to which the ill child reveals his *true feelings* about himself to others and his sense of being *distinctive*, or different—were also explored. In addition to analyses involving the self-image the ill and transplanted children were compared to others in terms of their overall levels of happiness and anxiety.

Adjustment of Sick and Normal Children. How does the child with chronic disease fare in terms of socioemotional adjustment?* The major differences between the ill and healthy children involve their body-image or satisfaction with their looks (see Table 4-2). Only along this dimension do the ill children appear to suffer. Thirty-nine percent of the chronically ill children are classified as "not satisfied" with their looks, compared to only 28% of the siblings and 22% of the Baltimore controls ($p < .05$ for the comparison of these three groups). This finding with regard to the importance of body-image is verified and discussed in Chapter 5 apropos of the transplanted children.

Other dimensions of the self-image appear to be *surprisingly undamaged* in the total sample of ill children. Self-esteem, self-consciousness, self-

* Although data concerning the transplanted children are presented in these tables, they are discussed in Chapter 5.

TABLE 4–2 SOCIAL-EMOTIONAL ADJUSTMENT

	Baltimore controls[a] (N = 621)	Sick children (N = 72)	Normal siblings (N = 44)	Post-transplant children (N = 52)
Happiness				
Low	42%	35%	40%	34%
Medium	46	51	44	43
High	12	14	16	23
	100%	100%	100%	100%
Self-image				
Self-esteem				
Low	37%	31%	41%	40%
Medium	29	37	25	34
High	33	32	34	26
	100%	100%	100%	100%
Self-consciousness				
Low	19%	44%	41%	50%
Medium	44	42	46	33
High	37	15	14	17
	100%	100%	100%	100%
				$p < .001$
Stability of self-picture				
Low	33%	35%	46%	47%
Medium	22	28	20	16
High	45	37	33	38
	100%	100%	100%	100%
Sense of distinctiveness				
Not different	11%	16%	5%	22%
Little different	26	33	27	22
Very different	63	51	68	56
	100%	100%	100%	100%

FOR SICK CHILDREN AND NORMAL CONTROLS

	Baltimore controls[a] ($N = 621$)	Sick children ($N = 72$)	Normal siblings ($N = 44$)	Post-transplant children ($N = 52$)
Body-image, satisfied with looks				
Not satisfied	22%	39%	28%	55%
A little satisfied	42	36	40	36
Very satisfied	35	25	32	8
	100%	100%	100%	100%
				$p < .001$
Relationship to others				
Show true feelings				
Not show	30%	26%	29%	22%
Show little	51	44	41	47
Show a lot	20	29	29	31
	100%	100%	100%	100%
Estimate of Popularity				
Not popular	8%	7%	7%	14%
Little popular	23	28	20	23
Very popular	69	65	72	63
	100%	100%	100%	100%
Anxiety				
High	11%	12%	14%	12%
Medium	54	53	54	54
Low	34	34	32	33
	100%	100%	100%	100%

[a] Using only white children, ages 10 to 18.

image stability, a sense of distinctiveness, felt ability to reveal true feelings, and estimates of popularity are all unhurt.*

For most of the chronically ill children, the level of happiness also appears no lower than that of the controls. Yet there are a few patients who show severe evidence of depression, according to their mothers or physicians. Four chronically ill adolescents made suicide attempts or threats. Among the four chronically ill suicidal patients were two youngsters heading for kidney transplantation, each of whom had watched a relative die after an unsuccessful transplant. The other two suicidal patients were among the 10 patients who had lupus erythematosis, a particularly severe disease affecting the kidney as well as other body systems. (The susceptibility of a few ill and transplanted adolescents to suicidal thinking was noted in Chapter 3 and is further discussed in Chapter 5.)

Factors Affecting the Child's Adjustment to Chronic Illness

Other than for a few extreme cases, is the psychological stress of chronic illness exaggerated? This conclusion would be premature before investigating whether subgroups of the population are more severely affected than others by the disease experience. Types of children who are more vulnerable to the stress of illness are identified in Figure 4-2, and the

Those with more severe illness
Adolescents
(Females)
Children from rural, lower-class, or large families
Children dissatisfied with their appearance
Children who take less responsibility for their own care
Children whose mothers are confused by the sick role

Figure 4-2 Children at greater risk.

following discussion is focused on factors that might be expected to increase vulnerability.

Effect of Disease Severity on Adjustment of the Chronically Ill Child. The first set of factors explored involved various definitions of the severity

* Table 4–2 does show that the Baltimore children are significantly more likely than any of the Minnesota groups to score high in self-consciousness. If a chi-square test is performed on the other three groups, eliminating the Baltimore sample, there is no significant difference.

of the chronically ill child's disease. The initial hypothesis is that children who are more seriously ill will show greater disturbance of the self-picture and a lower level of happiness. In Chapter 3 we indicated that transplanted adults with greater health problems showed less favorable sociopsychological adjustment. For this study of children, two objective and one subjective measure of severity have been correlated with the nine indicators of the child's adjustment. The two external judgments are those of the physician and the child's mother, one a medical and the other a family expert. The third measure of severity involves the child's own subjective perception of his disease.

Severity as defined by the physician was found to correlate significantly and negatively with three aspects of the child's adjustment (see Table 4-3). Severity as judged by the mother is associated at statistically significant levels with five measures of adjustment. Although the objective severity of the child's condition does affect the child then, several aspects of the self are unaffected.

TABLE 4–3 EFFECT ON CHRONICALLY ILL CHILD OF OBJECTIVE AND SUBJECT SEVERITY OF THE DISEASE (PEARSON'S CORRELATIONS AND CANONICAL CORRELATIONS)

	Objective definitions		Subjective
Child's emotional state	Physician's rating of severity	Mother's rating of severity	Child's own rating of severity
Happiness	−.18§	−.15	−.22‡
Self-esteem	−.01	−.18§	−.34†
Self-consciousness	−.02	.13	.38*
Stability of the self-picture	.11	−.14	−.18§
Sense of being distinctive, different	−.19§	.20§	.15
Satisfaction with one's looks	.03	−.12	.01
Showing true feelings to others	−.23‡	−.26‡	−.31†
Estimate of popularity	.08	−.32†	−.38*
Anxiety	.08	.18§	.43*
Canonical correlation	.37	.43	.59†
Common variance	14%	19%	35%

* $p \leq .001$. ‡ $p \leq .05$.
† $p \leq .01$. § $p \leq .10$.

The child's own definition of the severity of his disease, however, correlates more highly and significantly with almost all of the measures of adjustment in a negative direction (Table 4-3). Although there is a high correlation between the three definitions of severity, the highest correlation is between that of the mother and that of the child, and these two family definitions seem to have wider ramifications for the child.* In comparing the canonical correlations between each of the three definitions of severity and the nine adjustment measures, the child's subjective definition is found to account for more of the variance in the child's adjustment (35%) than the two objective definitions (14% explained by physician's definition and 19% by that of the mother). The fact that the child's *own* perception of his disease correlates most highly with his other self-assessments probably cannot be dismissed as simply a function of measurement consistency—that is, that responses from the same individual are always likely to correlate more highly than responses from different individuals. In fact, this pattern of a higher correlation among answers collected from *one* person does not always occur for these variables. For example, the *child's* definition of the severity of the disease is more important for the *mother's* self-reported adjustment than is her own definition of the severity of the child's disease. Because the true seriousness of the disease is frequently hidden from the child, his own interpretation seems to become more important than the reality, both for his own and his mother's psychological health.

However, with a one-point-in-time study (a cross-sectional design), we cannot be certain of this causal direction. Perhaps, as posited, children who perceive the disease to be a great problem react to this perception with a less-favorable self-image and level of happiness. If this is the major causal direction, we *could* conclude that the child's own subjective experience has more extensive and pervasive effects than the objective severity of his disease. However, children who previously suffered from low esteem and a low level of happiness could be the ones who are least able to cope with the disease and are most likely to perceive it as a major problem.

Effect of Age and Sex on Adjustment of the Chronically Ill Child. Other than differences due to disease severity, is the adjustment of these children related to background or status factors? In the Baltimore study Simmons and associates (1973b) found that disturbance in the self-image of normal

* Correlations of three definitions of severity: physician with mother, .32; physician with child, .28; mother with child, .57. Although the mother's and child's definitions correlate negatively with almost all dimensions of the child's emotional adjustment, the physician's definition is less consistent in direction.

children was related to their *age. Early adolescents* (aged 12 to 14 or 15) showed a negative drop in many scales, followed by a leveling or positive turn, especially for self-esteem, during late adolescence.

In our study of chronically ill children we found that age significantly affects three indicators of adjustment: depression, self-consciousness, and global self-esteem.* As in the Baltimore sample, depression and self-consciousness increase among the chronically ill children in adolescence, with the big increase occurring in the early teen-age years. The normal siblings also show greater depression and self-consciousness at adolescence.

Both the sick children and their siblings reveal a steady increase in self-esteem with age. In the Baltimore sample the transition year into puberty (age 12), when youngsters moved into junior highschool, was accompanied by a sudden short-lived dip in self-esteem. Because of the small numbers of children at any particular age among the chronically ill population, it was impossible to test for this decrease in self-esteem found for the Baltimore 12-year-olds. In any case, like the Baltimore children, the older adolescents demonstrate higher self-esteem than any other aged child. Thus, age-related changes appear to be similar for the chronically ill children as for normal groups of youth.

The sex of the child might also be expected to have an impact upon his or her self-image that is independent of the illness. Among the *adults*, females were found to adjust better to illness and the transplant than males (Chapter 3). Yet the suggested explanations for these results seem to lie in the adult roles of men and women. The male had to attain successful job rehabilitation to be self-content, while the woman could define herself as rehabilitated without leaving the home. Within the home the female's activity was so necessary for family order that she was presumed to be highly motivated to leave the sick role. However, these sex-role considerations are not relevant for adolescents and children—that is, the female child or adolescent should have no easier time than the male at defining herself rehabilitated, and her full participation within the family should be no more important than that of the male. Thus, if these sex-role explanations have any validity, the female children should not demonstrate higher adjustment than the males.

In fact, the Baltimore study of normal children indicates that in certain respects, females have a more difficult adolescence than males (Rosenberg and Simmons, 1975; Simmons and Rosenberg, 1975). The ill children seem to react the same way as do the normal youth. For both the sick children and their siblings, females are generally less well-off than the

* In general, throughout this chapter, if one of the nine scales is not mentioned there is no relationship in either direction between it and the relevant factor being considered.

male children in terms of stability of the self-concept and satisfaction with looks, but better off in terms of happiness. That females are less satisfied with their appearance is not surprising. In our culture good looks are more important for the female than the male; in adolescence, when appearance changes rapidly, the female is more liable to react negatively to these changes, whether she is ill or healthy.

In general, the effects of age and sex upon the self-image seem to reflect general developmental differences rather than to be a consequence of chronic illness.

Effect of Family Background on the Adjustment of the Chronically Ill Child. Family background factors also appear to have general consequences for children's self-images rather than specific effects for the ill child. In general, the urban middle-class family appears to be more beneficial for the self-image of both the ill children and their siblings than does the rural lower-class family. Even controlling for socioeconomic status,* and religion, rural youngsters (particularly the ill children but also their siblings), score lower in self-esteem than their urban counterparts and also more negatively along other dimensions of the self-picture (although the findings are not totally consistent). For example, the partial correlation between rural–urban residence and self-esteem is .32 (p=.008) for the ill children and .21 for their siblings (see Klein, 1975, for more detail). †

Several studies conducted in the 1930s and 1940s hypothesized that rural life would be *more* beneficial than urban life for the adjustment of the child (Mangus, 1949). Yet these studies did not show rural children scoring higher than big-city children in the California Test of Personality (p. 14) and our research also fails to show an advantage of rural life. In fact, at least in this population, a rural background is a disadvantage for the child. But why should rural residence be associated with lower self-esteem? We could hypothesize that it is due to the fact that rural families tend to be larger (our data do show the farm families to be larger). Perhaps in small families, which are more common in the city, children receive more parental attention to the benefit of their self-esteem.

Large family size does appear to be associated with detrimental self-image effects, although not totally consistently. Both sick children and their siblings are much less likely to reveal their true feelings if they live in

* As measured by the Hollingshead Two-Factor Scale (Bonjean, 1967).

† Moreover, when rural–urban residence is controlled, neither the children's social-class background nor their family's religious orientation have consistent effects upon their self-esteem in particular nor self-image in general.

a large family ($r = -.23$* and $-.33$*). Likewise, children from large families, especially if sick, are more likely to be highly self-conscious ($r = -.23$*). The *self-esteem* of the siblings is also negatively affected by being in a large family: 46% of siblings from large families† have low self-esteem, in contrast to only 33% from small families. However, the self-esteem of the ill children is unaffected by family size, and therefore the rural–urban differences in their self-esteem could not be due to family-size differentials.

Thus, in this population both the ill and healthy children from small urban families appear better adjusted on several, though not all, dimensions. These families seem to act as positive resources for all children in handling stress. Whether these findings will be replicated in other studies is an open question. In the Baltimore study there are no rural children to test (see Rosenberg and Simmons, 1972). That our findings are specific to children in families containing a chronically ill member seems unlikely but not impossible.

Satisfaction with Body Image: The Adjustment of the Chronically Ill Child. Apart from the severity of the illness and the background statuses of the child and his family, the child's appearance would also be expected to affect his adjustment. As the illness becomes visible, we would expect its effects to be greater. As indicated above, the most significant difference between the *chronically ill* and normal children relates to the ill youngsters' dissatisfaction with their body-image. Thirty-six percent of the ill children say the disease has affected their appearance. Thirty-nine percent perceive they are "too short," in comparison to only 23% of their siblings, a figure reflecting the retardation of growth caused by some kidney diseases. Furthermore, although the relationships are small, the chronically ill children who are less satisfied with their looks demonstrate greater instability of the self-picture ($r = .18$), a lesser ability to reveal true feelings to others ($r = .15$), and lower self-esteem ($r = .10$). Transplanted adults who were less satisfied with their looks also showed a less favorable psychological adjustment (Chapter 3). The impact of body-image upon transplanted children, which is even greater, is discussed in Chapter 5.

Impact of the Chronically Ill Child on the Family

In our society the family is the social unit most directly responsible for the care of its sick members. The effects of illness on the child cannot be

* $p \leq .05$.

† Families in which the ill child has three or more siblings.

understood without exploring the impact of the disease on his family and the amount of protection and support the family offers the sick child.

The diagnosis of a chronic disease in a child is often a "crisis" for the family. The immediate responses reported by the mothers to the diagnosis (of kidney disease) were characterized by pessimism, a felt lack of understanding and fear that the child might die. The mothers reported that their understanding and acceptance increased and their worry decreased over time. Although the disease was still perceived as a significant problem, it could be cognitively assimilated into the family's ongoing life.

A series of questions was asked of the patients and their mothers and siblings to explore what the child's disease actually meant to the family. These items were placed in a factor analysis which yielded three general factors: the *general* practical disruption caused the family, the *emotional* stress, and the *financial* burden. The general-impact factor deals with the level of disruption in the family—for instance, how much time and energy the child's illness had consumed or how much it had interfered with the family routine (see Appendix B).

The stressor event in each family is in general the same—the diagnosis of a serious and chronic childhood disease. The stressor does, however, vary in its seriousness; and severity should, hypothetically, be related to impact on the family. The data show that the more serious the child's disease (as defined by mother, child, and physician) the greater the general, emotional, and financial hardships for the family.

A crisis may be conceptualized as having various hardship aspects that differ in importance from one crisis situation and family to another. Although the stressor event was similar in each of the families studied, the way in which the family defined the event and the impact varied. The family carries with it certain recuperative resources—indexed by socioeconomic status, religious affiliation, family composition, and modes of family functioning—upon which it draws during a crisis. Some of these background factors are positive resources; others may increase the family's vulnerability. Furthermore, background factors may act positively or negatively depending on which of the three hardship dimensions is considered. Several factors that have been found to affect the family's response (Hansen and Hill, 1964) were examined in relation to perceived hardship.

Effect of Family Size, Structure, and Residence on Family Response to Chronic Childhood Illness. Overall family size is not either an advantage or handicap in meeting this crisis. Whether there is an older sibling at home is a related aspect of family structure. Having an older child in the home may, for instance, be a resource if the mother needs help. Although no differences are shown in terms of general disruption, there is some evidence that having older children in the home is a resource in alleviating the emotional hardship of having a child with chronic kidney disease. Where there is an older sibling in the house, fully 53% of the families report a low emotional impact, in contrast to only 37% of those without an older sibling. Thus, the sibling structure, not family size *per se*, is the important factor.

Rural families are more likely to show a high level of general disruption than urban families (33% vs. 16%), although there are no differences between rural and urban families in regard to emotional or financial impact. Just as the ill children and their siblings fared less well in a rural environment, the rural family appeared to find illness a greater stress. Further analyses, controlling for religion and family size, failed to destroy the relationship between rural residence and general disruptive impact. This difference may be explained in part by the demands of farm life which cannot yield easily to the needs of a disabled member. Greater distance from the medical center may also contribute to the difficulty.

Effect of Socioeconomic Status and Religion on Family Responses to Chronic Childhood Illness. If differences in family size do not explain the greater disruption for the rural family, socioeconomic status (SES) may, given the fact that rural families tend to be poorer. However, high or middle socioeconomic status, not lower, is associated with family difficulty along all three dimensions. For example, only 21% of those with high SES report a low level of general disruption in contrast to half of the lower-class families. This relationship holds when controlled for residence and religion. In terms of *financial* impact, the middle class is also more likely to report a greater impact. This disadvantage for the middle-class family may in part be attributed to the fact that they did not qualify for medical assistance and had to bear almost all the medical costs themselves. In addition, the middle class, in contrast to the lower classes, defines illness as more of an emotional or tragic crisis (Farber, 1960). Thus, socioeconomic differences cannot explain the greater problems for the rural families.

Religious differences do not explain the rural–urban findings either. Although Farber (1959) and Zuk (1959) found that the Catholic religion was a supportive factor in dealing with mental retardation, no significant differences in family impact in this study were found between Catholics and Protestants.

Effect of Family's Solidarity and Prior Experience. Quality of the family's functioning is expected to be related to the family's level of solidarity. Therefore, a scale of family solidarity was constructed from the mother's interview.* Families low in solidarity are more likely than families high in solidarity to report that the disease had a great general disruptive impact (50% vs. 17%). *Highly* unified families are, however, more emotionally disrupted by the child's disease, perhaps because of the emotional interdependence of its members (36% vs. 50% show a low degree of emotional impact). No consistent relationship between family solidarity and financial hardship was found.

Another aspect of the family's functioning expected to help in problem-solving is previous experience with similar problems (Hill, 1949). Our data suggest that previous experience is a resource in meeting the general and emotional aspects of the hardship. Of the mothers who reported that their families had experience with other serious diseases, 57% indicated a low level of general disruption this time (in comparison to 42% of the inexperienced), and 59% (vs. 39%) reported a low degree of emotional hardship associated with the child's disease. Experience is, however, a handicap with regard to the financial impact of the disease; those with previous illness reported greater hardship, suggesting the family's practical resources may already have been depleted. (See Chapter 5 for a somewhat different picture of families with two transplanted children.)

Characteristics of families at particular risk are shown in Table 4-4. Few generalizations can be made about the family at risk for all three aspects of the crisis. A factor intensifying one type of hardship—financial, emotional, or general disruption—may have no effect or may even mitigate another aspect of the stress.

* The items in the scale were:

> Do you think that the child's disease in any way brought the family closer together or in any way drew the family apart? Yes, together/Neither/No, apart.
>
> All families are different—some are very close and others are not. Would you say the people in your immediate family are: Very close/Pretty close/A little close/Not at all close to each other?
>
> How well do the people in your family get along together at home? Does your family get along: Very well/Pretty well/A little well/Not at all well?
>
> When a problem comes up in the family, how willing are the people in your immediate family to help out? Are they: Very willing to help out/Somewhat willing/A little willing/Not at all willing to help out?
>
> Compared to most families you know, do you think your family is: More happy/Less happy/About the same as other families?

Reliability and validity were satisfactory for this scale (see Klein, 1975).

TABLE 4–4 CHARACTERISTICS OF FAMILY AT RISK FOR HARDSHIP DURING CHRONIC CHILDHOOD ILLNESS

General disruptive impact	Emotional impact	Financial impact
Rural residence	------	------
Highest social class	Middle social class	Middle social class
------	No older children in home	No older children
Low family solidarity	High family solidarity	------
Lack of experience with similar crises	Lack of experience	Experience with similar crises

Impact of the Child's Chronic Disease on Family Members

Effects of the Disease on the Adjustment of Other Family Members. Chronic illness would be expected to affect the adjustment of individual family members as well as the family as a whole. In fact, maternal adjustment was found to be influenced by the child's disease. The mothers were administered the same scales used to measure happiness, anxiety, and self-esteem as those used in the study of adult transplant patients and their donors. The greater the severity of the disease as perceived by the *child*, the lower the mother's happiness ($r = -.20, p = .06$) and the greater her anxiety ($r = .15$) and guilt ($r = .31, p = .004$).

Severity of the child's disease as estimated by the mother was also found to be related to the adjustment of the normal sibling, although not totally consistently. Greater severity was especially related to lower self-esteem of the siblings ($r = -.23, p = .08$), a tendency to conceal true feelings ($r = .34, p = .02$), and a higher level of anxiety ($r = .33$). Furthermore, controlling for the severity of the disease,* we find that if the sibling reports he is very disturbed and unhappy about the disease, his overall level of happiness is likely to be low ($r = -.38, p = .02$). Either the specific anxiety over the disease renders the sibling generally unhappy, or the less-happy child interprets the illness in an especially negative light. In either case the child in a home where a brother or sister is suffering from a more severe chronic disease is likely to show an impaired self-image. The fact that a severe disease has emotional costs for the sibling as well as the ill patient helps to explain why there is not a greater difference between the self-images of the sick children and their normal sisters and brothers. However, the lack of difference between the ill

* Unless otherwise specified, we control for child, mother, and physician's view of severity simultaneously.

children and the Baltimore controls still remains to be explained (see Conclusion).

Sharing or Focusing the Burden of Childhood Illness. Many studies have indicated that of all the family members, the mother bears the greatest impact when one member is chronically ill (Litman, 1974). Is this pattern true in our population as well? We asked family members how upset and unhappy various family members had been by the disease (the emotional impact), how much each member had to give up, and how much the daily life of each had been disturbed by the disease (practical hardships). According to the mother *and the normal sibling*, the mother is more likely to bear the brunt of the *emotional* impact. Only one-third of the mothers saw themselves as relatively undisturbed emotionally, in comparison to their perception that 42% of the fathers, 53% of ill children, and 60% of the normal siblings were undisturbed. *Both* parents are seen as worrying more than their children, including the ill child.

Some interesting findings emerge when the practical and emotional aspects of the impact are differentiated. According to the mother, it is the ill child himself whose daily life is most disturbed on the practical level, and who has had to sacrifice the most: 54% of the children were seen as significantly affected by the disease in this way, compared to 40% of the mothers, 33% of the fathers, and 25% of the normal siblings. In terms of nursing care for the sick child, however, mothers assume the greatest burden, followed by the child himself. While other family members help with the housework, they appear to participate little in the care of the ill child, at least according to our data (for more detail, see Klein, 1975).

Unfortunately, however, in this and most studies of chronic illness in children, the father's perception has not been measured, and therefore we are relying for this information on the view of the mother, the sick child, and the normal sibling. Perhaps they underestimate the father's input.

Our initial hypothesis was that a family member upon whom the burdens of disease were focused would be maladjusted—that is, if one individual assumed the hardship himself or herself without family sharing support, there would be a mental health cost for that individual. There were few families (14 out of 72) in which the mother alone seemed to bear the burdens of care, however, and the effects on her adjustment seemed minimal.

To test the relationship between sharing of the burden and the ill child's adjustment, families were divided into three groups *according to the mother's perception*: (1) those in which the ill child does not share in the burden of care; (2) families in which the burden is shared by all members, including the child; and (3) those in which the burden of care is focused primarily on the sick child. Correlations with the nine scales of the child's adjustment show that the way the family manages the burden is somewhat important for the child, but for several scales in the direction *opposite* to the way predicted. Children upon whom the burden of care is *focused*, in contrast to those who do not assume a major burden of self-care, demonstrate *higher* stability of the self-concept ($r = .15$), lower anxiety ($r = -.19, p = .08$), are able to show their feelings more ($r = .36, p = .002$), tend to be more satisfied with their appearance ($r = .41, p = .001$), and are less likely to see themselves as different ($r = -.14$) even when severity of the disease and age are controlled.* Thus a strategy of giving the child sole responsibility for his own care seems positive for the child's adjustment along several self-image dimensions.

Further evidence of the benefit to the child in assuming responsibility for his own care is obtained from the child himself. If the child indicated in answer to several questions that he took care of himself when he was sick, he was more likely to demonstrate high self-esteem ($r = .29$, $p = .02$)† The way the family manages the burdens of the disease is important not only to the family members but to the child himself.

Mother's Tension in Managing the Sick Child's Role

The mother's management of the disease not only involves the extent to which the burden is shared, but also the level of emotional confusion or calm with which the sick role is approached.

Qualitative information from parents of ill and transplanted children suggests that certain dilemmas face the mothers, and mothers respond with varying levels of confusion. A major dilemma for the mother is whether to treat the child as "normal" or whether to make certain he receives special treatment. The danger of giving him special treatment is that he will become crippled psychologically. The above discussion indicates that the independent child who assumes responsibility for his own care is emotionally healthier than the child who does not. Yet if the child is treated as normal in all situations, his physical health may be placed at serious risk, as in the following case:

A 10-year-old girl received her father's kidney and was successfully transplanted. When she returned home, she did well and was able with some parental help to administer her own medications. A year later her parents decided to send her to camp, like other "normal" children. The medications at camp had to be adminis-

* These are partial correlations controlling for the severity of the disease and the child's age.
† This is a partial correlation controlling for the child's age and the severity of the disease.

tered through the camp nurse, and the nurse was sent these with instructions. When the child returned home, however, her blood tests indicated that she had started to reject the kidney. Upon questioning, the child indicated that when she went to the camp infirmary for her medications she could not find the nurse and did not receive her medicines for a week or more. The insidious chronic rejection of the kidney could not be halted and after a very stressful time period, the kidney had to be removed. The mother then donated her kidney to maintain the child's life.

This case is complicated by the fact that the "normal" child is not expected to handle medications. To escape the dependency of illness is difficult for the chronically ill child because he cannot evade the dependency of childhood. He is unnecessarily dependent for care upon busy adults who may fail to comprehend special needs. The parent feels compelled therefore to give him special protection to maintain his physical health. Yet some parents are very confused as to the proper course of action in this and other situations.

To investigate the consequences of maternal confusion in managing the child's sick role, we asked the mothers

> Do you generally feel you have been able to handle your child's illness well enough or do you feel it's been a problem for you?
>
> Parents sometimes feel confused about whether a child with this disease should be treated differently or whether (he, she) should be treated the same as other children. Has this been a problem for you—deciding how to treat your child? Has it been a great problem /Somewhat of a problem/A little of a problem/No problem for you?
>
> How much of a bother is the child's regular treatment? Is it a big bother/A little bother/No bother at all?
>
> How hard is it for your child to follow the doctor's orders? Very hard/A little hard/Not at all hard?

This index of tension in managing the sick child's role or the mother's difficulty in handling the child does not correlate significantly with measures of maternal adjustment. It is more important in understanding the child's adjustment, however. Controlling for the severity of the disease, on several of the nine scales, the mother's perceived tension in managing the sick child's role is associated with *negative* adjustment for the child. (On the other scales there is no difference.) The child's sense of being different and distinct ($r = .20$,* $p = .08$), his level of anxiety ($r = .26$, $p = .03$), the stability of his self-picture ($r = -.11$*), and the child's ability to

* These are partial correlations, controlling for the severity of the disease.

reveal his true feelings to others ($r = -.30$, $p = .01$) are affected by the mother's tension in managing the sick role. Although the correlations are not large, the importance of these findings is increased by the independence of the measures—the indicators of the mother's role-tension are derived from her own reports, while the measures of the ill child's adjustment are obtained from the child. According to these measures, if the mother is confused in her handling of the ill child, the child himself is at risk psychologically. The mother's conflict in handling the child thus provides a link between the coping of the family and that of the child.

SUMMARY AND DISCUSSION

The chronically ill children as a group appear to be quite healthy in terms of their self-image and socioemotional adjustment. Although they are more dissatisfied with their physical appearance, on the average they are not more disturbed than normal controls in regard to their levels of self-esteem, self-consciousness, self-image stability, sense of distinctiveness, ability to reveal true feelings to others, or perceived levels of happiness. These findings suggest a puzzle: Why don't the chronically ill youngsters demonstrate a more damaged self-picture, especially in view of the fact that adult patients on hemodialysis show significant damage along these same dimensions?

We can offer several hypotheses. First, the majority of these children were considerably less ill and less symptomatic than the pretransplant adults—only 9 of them were ready for hemodialysis or transplantation. And children who are suffering from more serious diseases do show greater socioemotional disturbance,* although their own definition of the disease appears to have greater correlation with adjustment than does the physician's definition.

Second, the child's functional role is not as vulnerable to illness as that of an adult. For the most part a chronically ill child continues with school whereas the adult may be unable to maintain a job or perform his family responsibilities. In fact the role of the normal child and the classic definition of the sick role (Gordon, 1966) are similar: Both the child and the ill person are generally exempt from social responsibility and are not expected to take care of themselves. Thus the deviations caused by disease are not so disrupting to the child as to the adult.

Third, parents can protect a child in ways in which the adult cannot be

* In their study of chronic illness, Haggerty and associates (1975) also find that on key adjustment measures differences occur primarily between severely ill children and other children, rather than between the moderately ill and normal youngsters.

protected. The parents can help the child *deny* the seriousness of his condition (Mattsson and Gross, 1966a,b; Salk et al., 1972). For instance, in comparing the way in which the ill child describes the personal costs of his disease with the descriptions given by his normal sibling and mother, some interesting discrepancies emerge. Most often the sibling reported that the illness had caused considerable sacrifices for the ill child whereas the sick child himself minimized these costs. The mothers' perceptions fell in between. For example, 30% of the siblings and 18% of the mothers but only 3% of the ill children reported that the ill child has had to give up "very much" ($p = .005$). For the child, the use of denial seems functional, allowing him to maintain a high level of adjustment.*

Along with this denial the parents abide by a philosophy, endorsed by physicians, to treat the child as normal (Collier, 1969; Davis, 1963; Mattsson and Gross, 1966a, b; Minde et al., 1972).

> I felt it was important for him to lead as normal a life as possible.
>
> We managed to put it [the disease] as part of family life. I tried to keep life on an even keel. . . .I preferred to have it something as normal as possible—Michael's going to the hospital and Bobby's going to school. It was just something he did. It was accepted as something 'normal' (mother of adolescent boy with chronic kidney disease).

The comments of this mother are characteristic of the attitude of most of the mothers interviewed. The mothers were asked: "Do you feel this child should be treated completely the same as other children, that (he, she) should be treated with some special consideration, or that (he, she) should be treated with a great amount of special consideration?" Eighty-two percent of the mothers responded with the ideology that the children should be treated the *same* as other children, and only 18% suggested some special consideration was appropriate. Yet, as indicated above, these children are at times very sick and require special care. The actual treatment of the child often conflicted with the labeling being given to behavior—the children were given extra attention to maintain their normalcy.

In addition to the ability of the parents to label the ill child as normal, they can also protect him or her with extra love and attention. Rosenberg (1965) and Rosenberg and Simmons (1972) have shown that the most powerful variables affecting children's self-images are the perceived opinions of significant others. If children believe that others rate them highly, they rate themselves highly. We have seen that the sick children

* The discrepancy between the ill child and the sibling may be due not only to denial on the part of the patient, but also because the normal sibling projects and exaggerates the plight of the sick youngster. The illness in imagination may be worse than in reality.

did not perceive themselves to be less popular with peers than did the normal controls. In addition, they were somewhat *more* likely than their siblings to report their mothers rate them highly. In answer to the multiple choice question, "Would you say your mother thinks you are a wonderful person/a pretty nice person/a little bit of a nice person/not such a nice person?" 43% of the sick children selected "a wonderful person," versus 36% of their siblings and 26% of the Baltimore controls. This favorable opinion of the mothers is undoubtedly protective for the child's self-image. Our data indicate that children who reported their mothers think they are "a wonderful person" scored more favorably on scales of self-esteem, self-consciousness, stability of the self-picture, satisfaction with looks, and ability to reveal their true feelings to others.

Furthermore, when asked to which family member they are closest, 29% of the sick children, in contrast to 18% of the siblings, chose their mother. They were also somewhat more likely than their own siblings to see themselves as the mother's favorite (14% versus 7%), whereas the siblings were more likely to choose the father as the closest (7% versus 20%). This evidence suggests the interaction pattern in the family may be altered, with the ill children perceiving a special alliance to their mothers. At any rate, the sick children do not appear disadvantaged within the context of the family.

Crain and associates (1966) did a similar study of the sociopsychological functioning of 19 diabetic children and 16 of their siblings. They too found that the functioning of the sick children did not differ significantly from that of their siblings. Furthermore, in trying to explain the lack of difference they showed that the diabetic children were closer than their siblings to the mother and that the mother's behavior was significantly related to the ill child's performance. Crain's study as well as our own suggests that there are costs for siblings in a family with a sick child and that closeness with the mother helps the ill child himself to compensate for the potential stress of chronic ill-health. That the sibling loses some maternal attention also helps to explain why the differences between siblings and ill children are not greater or always in the predicted direction.

We propose that the family of the ill adult does not protect him and his self-image in the way demonstrated by the mother of the ill child. Classic studies of the unemployed male during the depression indicate that even though the state of the economy was well-known, the male without a job lost considerable prestige within his own family (Angell, 1936). When the adult cannot perform his or her role and exposes the family to considerable stress, feelings of rejection seem more likely to occur than in the case of the child.

The effects of chronic illness on the child must be understood within the structure and functioning of the family. In this chapter the family's own coping as a unit has also been examined. Three aspects of the crisis for the *family* have been differentiated: general disruption, emotional stress, and financial burden. These factors have, in turn, been related to variables in the family's background which may be resources or liabilities in meeting the demands of a child's disease. The disease was found to have an impact on the adjustment and self-image of the child's mother and siblings. The more severe the disease, particularly in the child's eyes, the more negative the impact. The presence of an older sibling in the home, however, appears to reduce the emotional impact of the disease in the family.

One strategy for handling the sick child is to increase his or her responsibility for self-care. Where this occurs, regardless of the severity of the disease, the ill child shows a higher level of self-esteem. These data suggest that the ill child himself should share the burden of daily care with the mother. Of course with a one-point-in-time study we cannot be certain of the causal sequence. Children who have higher self-esteem prior to the disease may be the ones who will assume more responsibility for their own care, rather than that independence in handling their illness produces higher self-esteem. In either case there appears to be no psychological evidence to contraindicate giving the child a fairly high degree of responsibility.

Physicians involved in the treatment of these families should be aware that if the mother is confused on how to handle the sick role of the child, the child is likely to be at risk psychologically.

Despite these guidelines, the exact best balance for handling the child may be difficult to establish. The following two cases help describe attempts to achieve this balance, first in an unsuccessful case where the child is at risk, and second, in a case where the adjustment level is high.

The first mother has a 10-year-old-boy with chronic kidney disease. She reports, "We show no difference between him and the other kids." When the child is hospitalized at the university 200 miles from home, he is sometimes visited by his family on weekends. Although the mother acknowledges the boy is lonely, she expects the child to be very "mature." "He's very kind; he understands I can't be there." The patient himself voiced loneliness as his biggest problem in being sick. He was given *no special consideration* and was expected to understand that the family's needs outweighed his own need for support. Extreme denial of the seriousness of the boy's condition and complete responsibility by the child for his own care resulted, in this case, not only in psychological stress but also in poor disease control. Thus in some cases balancing of attention for the ill child against other family needs is difficult to achieve. This case suggests that problems can emerge when the child is given extreme responsibility unaccompanied by special emotional attention.

The second mother has a 16-year-old son who has had chronic kidney disease from age 2.

> I've tried to keep it as normal as possible, so it didn't seem like the attention was given because he was sick. He's had a lot of special attention but I don't want it to be something out of the ordinary. It's better to make it part of the daily routine. He may have to live with it all his life. . . .It [the disease] might have had a maturing effect—he's quite mature for his age. He's able to accept responsibility. . . .He organizes, carries through; he's very adult. He's had a lot of responsibilities from taking the medication; a lot depends on it—his life. It's a serious business; we never really talked about it, but we knew.

In this mother's account a need for special attention was recognized along with an effort to establish normalcy and responsibility. She alludes also to a positive personality gain or increased maturity attributed to the disease experience.

This increased maturity among the ill children was mentioned in several cases and should not be ignored as a possible effect of crisis. We asked the chronically ill children and their mothers and siblings what changes the disease had effected in the child. Although 14 siblings (32%) and 19 mothers (29%) mention negative personality changes (touchiness, irritability, withdrawal) in the ill child, 21 mothers (33%) commented on positive personality changes including increased maturity and appreciation of life. Among the children themselves, eight (11%) mention similar gains, although the more salient changes attributed to the disease were negative body changes, decreased energy, and activity restrictions. In terms of *personality* impact, however, the child and his mother tend to perceive the effects as more positive than negative. These feelings of greater maturity and a more fundamental appreciation of life due to the health crisis were also mentioned by adult posttransplant patients (see Chapter 3).

* * *

In conclusion, these results point to a surprising resiliency on the part of children faced with chronic illness. This resiliency may be due to some extent to extra protection and emotional support of the children by their families, a protection that is not afforded to chronically ill adults. Other factors leading to the relatively high adjustment of these children appear to be (1) the low visibility of kidney disease (those for whom the disease is more visible, whose physical appearance suffers, do show negative self-image damage), (2) the fact that many patients lack extensive symptomatology, (3) the continuing high opinion of significant others, and (4) a tendency toward denial fostered by the family. Evidence indicates that regardless of the severity of the disease, children who cope better are those who are allowed to assume more responsibility for their own medical care, whose mothers are not confused and overwhelmed by the necessary medical regime, and whose mothers are perceived as holding an extremely high opinion of them. The question now at issue is whether the children who have received kidney transplants demonstrate the same resiliency as these chronically ill children and as the transplanted adults.

5

PSYCHIATRIC ASSESSMENT OF THE ADJUSTMENT OF TRANSPLANTED CHILDREN

DOROTHY M. BERNSTEIN, M.D.

Although generally the death of a treatable child is unacceptable in our society, transplantation of children has been controversial (see Chapter 2). For example, as recently as 1974 a metropolitan newspaper reported the story of a rural family whose three sons died from a rare kidney disease ("Rare Kidney Disease," 1974). The doctors at a major midwestern clinic had told the parents that transplantation would but briefly delay death and recommended only that the parents help the children enjoy the remainder of life. Yet less than 100 miles away was the University of Minnesota with one of the largest pediatric transplant programs in the country. There is little doubt that these children would have been accepted for transplantation. Factors that have been cited as contraindicating transplantation for children include the possibility of only a short reprieve from death as balanced against the trauma of the procedure (Riley, 1964; Starzl, 1966b), the stressful side effects of the necessary medications and the retardation in growth that frequently cannot be reversed by the transplant. The child's emotional vulnerability and the stress to the family are also regarded by some as too costly to recommend the procedure. Yet these evaluations of the emotional effects of pediatric transplantation are not backed by empirical data.

Therefore the purpose of this chapter is to assess the emotional well-being and to document the physical status of children who have received kidney transplants. The reaction of children to this type of stress and to the restoration of health also has an interest above and beyond the policy issues under consideration.

Because of the controversy over the transplantation of children, relatively few of them received the treatment in the early years. However, with the development of new techniques and specialized equipment for young children, age of transplantation has been gradually extended downward over time in some centers. Najarian and his colleagues at Minnesota in 1968 established the basic protocols for patient evaluation, management of hemodialysis, techniques of kidney placement, and postoperative management in infants and children (Najarian et al., 1971).

At the University of Minnesota 105 children and adolescents from age 6 weeks to 18 years received kidney grafts in the time period from 1963 to 1974; approximately one-fifth of this group required a second or third transplant. If one excludes the four infants under 1 year of age, the probability of surviving with a kidney from a related donor was 86% at one year and 77% at 10 years (See Figure 5-1). When a cadaver kidney was used in the first transplant, the overall figures were 82% at one year and 63% at 10 years. As Figure 5-1 shows, after the second year of survival, patient and kidney loss were infrequent in this group. Thus the survival rate for children is quite high.

With the newer techniques, the rate of transplant function is as good as that for adults, and because children can be retransplanted after kidney rejection more easily than adults, the patient survival is even better than for adults (DeShazo et al., 1974; Fine et al., 1973). The question therefore becomes one of quality of life and psychological adjustment rather than one of survival. Particularly difficult physical problems, such as continuation of bone disease existing prior to transplantation, impairment of growth by complex metabolic processes, delay in sexual maturation, or Cushingoid appearance due to medication, can occur with children (Williams et al., 1969). The extent of these problems and the children's reactions to them are important to investigate.

Other psychiatric studies of small series of posttransplant patients

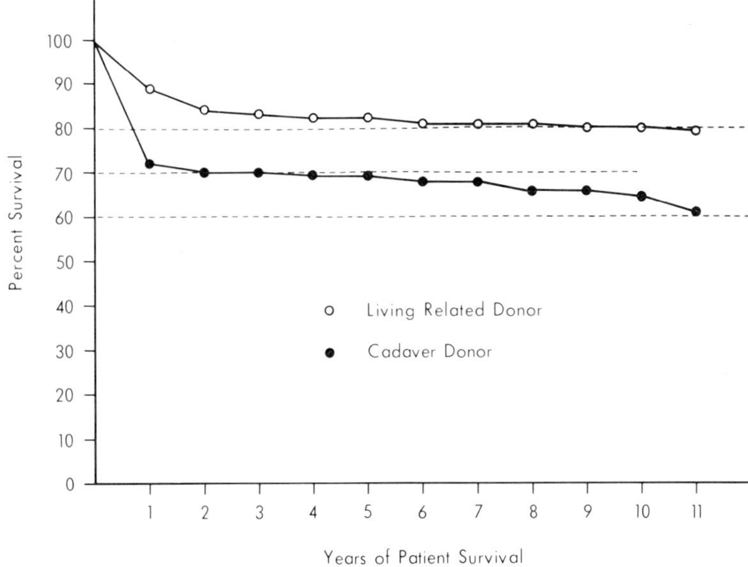

Figure 5-1 Children's survival following transplantation, by donation sources.

identified many socioemotional problems, although the likelihood of these problems varied among centers. Studying 35 transplanted children Korsch et al. (1973) reported that most children had returned to preillness equilibrium within a year posttransplant and that in the California Personality Inventory their overall adjustment scores did not differ from normal standard scores. However, their social adjustment scores were significantly lower than "normal" children's, and there was some indication that these patients might have lower self-esteem, although the control group used ($N = 8$) was too small to justify conclusions. More important, psychopathology was diagnosed in eight children, some of whom became depressed and failed to cooperate in their treatment. Khan et al. (1971) evaluated 14 children for social adjustment, emotional status, level of intelligence and self-concept after surviving a kidney transplant two to five years. Most of the children in the study had serious social and emotional difficulties. The most frequent findings were feelings of social isolation, excessive dependency on parents, and depression. Sampson's (1975) study of 14 posttransplant children (primarily adolescents) reported similar findings. The question arises to what extent negative adjustment will be found in the larger Minnesota series, and for which subgroups of children.

In considering the success of transplantation for either adults or children, the ultimate goal is returning the patient to normal life patterns and normal coping mechanisms for their ages. To evaluate these functions after a successful kidney graft, psychiatric and social-psychological studies of children and adolescents at the University of Minnesota have been conducted.

The focuses of these analyses are on the short- and long-term gains and costs for these children and upon the extent to which the tasks of growth and development are resumed in the physiological, psychological, and social spheres.

METHODS

The results of two discrete studies are reported in this chapter. The first, the bulk of the analysis, is the psychiatric evaluation conducted by the pediatric psychiatrist who is the author of this chapter. The second study involves the more quantitative data from Klein and Simmons' examination of the transplanted children. These latter data parallel that presented in Chapter 4 for chronically ill youngsters.

The Psychiatric Study

The coping responses and levels of adaptation of 100 children following their hospital discharge after a successful kidney transplant were examined in the psychiatric study. As a baseline, all of the children who had been transplanted in the past six years were examined psychiatrically prior to transplant as they entered the hospital for various procedures. They were also examined periodically as they progressed through the stages of dialysis and the surgery. In addition, they were seen six weeks following the transplant, at one year posttransplant, and then annually as they returned for follow-up in the Post-Transplant Clinic. For children transplanted earlier, retrospective data were gathered concerning emotional adaptation prior to surgery. For five children who died before the psychiatrist joined the staff, no such data could be gathered.

Population. The group was divided into younger children (aged 6 weeks to 11 years) and adolescents (aged 12 to 18 years) for purposes of comparison. Table 5-1 shows the characteristics of the study group population at the time of their first transplant.

Fifty-two percent of the cases fell into the pediatric group; 48% were in the adolescent group. The most frequently diagnosed renal disease lead-

TABLE 5-1 SEX AND AGE OF 100 CHILDREN AT TIME OF TRANSPLANT

	Age		
Sex	6 weeks to 5 years	6 years to 11 years	12 years to 18 years
Boys	11	19	28
Girls	4	18	20
TOTAL	15	37	48

ing to end-stage renal failure was glomerulonephritis (28% of the cases), followed by pyelonephritis (14% of the cases). Most often the diagnosis of kidney disease and failure to grow had been made by age 4 or 5. The children had been managed with medication and dietary restrictions as long as possible before transplantation became necessary.

At the University of Minnesota transplantation has been divided into two periods—before and after 1968. Since 1968 pediatric hemodialysis has been established and antilymphoblast globulin (ALG) therapy was initiated to help prevent rejection of the kidney. At this point transplants could be performed on children sooner after the diagnosis of end-stage renal disease was made. In the last two years, 34 transplants were performed on the younger age group, including four infants under 1 year. Although the infants were considered successes as far as the surgical procedures have been concerned, the lack of survivors has convinced the physicians that this group of patients is not currently suitable for transplantation.

In the population being studied, 22 patients (22%) have received more than one transplant since 1968. Of these, 19 are still functioning. Included in this group are 14 children who have received second transplants, three who received third transplants, and one who received a fourth transplant which is still functioning after two years, five months. Table 5-2 indicates that out of the cohort of 100 children seen by the psychiatrist, 85 reached a year posttransplant for evaluation, and 81 are currently surviving.

Procedures The procedure in the first study consisted of individual psychiatric evaluation supplemented by psychological testing procedures including the Draw-A-Person Test, Draw-Your-Family Test, and a designed Sentence-Completion Test. These tests and evaluations were conducted both prior to the transplant and at six weeks after the transplant during a visit to the posttransplant clinic. The parents were seen

TABLE 5-2 SURVIVAL OF CHILDREN TO AND AFTER 1 YEAR POSTTRANSPLANT IN PSYCHIATRIST'S COHORT

	Number of children	
Original cohort	105[a]	
Cohort seen by psychiatrist	100	
Deceased before 1 year	10	
Reached 1 year with functioning kidney	85	
Deceased after 1 year	9	
Currently surviving with functioning kidney beyond 1 year	76	81
Currently surviving; not yet reached 1 year	5	

[a] Five of these were children transplanted in the early 1960s who died before the psychiatrist joined the staff.

separately at this time and then yearly to gather additional information about the child's adjustment in the family and community.

Intellectual level of the child was assessed by the Draw-A-Person Test. Those at the upper and lower limits of normal were tested individually using the Wechsler Intelligence Scale for children. Intellectual assessment of the patient group revealed that three children were of borderline intelligence. The rest were in the normal range. Before transplantation, eight of the adolescents had been diagnosed as having psychiatric disorders, and six other children had a diagnosis of transitory adjustment reactions at some time before the transplant.

The Social-Psychological Study

A subgroup of the above pediatric transplant patients received virtually the same interview questionnaires as the chronically ill children described in Chapter 4 by Klein and Simmons. All children, aged 8 to 20, who had received a kidney transplant at the University before June 1973 and had maintained it for at least a year were measured with the same quantitative questions that had been administered to the chronically ill children, their siblings, and the normal control group from Baltimore. Thus the adjustment of the posttransplant youngsters can be compared directly to these other groups.

This part of the study involved 52 children who were an average of two-and-a-half years posttransplant. Although these measures allow a comparison of children who have received the therapy of transplantation to those with chronic *kidney disease*, the results are not directly analogous to the studies comparing adults pre- and posttransplant (see Chapter 3), because the chronically ill children by and large are not as ill as the pretransplant adults.

The psychiatric and social-psychological studies of the transplanted children are meant to complement and validate each other. While the quantitative measures allow precise comparisons between different groups of children along a variety of dimensions, the psychiatric evaluation permits an in-depth, holistic view. In addition, while the quantitative measures were administered at one point in time, the psychiatric evaluation was a continuing one over time and therefore allows one to compare the children to themselves pre- and posttransplant. Finally, the psychiatrist was able to evaluate those children under age 8 who were too young to answer the quantitative questionnaire.

FINDINGS

Physiological Gains and Losses

Physical Vigor and Feelings of Physical Well-Being. In the findings of these studies, biological gains and losses after the transplant were evaluated. Klein and Simmons (see Chapter 4) have reported that tiredness and lack of energy are among the major costs of chronic kidney disease. The gain noted most prominently by parents after the transplant was *increased physical vigor*. Sixty-four of the 100 parents in the psychiatric study and 48 of the children rated this as the most prominent change in the post-transplant child. This increased vigor was as apparent in the younger child as in the adolescent. If no complicating factors in the function of the new kidney occurred, this change in energy level was apparent within a few days after the transplant merely by observing the child.

Typical of this change is the history of a 3-year-old male child with congenital malformation of the kidneys. Due to weakness he never crawled. At 1 year he made attempts to walk; but as his physical condition deteriorated, he made no further attempts to stand or walk unaided. Muscular coordination was poor and he showed little activity when awake, and his usual activities consisted of sitting in a stroller 14 to 16 hours each day when he was not sleeping. At age 2, he was transplanted with a kidney from his mother, and the day after surgery he displayed increased energy. Within seven days after the transplant he not only had learned to walk but was running as well. When seen in the Post-Transplant Clinic after one year, this child showed a very active pattern of physical activity—running and climbing. In addition, he showed a pattern of improved fine and gross muscular coordination. He was now able to pile blocks and dress himself. He attended nursery school three times weekly and was able to participate in all physical activities at a normal age-expected level.

Adolescents also noted increased physical vigor and a feeling of well-being soon after the transplant if the transplanted kidney was functioning well. At a year following the surgical procedure their capacity for physical activity usually equalled or exceeded their preillness levels. Five of the male adolescents became active in athletics whereas prior to transplantation they had been unable to participate in sports. For young children or children with long-standing chronic renal malfunction, this kind of change represents a level of vigor surpassing the preillness state.

At the one-year examination, compared to the 6-week posttransplant examination, the only children with decreased physical vigor were those who showed a complicating factor in the function of the transplanted kidney. Seven children were in this category.

Diet. Another important physical gain in the daily follow-up examination was that the child showed an increase in appetite and was beginning to eat a normal diet. Prior to the transplant the child was usually on a diet highly restrictive of fluids and foods containing salt. Many pretransplant children had found this to be an oppressive restriction. Some children had difficulty adhering to these restrictions and would surreptitiously seek salty food or liquids while at home. An example was the case of a 16-year-old boy on dialysis who continued to retain excess fluid and gain weight, although he was on a special diet that would have brought these factors under control. The physicians suspected that he was not adhering to his diet, but the boy denied it. It was later confirmed that he was eating salted popcorn and potato chips while with his friends. This was a move on his part to live the life of a "regular teen-ager" and conform to peers. He was unable to acknowledge differences in himself. Some parents also failed to provide the correct diet for the pretransplant child at home.

At a year posttransplant with a functional kidney, most children were able to eat a normal range of foods with little restriction. For those children who had a long history of chronic illness preceding the transplant, this often meant being introduced to and learning to eat foods they had never known before. With a normal diet, children who before were malnourished showed a weight gain and improvement in physical appearance.

Physical Appearance. The appearance of some posttransplant youngsters has been one of the main arguments against transplantation for children. Although both adults and children may become very full-faced (Cushingoid) in response to the steroid medication, particularly when threatened kidney rejection requires high steroid doses, the adolescents tend to look more abnormal even at lower dosage levels. In particular, the growth retardation associated with their previous kidney diseases, plus the protuberant abdomen and prominent jowls associated with the Cushingoid state make them look more bizarre. Girls who are developing figures but not growing as tall as normal, appear more abnormal when their faces and waists are swollen. In most patients with successful kidney transplants, these problems abate with time; and most adolescents, though still short, appear increasingly normal four to five years after transplantation. At the time of the psychiatrist's one-year posttransplant examination, 14 girls and 9 boys appeared Cushingoid (27%), and currently 16 out of the 81 survivors (20%) exhibit this cost of transplantation (see Table 5-3).

The growth retardation of severe kidney disease is somewhat reversed by the kidney transplant,* but in many cases growth during the ado-

TABLE 5-3 CURRENT PHYSICAL CONDITION OF 81 SURVIVING TRANSPLANTED CHILDREN

	Current age				
Physical disability[a]	0–5 years (*N* = 5)	6–11 years (*N* = 15)	12–18 years (*N* = 30)	19–24 years (*N* = 31)	Total
Deafness	0	3	1	0	(4) 5%
Bone disease	1	0	2	0	(3) 4%
Cushingoid appearance	1	3	10	2	(16) 20%
Short stature	1	5	14	10	(30) 37%
Delay of sexual maturation			6	1	(7) 9%

[a] Children may appear in more than one group.

* The sample of chronically ill children described in Chapter 4 contains many youngsters whose type of kidney disease is not severe enough to retard growth.

lescent years is suboptimal. Some children grow rapidly immediately after the transplant; some grow poorly. Some who grow poorly during their first few posttransplant years may spurt later. In fact, some children who do not grow for the first few years after the transplant may grow several inches in the early 20s. In general, however, girls grow less well than do boys. This is particularly striking for girls in early adolescence.

In 1974 among all the adolescents who were transplanted before age 19, who currently were age 15 or older and who had reached 10 months or more posttransplant, 20% of the boys (3 out of 15) had not yet attained five feet in height and 53% were below 5½ feet. Four girls (21%) (4 out of 19) were 4½ feet or less in height, and 53% were below five feet.

In short, growth is variable and frequently disappointing. Failure to grow is related not only to preexisting disease and dose of steroids, but also appears to be related to the amount of imperfection in the function of the new kidney. A degree of renal compromise that would allow for apparent perfect health in an adult does not support the continued normal growth of the adolescent (De Shazo et al., 1974; Najarian et al., 1971).

Although increased growth is an immediate or long-run physiologic gain of transplantation for some children, for others this cost of kidney disease is not reversed.

For a few children muscular and skeletal abnormalities further compromised their appearance. There were three children who prior to transplantation had developed renal rickets. Although this condition was much improved by the transplant, some remnants of the problem still remained a year afterwards. In addition, there were four cases of aseptic bone necrosis (a form of arthritis). Implications for the behavior of these children lay in the reaction of peers. Adolescents particularly were subject to teasing and jesting.

Although growth retardation continued to be a cost for many of these patients, the majority of children showed normal sexual maturation in the period they were followed in this study. Nine percent, however, still show a lag in developing secondary sex characteristics or in beginning to menstruate (see Table 5-3 for information regarding current long-term survivors).

In three cases of delayed sexual maturation, a psychological reaction resulted. One 15-year-old boy who lacked pubic and axillary hair refused to take physical education or shower at school. A 16-year-old girl became isolated from peers because she thought that boys would find her different.

Medications. Another physiological factor reported by some children as difficult to manage was continued maintenance on the medications necessary to preserve the kidney—steroids, immunosuppressive drugs, and so on. One young child had difficulty leaving his mother to visit peers because of the complicated task of taking 27 dosages of medications per day. There were five instances of adolescents who became rebellious about the regime of taking medications and either skipped dosages or stopped their medication for varying periods of time, with the resultant possibility of acute rejection of the kidney. One 17-year-old boy on three occasions ran away from the hospital, went off his usual medication schedule, and engaged in episodes of illicit drug abuse. When symptoms of a kidney rejection reaction appeared, he returned to the hospital.

However, the majority of children learned to manage their own medications with proficiency. They assumed responsibility for telephoning their interim laboratory blood values to the University Center if these tests were performed by a local hospital. Children who were old enough to read were instructed on discharge from the hospital about their dosage schedule. Parents acted as a backup in seeing that the child carried out the instructions. Klein and Simmons' data suggest that responsibility for self-care is important to the child's adjustment (Chapter 4).

Alterations in mood due to steroids or other medications were found in five children. Three children manifested mild euphoria or depression while on high doses of steroids. Two teen-agers experienced mild hallucinations due to their medication and a 5-year-old boy became disoriented after treatment with monoxidel. All of these reactions disappeared with decreasing drug dosage or discontinuing the drug when possible. Marked depression or elation states, which are said to occur with the use of steroids in adults, were seen infrequently.

Four children showed hearing loss after the transplant due to a side effect of the combination of particular medications. After this tragic side effect was identified in this group, the dosage levels for the other patients were adjusted successfully, and hearing loss no longer occurs.

Psychological Gains and Losses

Psychological factors were evaluated for gains and losses. For many children, particularly those who had been chronically ill with renal disease for many years preceding the transplant, an improved level of emotional adjustment was seen on examination one year after the transplant. As one 14-year-old boy stated, "I had 13 years of needles and feeling lousy before my transplant. Now I can go ahead and be myself."

Psychiatric Assessment of Personality and Cognitive Development. According to the psychiatrist's examination, striking development of personality traits, together with cognitive growth, was most prominent in the *young children* who had been chronically ill since birth or shortly thereafter. When examined before transplantation, they were found to be lagging developmentally. An example is the 3½-year-old boy with a history of progressive renal failure since three months of age. When examined before his transplant, he was just learning to walk. He could master only six or seven steps. According to his history, he had not begun to sit alone until one year of age. He was not able to throw or catch a ball or balance a tower of cubes. He was unable to draw even a scribble. He knew only two or three words other than "mama" or "dada" and could not recognize colors. He could drink from a cup but was unable to use a spoon. He spent most of his time watching television in brief episodes. He related poorly to the examiner. Some of these findings could be accounted for by weakness; however, there was evidence of a general lag in development. When rated by the Denver Developmental Screening Test before his transplant, he was classified at a level of 11.6 months in gross motor development, 1 year in fine motor development, 1.1 year in language development, and 11.6 months in personal-social development.

One week after the transplant he became very active in motor function and began to run. When reexamined at one year posttransplant, he continued to be very active. He gained 11 pounds and grew five inches. He could pedal a tricycle and balance on one foot for one second. He could copy a rudimentary circle. He could combine words into sentences, use plurals, and recognize eight colors. He was able to dress himself with supervision, except for tying his shoes, and now played interactive games with his siblings. At this point his rating was 3.0 years in gross motor development, 2.9 years in fine motor development, 3.0 years in language development, and 3.1 years in personal-social development. Fourteen other small children under 6 years showed a similar pattern in developmental growth after the transplant.

Many *preadolescent children* showed developmental psychological growth as well. There were eight preadolescent children for whom hospitalization, transplantation, and then return home and school became a corrective emotional experience. They were more reactive on an interpersonal basis and less shy and withdrawn. They became less dependent on their parents and took responsibility for handling their medications and transmitting results of their laboratory values to the University Center. They interacted with moderate openness with their peers about their transplants. If schoolmates were curious about their shunt sites, they explained the process and did not dwell further on it.

The *adolescents* showed development in personality but not so strikingly as the very young children. A few older adolescents were philosophical: They regarded the transplant as a second chance to live and believed it had sharpened their perception of life. The experience of the crises they had weathered had a maturing effect from their point of view. Four adolescents expressed a desire to engage in occupations that aided others, such as work with the handicapped and underprivileged. They linked such feelings specifically with their renal failure and subsequent transplant experience. Other children identified with the medical staff and vowed to become doctors, nurses, or laboratory technicians in the future.

As noted earlier, the crisis of severe illness produced similar effects both for the adult posttransplant patients (see Chapter 3) and the children chronically ill with renal disease (Chapter 4). A feeling of being more in touch with the important values of life appears to be one consequence of a brush with death, particularly from late adolescence on. Among the transplant patients, most younger adolescents did not report this gratitude at restoration to life. They had expected to be rescued by their parents.

Emotional Problems Diagnosed Psychiatrically. Following transplantation, diagnosable emotional adjustment problems, including suicidal thinking, were seen more frequently in the adolescent age group than the pediatric group.

When examined at one year posttransplant, 9% of the pediatric group (4 out of 44) showed significant emotional problems, as did 12% (5 out of 41) of the adolescents. These emotional problems consisted of anxiety, depressive reactions and a compulsive reaction, and phobic reactions. In all cases these emotional reactions were associated with an episode of acute or chronic kidney rejection or other complications at that time.

Thus, severe emotional reactions at a year posttransplant are relatively infrequent and seem to be triggered by anxiety related to medical difficulties. Does this picture change if we examine the entire cohort of 100 children and explore the frequency of emotional problems *at any point* in their posttransplant history? Table 5-4 presents the relevant data. It is clear that serious psychiatric problems are rare when kidney function is adequate. Almost all of the surviving children have experienced *adequate kidney function* for sizeable time periods during their course, and this is the normal long-term physical state for the majority of these survivors. Out of all these youth, only three demonstrate diagnosable emotional difficulties when they are this healthy. However, temporary episodes of threatened rejection and other medical complications are not infrequent, and they seem to account for the bulk of emotional problems. Twenty-two of the

TABLE 5-4 TOTAL NUMBER OF CHILDREN EVER DEMONSTRATING MAJOR PSYCHOSOCIAL PROBLEMS

	Current age				
	0–5 years ($N = 9$)	6–11 years ($N = 23$)	12–18 years ($N = 35$)	19–24 years ($N = 33$)	Total number ($N = 100$)
At time when renal function is adequate					
Anxiety reaction	0	0	1	1	(2) } 3%
School phobia	0	0	1	0	(1)
At time when there is threatened renal failure					
Anxiety reaction	1	2	3	0	(6) } 22%
Depressive reaction	0	1	4	1	(6)
Suicidal reaction	0	0	4	1	(5)
School phobia	0	1	2	0	(3)
Psychotic reaction	0	0	2	0	(2)
After renal failure[a]					
Anxiety reaction	0	1	0	0	(1) } 4%
Depressive reaction	0	0	1	0	(1)
Suicidal reaction	0	0	0	1	(1)
Completed suicide	0	0	1	0	(1)
Total number	(1)	(5)	(17)	(4)	(29)
Percentage of children demonstrating problems	11%	22%	49%	12%	29%

[a] Out of the 100 children 22 rejected their kidneys and returned to a condition of renal failure before retransplantation or death.

youngsters reacted to a recurrence of medical complications with anxiety, depression, psychosis, or school phobias; and four more responded similarly when their kidneys were rejected.

Although differences among children of various ages in rates of kidney rejection are not evident, there seem to be marked age discrepancies in severe emotional reactions. Youth who are currently adolescent (aged 12 to 18) are much more liable than younger children or than older post-high school youth to have demonstrated significant psychiatric symptomatology. The adolescent appears to be at greater emotional risk than other age groups.

One of the most severe reactions, suicidal thinking, occurred only among adolescents. As reflected in Table 5-4, three adolescent girls and four adolescent boys (7% of the total cohort) had at intervals revealed suicidal thinking. One of these boys completed a suicidal act. Again, suicidal thinking usually occurred at the time of a complication or management problem of the transplanted kidney. Three of these teen-agers were from disrupted families that failed to give the teen-ager emotional support as he or she faced a crucial medical complication. The teen-agers involved came to feel that the outlook for normal kidney function and normal living was hopeless. One example was an 18-year-old girl who after a successful kidney transplant left home due to conflict with her father who was the donor. She attempted to establish an independent style of living, obtained a scholarship, and entered college. However, she became ill with an early kidney rejection reaction and was forced to return to a tumultuous family setting. Her father who had previously ousted her from the family lavished her with affection. However, he discovered that she had been using illicit drugs. The patient felt guilty about her drug use, which she associated with the rejection reaction involving her father's kidney. She feared her father might turn her over to the police as had been done to a brother in the family. She became confused and suicidal in her thinking, hopeless in her outlook, and depressed about the loss of the kidney.

Though most episodes of kidney rejection could be reversed, total rejection of the kidney sometimes required surgical removal and return to hemodialysis. When total rejection occurred, many teen-agers unlike younger children, reacted with guilt feelings that varied from mild to severe and might be accompanied by depression. As one 17-year-old stated, "My brother gave me a perfectly good kidney and it's ending up in the ash can." There were cases in which the donor overtly admonished the recipient after the transplant, "Wear your rubbers. Keep your muffler on. Don't get into a fight," with the implication, "Take care of my kidney." When kidney rejection occurred, usually the cause was not directly connected to behavior and was beyond the control of the recipient. Nevertheless, the patients blamed themselves for the rejection.

There *were*, however, cases in which actions of the teen-ager did directly affect a well-functioning kidney. Examples of such actions were running away from the hospital, stopping prescribed medication, eating restricted salted foods or excess fluids and failing to keep follow-up clinic appointments. Four boys and one girl who were on low-sodium and low-fluid diets did not adhere to their diet. Surreptitiously they sought salted French fries, potato chips, and soda pop. Three teen-age boys and three girls whom we know of stopped their medications either intermittently or completely. One of the teen-age girls subsequently died. For the others, an episode of acute rejection usually followed and required hospitalization and treatment. The teen-agers' withdrawal from necessary medication seemed to have one of two motivational bases—either it was derived from a need to test the limits of living like other teen-agers or from a depression associated with disruption of interpersonal relations and lack of emotional support within the family. In some cases the behavior was definitely suicidal; in others it was not. In either case the life of the adolescent was endangered, and when kidney rejection resulted, the adolescent frequently demonstrated severe emotional problems.

In general, anxiety about the possibility of rejecting the transplanted kidney remains the primary psychological as well as surgical problem of transplantation. This is true even though a patient can return to hemodialysis if the kidney is rejected. In general, young children who have been returned to hemodialysis have adjusted well, but the adolescents often have reacted to the restrictions of hemodialysis with psychological maladjustment reactions.

Quantitative Social-Psychological Measures. Thus, according to psychiatric judgment, many of the children with successful kidney transplants demonstrate personality or cognitive gains, and few exhibit significant emotional problems except at times of threatened rejection of the kidney. Do the quantitative measurements also indicate a high level of adjustment overall?

As can be seen in Table 4-2 (p. 98), the transplanted youngsters score as high in social-emotional adjustment as the normal controls (both siblings and the Baltimore control group) along all but one dimension measured. Their levels of happiness, self-esteem, levels of self-consciousness, stability of the self-picture, sense of distinctiveness, ability to reveal their true feelings, estimates of popularity, and the levels of anxiety are as favorable as those of the control groups. There is also little difference between the adjustment of the transplanted youngsters and those children who are chronically ill with kidney disease. In Chapter 4 the possible reasons why the chronically ill children scored so high were discussed. At this point the issue to be noted is the perhaps surprising overall adjustment of the transplanted children.

Also to be noted, however, is the one dimension along which the transplanted youngsters fare badly—that is, their satisfaction with their appearance. The chronically ill children also scored unfavorably along this dimension in comparison to normal control groups. Over half (55%) of the transplanted youngsters are classified as dissatisfied with their looks, in comparison to 39% of the chronically ill children, 28% of the normal siblings, and 22% of the Baltimore controls ($p < .001$). The transplanted children are undoubtedly distressed by the side effects of the steroid medication, the Cushingoid moon-face, and by their lack of growth. In fact, 80% of the transplanted children perceive themselves as "too short," in comparison to 39% of the ill children and 23% of the siblings.

Impact of Dissatisfaction with Appearance. For some children, their handicap, a kidney transplant, has become visible in terms of an altered appearance, while others maintain their normal looks. In Chapters 3 and 4 we noted that both transplanted adults and chronically ill children whose appearance was a problem were less well-adjusted generally.

How significant for the transplanted child's adjustment is the dissatisfaction with looks? In general, dissatisfaction with one's appearance is detrimental to the psychosocial adjustment of the child as it is for the adult. Posttransplant children who are *satisfied* with their appearance are found to be at least as well adjusted and more often better adjusted than the normal controls on the nine scales administered. The satisfied children fare so well that they statistically balance the dissatisfied, allowing us to conclude that transplanted children as a whole are not psychologically harmed.

Transplanted children who are dissatisfied with their appearance are vulnerable. They tend to exhibit lower self-esteem than those who are satisfied ($r = .43, p = .005$); they rate themselves as less popular ($r = .27$); they feel more distinctive ($r = -.22$) and self-conscious ($r = .34; p = .03$). In contrast to children who were satisfied with their appearance, the dissatisfied show higher anxiety ($r = -.33$, $p = .03$), lower levels of happiness ($r = .28, p = .05$), and more instability of the self-concept ($r = .30$, $p = .05$).*

Extreme Cases. The negative impact of the Cushingoid appearance was evident also upon psychiatric follow-up. The problem appeared to be

* Similar results are shown if we correlate the child's self-picture with the interviewer's rating of the child's appearance. Those children who appeared to be more Cushingoid to the interviewer demonstrated lower self-esteem ($r = .21$), greater self-consciousness ($r = .23$), more instability of the self-picture ($r = .31, p = .05$), and a lower estimate of their own popularity ($r = -.09$). However, they also were more likely to reveal their feelings to others according to our measures ($r = .30$, $p = .04$).

more extreme for girls than for boys. For example, one 15-year-old girl with a chronic kidney rejection pattern required frequent rehospitalization and institution of high doses of steroids. In addition to stunted growth, she now had a pronounced Cushingoid appearance. She became withdrawn and isolated herself in her room and refused to go out of the house and attend school because of her looks. Another 17-year-old girl with a pronounced Cushingoid appearance stated that her friends did not recognize her. She ruminated, as did other girls, that no one would ever marry her, and she became depressed. Periodically she altered her dose of steroid medication to decrease her Cushingoid facial appearance. Still another 16-year-old girl could not tolerate her appearance. Unknown to her physician, she discontinued her medication, and eventually, as mentioned earlier, she died.

The Transplanted Kidney Itself and Body Image. One factor that was examined by the psychiatrist at the end of a year posttransplant was the child's concept about possession of the new kidney. Immediately after the transplant, most youngsters felt as if the new kidney were a foreign body. One 10-year-old child stated it thus, "I thought I had swallowed half a turkey with mashed potatoes." Abdominal distension by the implanted kidney accounted partially for her concept. During the time that postoperative abdominal pain was present, the child rejected the concept of owning a new kidney. When the kidney became functional and the surgery was no longer a source of discomfort, the child began to be more certain but was still ambivalent about the new kidney. For the first three months usually the child "thought about the kidney a lot" and at times wondered "if it would stop." At a year most children felt the kidney belonged to them and were not consciously aware of its function. One adolescent said, "I don't think about it unless someone tries to hit me in the stomach. It's mine—in fact, I like it better than the old one."

Most often the patient's own kidneys were removed either before or during the transplant operation. Children after transplantation did not appear to mourn the loss of their original kidney as do patients who have lost a bodily organ or appendage in surgical procedures, as for example, amputation of a limb. There was little inquiry about what happened to the kidney removed. Children who did express fantasies about what happened to their kidney stated, "It was no good. They put it in the garbage can." The children appeared to focus in compensatory fashion on the new substitute organ. This attitude may account for the excess hopelessness and guilt that develop if the new kidney becomes nonfunctional. The child would then feel responsible for a dual kidney loss, and this involved accountability to a more powerful figure, usually the parental donor.

The success of the child or adolescent in integrating the new organ into his or her body-concept or image was examined early and at the end of a year. Because of better results that are obtained using living related kidney donors rather than cadaver donors, this is the preferred choice at the University of Minnesota. This may introduce relationship problems because donors were most often parents and siblings. Unresolved family conflicts existing prior to the transplant may be exacerbated.

The younger child was nonspecific about his body-image concept. He often had gross concepts that his body might have been damaged in some way during the surgical procedure. Small children sometimes questioned how the large organ of an adult would fit into their small bodies. Four of the pediatric group had a concept of being overpowered by the adult. Other children felt stronger and more powerful than peers. Several became more aggressive and engaged in more fights with peers.

An example was a 5-year-old boy who behaved aggressively because he thought the surgery had made him more powerful—"like Frankenstein." Three young children thought that the surgery had specifically altered their sex organs. One of them, a 5-year-old girl, received a transplant from her older brother. She began to wonder if she were now "half-girl/half-boy."

Teen-agers focused specifically on their abdominal surgical scars as evidence of bodily change. They sometimes concealed them from peers and attempted to deny their existence. Others, especially boys, used bravado explanations for the surgical scars such as the 16-year-old boy who related to his peers that he had been "knifed in a gang fight" and the 15-year-old boy who told his friends that he had incurred the scar after crashing in a drag race. One 16-year-old boy thought his sex organs were malfunctional because his own kidneys were proven so. When he was not sexually responsive with his girl friend, he felt he would never be so because he was a transplant patient. A few teen-age girls thought they would never be able to bear children in spite of being told that a number of adult patients have carried pregnancies to term with success.

For the most part, however, the integration of the transplanted kidney and the acceptance of the status of transplant patient was not a major problem. In terms of the body-image, the issue was primarily one of adjusting to a less attractive and less normal external appearance in those cases where looks were unfavorably affected.

Social Gains and Losses

The Family. In addition to the evaluation of the child's physical and psychological well-being, the child's social adjustment was examined.

After hospital discharge, the first transition the child faced was to return home and assume a healthy role whereas before he had occupied a sick role. Kemph (1967) has pointed out that for adults this often results in a change in family dynamics. Family equilibrium is altered for the child as well.

The family is now responsible for the care of the new kidney—a situation that had required the efforts of a complex team at a major medical center. Parents are often apprehensive about preparing the required diet and handling the medications. This apprehension occurs even though the parents and children aged 6 and above were instructed before leaving the hospital regarding the medication regime. Parents were also told by the physicians that the child could return to school within a month and could engage in any physical activity he wished, including strenuous sports such as football.

In spite of these instructions, the parents had a high level of anxiety about their role. Klein's research (1975) indicates that if the mother persists in anxiety and confusion about the family's medical handling of a chronically ill child, the self-image and adjustment of the child is in jeopardy (see Chapter 4). The usual finding here was that parents handled the transplanted child gingerly at first. They often hesitated to pick up a young child for fear of damaging the new kidney, although they had been told by the surgeons that the transplanted kidney was placed in a more protected position than the original kidney. They showed overconcern and uncertainty about what limits to place on the child. Sometimes the usual family rules were suspended for the transplant child. As one 14-year-old girl stated, "When I went home they wouldn't let me do anything—not even walk up the steps. If I wanted something, I got it fast. They wouldn't even hit me if I did something far out. I didn't like it that way." Other children capitalized on the secondary gain. Problems in management of the child's behavior then arose.

Siblings showed envy of the transplant child. Often the mother had been separated from the family for several months while the child was hospitalized at the transplant facility located in the metropolitan center. In three families who came from another state, the siblings were sent to relatives in different states while the mother accompanied the transplanted child. The 9-year-old brother of a young transplant patient expressed his rivalry, "I'm sorry I have two kidneys. I wish I could have a transplant." There was one family that handled the separation more skillfully. Both parents and the two siblings accompanied the child to the transplant center from a distant state, allowing the siblings to be involved in all stages of the transplant procedure. The family lived near the hospital and the siblings attended school. One of the siblings, a 10-year-old girl, walked in her sleep one night. Her destination was the University Hospital where she sought to care for her sister.

There were four families at the University of Minnesota in which more than one child in the family had received transplants. This occurred in families with hereditary renal disease. They had more adjustment problems with the second child than the first. They had not fully resolved their anxieties about the first transplant when they were faced with a second major procedure and attending financial and economic stress. One factor that was found was a competition by the children for the mother. When one child had to be hospitalized for investigation of an infection or other problem, the mother usually accompanied the ill child. The second child at home reacted with behavior or management problems. When her older sister was returned to the University Center for treatment of a kidney complication, one 8-year-old girl began to increase her sodium intake while her mother was away. The situation was an expression of anxiety on the child's part involving not only competitive dependency on the mother but identification with the rehospitalized sibling.

Between the siblings themselves was seen a similarity of symptoms usually more pronounced in the second child. When a 15-year-old boy underwent transplantation, his 12-year-old sister complained of similar symptoms three weeks later. This behavior occurred even prior to the manifest progression of the sister's familial renal disease. After both siblings received transplants, the second child often had complaints simultaneously or similar to the first child's. Both children checked the results of the blood tests of the other and became anxious if there were slight changes in the creatinine level (a measure of kidney function).

The families with two transplanted children were not the only ones worried about the blood tests. For the first three months following hospital discharge, all transplanted children had to have blood tests three times weekly at a local hospital and report the results to the University Center. They came to the University Center Post-Transplant Clinic to be checked once a week. Most families and children showed a high level of anxiety during that time and feared every phone call would bring adverse news about elevated laboratory values. At the end of that time, however, reports to the University and check-up visits to the Post-Transplant Clinic were not so frequent. Family anxiety began to diminish. At the one-year check-up visit, in the majority of cases the child had reintegrated into the family well. He or she was no longer being treated as unique, and the precautions being taken seemed reasonable. Anxiety was generally at a low level. It became aroused if a specific problem arose but was no longer constant.

Adjustment to School and Peers. While the child was readjusting within his family after his transplant he also encountered neighborhood and school peers. The *young child* readjusted to peers quickly. Other children were awed and curious about evidence of the transplant such as the scars of the shunt site on the forearm of the transplanted child. They asked what happened but were easily satisfied by a cursory explanation without undue anxiety. Peers had usually heard about the transplant from their parents and were protective of the transplant child. They did not allow the transplanted child to engage in strenuous play even when the child was so inclined. At the end of a year, however, peer activity was usually normal. Five children remained overprotected by peers. In each case it was because he or she was receiving secondary gain by prolonging the situation.

Adolescents had more difficulty than younger children in readjusting into neighborhood peer groups. They concealed evidence of operative scarring. They did not spontaneously bring up the subject of their transplant experience except to their most intimate friends. The peer group was not protective. Differences in the transplanted adolescent from other teen-agers seemed to arouse their anxiety. There were three instances in which teen-aged transplanted boys in quarrels with peers were deliberately struck in the kidney area inflicting trauma to the kidney. These attacks required rehospitalization and treatment of the patient. One 12-year-old boy complained, "The other kids know my weak spot and they hit me in the stomach every time."

Return to school after the transplant took place quickly in most young patients. There was a difference in children transplanted recently and those earlier. With improved methods of treatment, the recent trend is to discharge the patients quickly if no complications take place. Recently four children were discharged two weeks after a transplant took place, and one 12-year-old child returned to school in another week. By the end of a month he became active in sports and had joined a team. His previous history had been that of a chronically ill fatigued child who often missed school and was unable to be active in sports.

In the early days of transplantation a child may have been isolated one to two weeks and then kept in the hospital four to six weeks longer. Return to school was not accomplished for three to four months. Several problems in reception of the child at school arose with these patients. In many instances the child felt well and active, but the school nurse or teacher was apprehensive about how to deal with the transplant child and placed undue limitations on him or her. For example, a teacher insisted that one 8-year-old girl take a nap every day after lunch when the child herself did not feel she needed it. Often the physical education teacher was overly cautious about the child, making the child sit on the sidelines when any vigorous activity took place. As one parent later stated, "It took six months and several long distance calls to the University before the gym teacher was convinced about allowing activity."

At school, as in the neighborhood, the peers of younger children protected them. At times other children would not allow the transplant child to run or jump. One 8-year-old boy stated, "I had new tennis shoes and wanted to run. But the kids would only let me be in the circle and not use the tennis shoes." Adolescents were not protected by school peers. In fact, they were often subjected to teasing. When one 16-year-old, obese, Cushingoid-appearing girl returned to school, a rumor spread that she was pregnant. Adolescents were also singled out because of their short stature.

At the end of a year, however, all but three of the 85 children and adolescents were attending school regularly without major problems. Of the three children who were having difficulty at school, one was a 7-year-old girl who still assumed a sick role at school in spite of a well-functioning kidney. She sat just below the teacher's elbow even if asked to move elsewhere. She went to the school nurse frequently with physical complaints that could not be accounted for. Another was a 12-year-old boy who refused to attend school because of his short stature and had to have a tutor at home. He was shorter than his 6-year-old brother, although he later began to grow. The third was a 14-year-old girl who complained she was too weak to walk up the stairs in school and would attend only 2½ hours a day. She had a well-functioning transplanted kidney, and no physical problem could be regularly demonstrated. These children needed a longer period of time than the rest of the children to cope but they did eventually adjust and return to school.

Currently the children and school-aged adolescents are all in school with the exception of three children who have lost quite a bit of school due to serious medical problems, such as chronic rejection of the kidney, and two teen-agers who are in good health but have dropped out of school due to poor school motivation.

In school only 8% of the transplanted children answering the quantitative questionnaires currently report they need a tutor, in comparison to over half of the chronically ill youngsters. However, the average grades of the transplant children seem relatively low: Only 16% of the transplanted children receive an average grade of B or better, in contrast to 77% of the chronically ill students. Thus, while the transplanted youngsters appear able to attend school and engage fairly normally in activities, their past or present condition seems to have had an effect on school performance.

Impact of Satisfaction with Looks upon Social Adjustment. It was noted earlier that those transplanted children who are dissatisfied with their appearance are particularly vulnerable in terms of their psychological adjustment. According to the information on the quantitative questionnaire, these children are also less well-adjusted socially. They have fewer friends of the same and opposite sex—for example, 50% of those who are satisfied with their appearance report having a friend of the opposite sex, in contrast to only 25% of those who are dissatisfied. In describing their after-school activities, 47% of the satisfied children, in contrast to 26% of the dissatisfied children, mention socializing with peers. The interviewer's objective rating of the extent of Cushingoid appearance in the child is rated similarly to the child's sociability. Most of the children, whether satisfied or dissatisfied, however, do report they have a "best friend" (94% vs. 80%).

Reaction of the General Community. The transplant child has been well received within the general community. A child returning to his community after transplantation often is preceded by newspaper coverage. When walking down the street of his home town, he is often greeted by strangers. He could be a celebrity. Young children liked this, but adolescents reacted with ambivalence and did not like being singled out. Since the news of the first heart transplant was published as a lead headline story, advances in transplantation in general have received a great deal of public interest. But in spite of this publicity, problems have arisen within the community due to inadequate information about the individual transplanted child, resulting in the child being treated as a curiosity. The recent increase in publicity about transplantation has affected the attitudes of patients themselves when they first learn of the need for this therapy.

Early in this study, when children were asked about their first reaction to the news that they were going to have a transplant, the most frequent response was one of anxious disbelief. They expressed amazement such a procedure was possible. One child stated, "I almost fell through the floor when I first heard about it. I thought it was an awful idea." Recently, however, urban children coming to transplant seem less anxious about the procedure. Many stated that they had already heard about it in their health education classes at school. Children and parents coming from rural areas appear bewildered both by the idea of transplantation and the complexities of a huge medical center.

Children Who Have Become Adults. In the current cohort are 33 patients who were transplanted as children but now have reached the adult age of

19 to 25. Among these patients are some of the longest-term survivors. For the most part their social rehabilitation is good. Twenty-five of the 33 are either in college, vocational schools, have jobs, or are homemakers. Four are unemployed, although they are in good health; and four are not well rehabilitated because of kidney rejection episodes.

An interesting example of a long-term survivor is the young woman who was transplanted 11 years ago at age 12. Following the transplant, her mother overprotected her as is typical in the early stages. For instance the patient was frequently reminded to "wear your boots and don't get chilled." However, currently the patient appears free from anxiety about her transplant. She is amnestic about her original surgery and cannot even recall the date accurately. She works in a clerical position and has been leading a normal productive life in the community.

Parental Reaction to Transplant

At a year's follow-up in this study, the parents were given the opportunity to list the most significant gains and losses of transplantation from their point of view. The majority of parents did not hesitate to list as the most important gains the prolongation of the child's life.

When the transplant process had been uncomplicated and resulted in good function, there was no doubt in the parent's mind as to the value of the process. As one mother put it, "My child had a rebirth. There was no doubt she had a second life."

When there were severe complications and poor results, the parents often had ambivalent feelings regarding the procedure. This was seen in three sets of parents. One mother was very hostile and uncooperative with the medical staff because she had the covert belief that the child would not survive in spite of transplantation. The sacrifice in donating her kidney would thus be too great. A great financial burden on the family would ensue as well. A second mother who donated her kidney to her 15-year-old daughter became depressed when faced with the decision regarding a second transplant in the child. The first kidney had been functional only one month before it began to fail. The mother was unprepared for failure, having had unrealistic expectations that the transplant would be a certain success. She reacted with disillusionment concerning the entire process and struggled with her own feelings as an older son offered to donate his kidney to his sister. The conflict was intensified, because she knew that her daughter's chances for a well-functioning transplanted kidney were greater with a living related donor than with a cadaver donor. Another family decided to discontinue treatment for their child after the first transplant failed. They came to this decision when the child resisted going back to hemodialysis. This case raised the issue in the minds of the staff of whether a child or adolescent should be allowed to make such a decision.

Second to prolongation of life, parents listed the increased well-being of the child as a major gain of the transplant. They noted the increased vigor, activity, and health of the child. They rejoiced as they saw him play with peers and attend school regularly. Parents perceived the change to be great with a successfully functioning transplant.

In all groups strengthening of the donor-recipient relationship was the general rule. Explicit gratitude was often expressed directly to the donor (see Chapter 6). When a donor-father was asked how his 10-year-old son felt about the donation, the father replied, "He's very pleased. I suppose there's a little hero worship there." Most often donors were parents or siblings. Parents were unhesitating donors who usually gave without reservation. Often they struggled with their own feeling of loss of an organ but felt a compensatory gain as they acknowledged giving their child "another chance." A number of parents volunteered the information, "This was like a rebirth experience for me. I felt I gave my child a second life." One father of a 13-year-old boy experienced maternal feelings. He dubbed donating his kidney to his son as the most significant act of his life. To the chagrin of the teen-age boy, his father now wanted to protect his every move and hold the boy on his lap.

There were only four cases in which a hostile dependency relationship ensued and the recipient felt controlled by the donor. As one 13-year-old boy put it, "My grandfather gave me a kidney. Now he wants me to cater to him all the time." When another 16-year-old girl became sexually active, her donor mother complained repeatedly, "I'm sorry that I gave you a kidney if this is the way you are going to be."

In Chapter 3 we noted that there were no differences in the psychological adjustment of adults who received kidneys from cadaver-versus-related sources. Similarly, according to the quantitative data, the source of the organ had no effect on the adjustment of children, although only a few youngsters (20%) obtained kidneys from cadavers.

In general, in spite of the numerous problems that may arise from a major process like a kidney transplant, there were many instances in which the transplant and the related donation seemed to bring families together in what was described as a unifying human experience. For example, teen-agers who were previously not close to their siblings formed a closer bond to the sibling who came forward to donate (see Chapter 6). Positive family gains from this joint experience with crisis were not uncommon.

CONCLUSION

Transplantation represents an instance in medicine when a child returns from a terminally ill state to an active state of health. As Abram (1969) comments, "It is a return from the dead to the living." At the University of Minnesota children have not been found to be an unusually high-risk group as to kidney loss or loss of life with immunosuppressive therapy available after the transplantation. For the first three months following the transplant, the anxiety level of the children was high. There were adjustment problems in returning to the family setting, to the peer group, to school, and to the community at large.

During the next nine months, children became more confident about survival and function of the kidney. At a year posttransplant the majority of children and adolescents were adjusting well in spite of the additional tasks with which they might have to cope on an everyday basis such as the required maintenance medication, delay of growth, and Cushingoid appearance.

Anxiety was activated, however, if there was a threat to the function of the kidney. The child and even the adolescent's perception is often an "all or none" one. He views a rejection threat as an untreatable medical problem.

In this study, at a year after a transplant nine out of 85 children (10%) manifested behavioral or emotional problems of sufficient magnitude to require treatment—depressive reactions, anxiety reactions, phobic reactions, and a compulsive reaction. They were associated with an inability to cope emotionally when a complicating factor associated with the kidney function arose. Adolescents from disrupted families had more difficulty adjusting.

The most vulnerable children, then, appear to be adolescents and those undergoing significant health problems, such as threatened or actual rejection of the kidney. Another major point of vulnerability for the transplanted children as well as for the chronically ill youngsters lies in their satisfaction with their body-image. Objectively, a substantial minority of these children are either very short due to prior kidney disease or they exhibit the Cushingoid moon-face and rotund figure that results from necessary steroid therapy. The subgroup of children who are dissatisfied with their physical appearance indicate a lower level of sociability as well as damage along a variety of dimensions of the self-image. A disease that becomes grossly visible appears to have more significant consequences than the same disease when it does not compromise the physical appearance.

Another of the problems for these children was seen in the community itself. Although the public has become fascinated with the concept of rebuilding modern man, individuals in the community dealing directly with the child often do not possess adequate factual knowledge about transplantation. The result is that they approach the transplanted child timidly. The peers of transplant adolescents note their differences in appearance or history and react with anxiety which makes it difficult for transplanted adolescents to reenter peer groups. Transplant adolescents sometimes tend to withdraw because they feel different from the mainstream group.

CONCLUSION TO PART II

Several significant themes have emerged from Chapters 3, 4, and 5. In general, both children and adults are able to make a healthy emotional adjustment to posttransplant life. Vital to this adjustment appears to be the persistent comparison patients and families make to the earlier pre-transplant period when the patients were dying of end-stage renal disease or on hemodialysis. Their reference point tends to be the period of greatest stress rather than their earlier life of health (if there was such). Thus at least within the first year after the transplant, the patients and their close relatives are acutely aware of the positive gains of restored health, and their emotional adjustment reflects this awareness. In fact adolescents and adults often report a positive growth in maturity and a greater appreciation of the important values in life because of the crisis they have experienced.

However, the patient's level of adjustment is affected by his developmental stage. *Preschool children* show tremendous physical and personality gains. *Preadolescents* cope very well both with chronic illness and the transplant experience. While the majority of *adolescents* also cope well, they are at greater risk for severe psychiatric and suicidal reactions both to chronic illness and to posttransplant difficulties. Whereas dissatisfaction with appearance has an important negative influence on the overall self-image of all patients, the significance of this factor appears greatest for adolescents. The steroid-induced Cushingoid appearance and failure to grow render the adolescent more different from his peers than are other age groups. The toleration of any differences from peers becomes especially difficult in the teen-age years. In general *adults* show extreme negative reactions to chronic illness in terms of their self-image and just as extreme positive responses to the restoration in health that occurs with a transplant.

Finally, emerging from all three chapters is evidence that family support is very important in protecting these patients. Children appear to be able to withstand the impact of chronic illness surprisingly well, probably in part because of the extra familial attention and love they receive. Where the mother is confused about how to care for the ill child, the child is at risk emotionally. Posttransplant suicidal children frequently have been rejected emotionally by their families and therefore cannot cope with medical complications. Adults who feel rejected or less close to their families before the transplant are also at greater risk at a year posttransplant in terms of their self-image and feelings of well-being.

III

THE IMPACT OF THE DONOR SEARCH

From the point of view of most recipients, whether adult or child, the transplant represents a crisis and stress successfully managed. The outcome of the crisis for the majority of patients is physical and mental health with evidence of major gain and psychological maturation in many cases. The patient, however, is only one of the persons affected by this unique therapy. He is the recipient in a gift relationship that involves many others as potential donors. The need for a donor implicates the entire family of the recipient and may also affect a family of a cadaver donor. Frequently these families are already subject to severe stress: The close relatives of the recipient must cope with his illness and the threat of his death; the family of the cadaver donor is reacting to the shock of an unexpected death of a generally young healthy family member. The basic issue here is whether the added stress of the donor search is excessively costly for these families and family members.

As noted in Chapter 2, the use of related donors is controversial and is likely to remain so as long as the success rate of transplantation with related donors is superior to that with cadaver donors. Centers vary dramatically in their encouragement or discouragement of related donors. In Chapter 6 we examine the costs and benefits of related donation for the donor himself. His emotions during both the pre- and post-transplant periods are explored in some depth. Chapter 7 is focused on the nondonor, who is defined as that family member who is eligible but did not volunteer to donate. At issue is the question of whether there are any predictable differences between donors and nondonors. In Chapter 8 the actual decision-making process of nondonors, donors, and volunteers who were not selected for donation is analyzed to further evaluate the implication of the donor search for the parties concerned. Finally, in Chapter 9 the family is examined as a unit, with particular attention to the sources and degree of family stress and to family communication during the decision-making process.

Chapter 10 is focused on another family, the grieving family of the cadaver donor. The experiences of 15 such families are examined in an initial attempt to determine the benefits and difficulties of cadaver donation.

In the transplant situation certain fundamental social-psychological processes stand out in clear relief. The transplant setting thus provides a valuable research site for the analysis of interpersonal altruism and gift exchange, of family help-giving and communication in seeking help, of individual and family decision-making processes under stress, of the consequences of crisis-management and altruism for the self-image, of family grieving processes. It is hoped that this section of the book will provide fruitful insights into these important theoretical areas.

METHOD

Chapters 6 to 9 all relate to data gathered between October 1970 to June 1973. During this time all related donors at the University of Minnesota, all available nondonors, and as many members of the recipients' families as possible were studied. Both quantitative and qualitative in-depth interviews were utilized. The quantitative measurements used paralleled and repeated exactly the same measures and scales used in interviews of recipients during the same period (see Chapter 3). The first quantitative measurement of the *donors* took place during the three-day work-up, before the donors knew whether they would pass the necessary physical examination. At this time brief self-image and personality questionnaires were administered. In addition, the subpopulation of 100 potential donors "worked-up" between January 1971 and July 1972 were given Minnesota Multiphasic Personality Inventories (MMPIs). All quantitative measurements other than the MMPI were secured for the entire time-period of the study and for the total population of donors. Two days before the transplant an hour-long interview which contained both multiple-choice and open-ended items, with a predominance of the former, was conducted with donors. Five days after the transplant before hospital discharge, a second interview with a similar questionnaire was conducted. The brief self-image questionnaire was also readministered. Finally, at a year posttransplant the third interview and self-image questionnaire were administered to these donors, if the transplanted kidney was still functioning.

All together, the hour-long quantitative questionnaires were obtained for 130 donors pretransplant,* 128 donors at five days posttransplant,† and 111 at a year posttransplant. There were only seven refusals to be interviewed at any one point in time, involving only 10 different donors. Nine MMPIs were not completed, although in some cases the problem was less a matter of refusal than a difficulty in fitting the MMPI into a busy schedule of physical tests. Most donors were more than willing to talk to the interviewer about their feelings and experiences. Two of the donors who did not wish to complete one of the pretransplant questionnaires had spoken with us in a more open-ended fashion, and a third would have accepted the questionnaire if her husband could have remained with her during the interview.

One hundred eighty-six nondonors (i.e., eligible relatives who had failed to volunteer) as well as some other family members received quantitative questionnaire interviews approximately one month after the transplant after the patient was discharged from the hospital. Because nondonors were the family members who had declined to donate a kidney, we felt they might be unwilling to undertake more than one such multiple-choice questionnaire. Therefore, a time was chosen after the completion of the donor search at a time posttransplant when almost all patients would be doing well. At one-month posttransplant for recipients who have been discharged from the hospital, there is a relative "golden period" before complications or definite rejection are liable to occur. Because the donor search for a recipient who receives a cadaver kidney is not clearly over until the transplant, this interview had to take place after the transplant. In addition to multiple-choice items, this interview also contained qualitative in-depth sections to reconstruct the donor search from this family member's viewpoint. More detail about the nondonor population is presented in Chapter 7.

* In the four cases where the same recipient had more than one transplant and more than one related donor in the three-year period, the above figure includes only the last of these donors for purpose of this analysis.

† A few recipients had hyperacute rejections and the kidneys were no longer viable at five days.

In addition to quantitative measurement, a *second* source of data involved qualitative in-depth interviewing with as many family members as possible throughout the donor search and transplant period. All families seen by the transplant service from October 1970 to September 1972 (205 families and 114 donors) were followed in depth. Not all of the potential recipients concerned reached transplantation—some were not ready because they had not yet lost all kidney function: some remained on dialysis; and others died pretransplant.

The qualitative interviewing yields information on almost all of the donors and nondonors in these families. In practically all cases donors were interviewed at least once prior to their being definitely selected as donors and prior to the questionnaires. Recipients, their spouses, and as many members of the extended family as possible (including all potential donors, their spouses, and even sometimes in-laws) were interviewed repeatedly to clarify participants' emotions and to help us follow the donor search and analyze communication and decision-making events. A focused interview guide was used in these instances. More than 900 individuals were interviewed in connection with this aspect of the study.

Two independent coders were asked to classify and categorize much of the case material stemming from these in-depth interviews. Reliability was generally satisfactory and is discussed as it is relevant.

The detailed interviews of many involved and less-involved persons helped us to reconstruct in detail the family process of donor selection. Thus although the memory of nondonors on the questionnaires at a month posttransplant might be expected to be somewhat distorted, the repeated qualitative interviews of many family members prior to the transplant allow us to identify and analyze some of this bias.

All respondents were assured that all material expressed in these interviews was completely confidential and would not be repeated either to other family members or to the medical staff.*

* Identifying details are changed in these case reports, although all material is accurate otherwise.

6

LIVING RELATED DONORS: COSTS AND GAINS

Critics of the use of living related kidney donors question the fundamental willingness of relatives to make this type of sacrifice. Donors have been viewed by some as victims of family blackmail (Brewer, 1970), ambivalent about the loss of a body-part but donating because of family pressure or internal guilt. Kemph (1967) has noted postoperative depression on the part of many donors as a result of losing a major body organ. In a preliminary report we observed that the donor search generated significant stress in 25% of the families studied up to that point (Simmons et al., 1971a, b).

However, Fellner and Marshall (1968, 1970) and Eisendrath (1969) claim that donors experience long-term gains in their levels of self-esteem by donating, and in our earlier work (Simmons et al., 1973a) we have shown that the great majority (67%) of all relatives who are eligible to donate actually volunteer to donate (see Chapter 7). With the larger population of 130 donors and 205 families studied intensively, we can document the costs and gains of donation for donors. First the possible negative aspects are explored rather extensively both for the pre- and posttransplant periods. We then turn to a discussion of positive gains.

PRETRANSPLANT COSTS

Ambivalence

The University of Minnesota Transplant Center strongly encourages related donation. Except for minors, potential donors do not routinely receive psychiatric examination. In cases where strong ambivalence is expressed to the special physician assigned to the donor service, the potential donor is given a false medical excuse so that family members will be unaware of his unwillingness to donate. In several cases, however, donors have understated their concerns to the donor physician but revealed them to the researcher who had promised them complete confidentiality.

Extent of Ambivalence. In such a setting are the actual donors likely to be so ambivalent ahead of time that their donation must be regarded as an ethical transgression? We have two sources of data upon which to base our conclusions. First is the overall qualitative judgment of two independent coders based on case material, in-depth interviews. The coders were asked to classify donors into four categories—those showing no ambivalence or worries, those with some worries but no real ambivalence, ambivalence, and those with extreme ambivalence. The independent coders agreed 85% of the time in this coding. The second source of data involves a series of multiple-choice questions from the questionnaire administered to the donor prior to the transplant shown on Table 6-1.

The coders who utilized all qualitative information from the case to classify the donors have agreed in rating 7% of the donors (8 out of 114) as demonstrating considerable ambivalence, and 14% more (16 out of 114) as indicating some ambivalence. Thus the majority (67%) are coded reliably as free of fundamental ambivalence, although not without some fears or worries.* The estimates of ambivalence from the multiple-choice items are very similar—that is, a small percentage exhibit *extreme* ambivalence, and a sizeable minority express *some* real doubts as to their desire to donate (see Table 6-1). One-quarter of the donors agree with the statement "Sometimes I feel unsure about donating," and 5% agree "a lot" with the same statement. Twelve percent of the donors agree that they would be relieved if they were not able to donate, and 1% would be "very relieved."

The overriding finding, however, is that on each item 3/5 to 3/4 or more

* For an additional 13%, the coders indicated either unreliability of coding or a feeling that the information provided was not adequate enough to code.

TABLE 6-1 AMBIVALENCE OF DONORS PRETRANSPLANT ($N = 130$)

	Agree a lot	Agree a little	Disagree a little	Disagree a lot
I sometimes feel unsure about donating.	5%	21%	5%	70%
I sometimes wish the transplant patient were getting a cadaver kidney instead of one from me.	2%	11%	7%	79%
I would really want to donate myself even if someone else could do it.	60%	26%	8%	6%
	Very disap-pointed	A little disappointed	A little relieved	Very relieved
How would you have felt if you found out that you couldn't donate for some reason?	65%	23%	11%	1%
	Very hard	Somewhat hard	A little hard	Not at all hard or "It was no decision"
How hard a decision was it for you to decide to donate?	4%	10%	13%	72%
	Knew right away		Thought it over	
Did you know right away you would do it or did you think it over?	78%		22%	
	Yes	No		
Many donors have doubts and worries going into the transplant operation, even though they go through with it. Did you ever have any doubts about donating?	36%	64%		

of the respondents who later give a kidney rate themselves as positive toward donation and free of far-reaching doubts before the transplant. Indeed, 65 percent of the donors pretransplant say they would be very disappointed if they found they could not donate, 60% "agree a lot" that they would want to donate even if someone else were available to do so, 72% report that it was not at all hard to decide to donate. The decision-making process of these donors, as discussed in Chapter 8 also indicates, as does Fellner and Marshall's data (1968, 1970) that the majority of donors make an immediate decision to volunteer their kidney upon hearing of the need, without rumination or further investigation.

What are the major sources of the ambivalence and worry that do exist? Fear of the surgery is admitted by many donors, even those who report no basic doubts about the donation—20% "agree a lot" that surgery frightens them, and 31% more "agree a little." One-third of the donors in the in-depth interviews express concerns about their future with one kidney—they worry about their long-term survival chances or about possible future restrictions. Almost two-thirds are worried about the patient's prognosis—the possibility that he will reject the kidney that they have sacrificed in his behalf. Between 10 and 20% of the donors express concern about either the length of the recovery period, the particular personal inconvenience caused by the timing of the operation, the financial sacrifice involved, or a conflict felt between their obligations to the recipient and those to their own immediate family.

Although the majority of donors do not indicate any great emotional distress with their decision, for those few who were ambivalent the level of stress was extreme. The following cases illustrate the problem for four of the most ambivalent donors pretransplant.

Donor 1 (a brother donating to his sister)

BROTHER. I don't know what to do. It's my conscience against my body. My conscience says I have to do this, and my body says no. I don't want to. Like when I called Gwen yesterday after I got here I was going to tell her better about the conflict I feel. She said, "You don't have to do it." I said, "I know I don't have to," and I said, "Gwen, I don't want to do it. No one really wants to." She started to cry then and said, "Then don't. I'll just die." God! What can I say??! I told her I'd never let her die, but I thought Bill [patient's son] should be first. He could do it. . . .

Donor 2 (a son donating to his father)

I have to face the problem. It's my risk, and it's a lonely feeling. I'm smart enough to see through those chivalrous sayings people have about it being "a great thing," and "it's no more than an appendectomy. . .it's nothing." It scares me, and I have to live with myself. No one can help me. They can talk, but I'm the one who volunteered to give, and I'm the one who's a damn fool. Frankly, you do think things like that. You voluntarily are maiming yourself for life, and you kind of resent a person putting you in that position. Although I have a great respect for a person's desire to live. . .I guess I don't have any resentment. I have enough empathy and respect for his position. It's a hopeless position and helpless. He wants me to give. He has the urge to live. . .and that is important. He's never asked anything of me before. . .consciously anyway. Although he's given me a lot. And it's very uncomfortable for him to do this. The mere fact that he could ask, being so uncomfortable in it. . .that he's frightened enough and yet strong enough to ask me. . .he overcame his pride. . .I could never say I won't.

Donor 3 (daughter donating to her mother)

INTERVIEWER. How did you feel when they asked you to call [for the blood test]?

DONOR. I don't know. It's hard to say really how you feel. One minute you want to, then next you wonder, and you feel you have to. I'd feel terrible if I didn't and she couldn't live without it. I guess you wouldn't know how it feels if you haven't had the opportunity to face the situation of being a donor. I don't know how to say it.

Donor 4 (daughter donating to her father)

DONOR. This has been just a continuous long period of mental anguish. I've had an albatross around my neck. . .and now I'm going to settle it one way or the other.

INTERVIEWER. Do you feel you've been pushed by your family?

DONOR. Not pushed. It's something you feel yourself. I feel like I had to do it. . . .I've thought like. . .what if an embolism occurs during the operation? There are complications that arise after the operation too. . . .You think of these things. . . .What if he rejects. . .then I'd have one and he'd have none again. I have to think of the future of myself too! I guess I'm a big chicken. . . .I feel I don't want anything to happen to him. I love him. When it comes to a decision like this. . .it's a strain on your mind. You don't know what to do. People can go crazy making decisions when they don't know what to do. . . .

Dramatic statements like these are infrequent but cannot be ignored. We may be underestimating the level of ambivalence or degree of anxiety in this population as a whole. Yet our impression was that donors were quite aware that the sociology research staff would not repeat any information given to them and were grateful to use the interviews to ventilate anxieties and worries that could not be expressed to the recipient. In as many cases as possible we also spoke with donors' spouses and other family members, and all of this information has been utilized in classifying donors.

Family Pressure

A major ethical issue concerns the extent of family pressure upon the donor. Much emphasis has been placed on the question of whether the donor's decision is voluntary or whether it is unduly influenced by family pressure. Some of the ambivalent donors cited above clearly experienced pressure from the recipient or family. The question facing us at this point is whether this pressure is widespread.

The issue is complex and has several subdimensions: (1) How much blatant, direct, and conflictual pressure exists within these families? (2) To what extent do subtle situational pressures exert influence? (3) how much does internal guilt and fear of family disapproval motivate the potential donor? And (4) How great a role is played by feelings of family obligation and duty?

Open Pressure. Our coding ratings based on in-depth open-ended material indicate that 6% of donors *perceived themselves* as subject to undue family pressure. Regardless of the donor's own perception, the coders rated 11% of the donors (13 out of 114) as under significant family pressure. In the vast majority of cases open direct pressure does not appear to be a major problem. But it certainly does exist in some cases:

(Son volunteered to donate to father, but was not used as a donor)

VOLUNTEER. Of course my father is so obsessed with the idea if he gets this kidney he's going to be 32 again.

INTERVIEWER. Is he quite obsessed with that?

VOLUNTEER. Yes, he is. He didn't even wait to think in asking his son that it might put him in danger. . .he wants it so desperately. He just doesn't let himself think about my side of it. He cried. When I grew I never saw my father cry. . . .When I saw him sick and heard him cry. . .it just killed me. . . .I guess his physicians, the doctors that consulted [said he said] he'd commit suicide if he couldn't have the transplant.

VOLUNTEER'S WIFE. I don't think [the potential recipient] thinks of the point. . .he fails to recognize his years. He doesn't comprehend others' lives. We're trying to make a family, and BOOM! One thing I think he doesn't feel he asked my husband. He thinks John's offered. That's eased his mind a lot. He doesn't realize he's been driven there on his pushing. My husband hasn't ever said much. . .other than he can't say no. Apparently that's enough for [my father-in-law] to feel John wants to do it.

Many of the donors who report this type of open pressure are among the most ambivalent of the donors.

Subtle Situational Pressure. As one would expect, subtle situational pressure from the family is much more difficult to document than is direct open pressure. The manner in which the donor is informed of the need for a related donor may make it difficult for him to resist volunteering. Some immediate volunteers, even those who are positively motivated toward donation, may have responded more rapidly because of the manner in which the donor need was broached.

There are more and less direct ways of asking a donor if he wishes to donate. The detailed analysis of this type of communication is presented in Chapter 9. At this point, however, we should note that a relative (1) may be told he is obligated to donate; (2) he may be asked directly if he wishes to donate; or (3) the general need for a donor may be presented without directly questioning the relative about his specific intentions. If the family member is asked directly by a loved one or ordered to donate, it becomes difficult to avoid committing himself without hurting the already vulnerable patient. If no direct question is posed and the need is presented in a statement instead, a direct answer can be avoided until the donor has had time to deliberate. There is a basic but subtle difference between the three following methods of informing a relative of the recipient's need:

You'll have to donate. I think you should donate.

Would you donate?

He needs a donor. Relatives can donate and he is twice as likely to do well if he receives a kidney from a relative.

Based on the stories told by the donor, the recipient, and other witnesses, we attempted to code the directness of the initial "request" for a donor if it was made by a family member. Clearly despite careful comparisons of multiple stories of the same event, this coding is difficult and must be regarded as tentative. In fact in nearly half the cases such classification either was not relevant or could not be done reliably—that is, in 13% of the cases the donor was not informed of the donor need first by a *family* member, in 16% the coding was unreliable, and in 20% our information is too scanty for coding.

For cases in which the donor was first informed of the need by a family member and in which the information is clear enough for reliable coding, we find that about 12% were told in a way that would make refusal difficult—2% were in effect ordered to donate, 4% were asked directly if they would donate, and 6% heard statements that would be difficult to avoid: "If you'd donate, you'd save me," "John needs a transplant, you're the only one with the right blood type." However, most of the donors were informed of the need for a transplant and donor without a direct question being posed. Thus a direct answer could be avoided. In fact in many of these cases (42% of the total group) the need for a donor itself was not specifically mentioned; rather it was implied when the relative was told of the necessity of a transplant.

As far as we can determine, over time approximately half of the donors were always approached in an indirect manner. No immediate answer was ever required. The other half were approached more directly at some point: Some of them were asked directly right from the start; while approximately 1/3 of the donors were solicited initially in an indirect manner, but as time went on the request became more direct.

It is not our contention that an indirect statement of need or a hint cannot carry with it great moral weight, but a response to such a statement can be gracefully avoided (see Chapter 9). Our purpose at this point is to explore the force of the specific situation in which the request is made, rather than the pressure engendered by the general need for a donor. When a direct question is formulated, the situation itself becomes structured so that avoidance is difficult and there is a pressure to respond. Half the donors have been in this type of "pressured" situation at some point. However many of these donors probably did not perceive the situational pressures as such.

The parties present at the time of such a request may also exert situational pressure on the donor. If the recipient himself is present when the issue is raised, refusal or delay of decision-making becomes more difficult. The donor who wants to avoid hurting the patient will not wish to indicate reticence when he is "asked" for help, especially if his instantaneous reaction is to offer to donate. The presence of other family members who make their own willingness evident also make avoidance difficult.

If we examine the occasion when the donor *committed* himself to donate, at least 36% of all the donors for whom we have clear information might have been influenced by the presence of key family members. These donors did not seek out the occasion to volunteer, but as the situation unfolded they did volunteer and at a time when either the recipient or another family volunteer was present. Thirty-four percent of all the donors on whom we have information volunteered when the recipient was there, and an additional 2% committed themselves in the presence of prior volunteers. In addition, 11% more volunteered at the same time other family members were offering, although the exact order of the offers is unclear. In some of these cases the donor may have been the first to offer and therefore may have been unaffected by other family members.

If we cumulate those cases in which the interpersonal aspects of the situation clearly appear to have a compulsory quality, 54% of the donors would be affected. That is, those donors either were asked to donate directly, or the situation in which they committed themselves to donate was not one they had initiated themselves with the purpose of volunteering but was one in which the recipient or another prior family volunteer was present. Fifty-four percent of the donors either were subject to this type of pressure *or* to the more direct family coercion discussed earlier, and the proportion of ambivalent donors in this group was higher than among the remainder of donors (38% vs. 9%).

However, to conclude that the majority of donors who reacted to a compelling situation were less then eager donors would be inaccurate. The above data indicate that 62% of donors under situational pressure were free of fundamental ambivalence.* Frequently donors who are closest to the recipient and least ambivalent about donation are the ones the recipient feels free to approach directly, and they often volunteer immediately in his presence. If we check to see whether the donor was first informed of the need for a kidney by the recipient himself or by someone else, we find that those to whom the recipient feels closest are indeed the ones he approaches himself, leaving the rest to be solicited by others. Forty-eight percent of the donors to whom the recipient felt "very close" pretransplant were first informed of the donor need by the recipient himself, in contrast to only 14% of those who were less close.

Internal Guilt and Fear of Disapproval. Family pressure can originate from external sources either in a direct or subtle unintended form. It can also originate from internal feelings of guilt or fear of family rejection. Several

* According to the coder's classification.

writers have documented cases of "black sheep donors"—that is, donors whose motivation to donate could be interpreted as an attempt to compensate for past family wrongs and to restore their position in the family (Eisendrath et al., 1969, Kemph et al., 1969, Wilson et al., 1968).

A substantial minority of donors in our sample could be characterized as "black sheep donors," at least in part. Twenty-nine percent of the donors agreed that they "had done something major in their life that their family did not aprove of." Twenty percent reported that there was a period in their life when they and the recipient did not get along well, although only four donors (3%) of the total pool of donors answering the question indicated that this lack of closeness involved a *major* problem with the recipient. In addition, one-quarter of the donors agreed and 5% agreed a lot, with the statement in the questionnaire "Donation may be one way to make up for the wrongs we may have done to others in our lives."

Also in cases in which the donor was the patient's sibling or child, he was asked

> In many families there is often at least one child who is thought of as being difficult for the parents—a child who is harder to handle than the others, at least for a period of time. Thinking of your own parents, yourself, and your brothers and sisters, has there ever been a child who raised particular difficulties for your parents?

Seventeen percent of all donors and volunteers in these families were identified as "the most difficult child."

Yet questions aimed specifically at the *recent past* fail to uncover much "black sheep" motivation. When asked whether parents and siblings "during recent years have been generally approving and accepting of you and your life, or not generally approving," 94% claimed they had been generally approving. Furthermore, only 7% of the donors say that before the transplant problem arose they were "not very close" or "not at all close" to the recipient.

Thus it appears that a substantial minority have some problem in their past with the family or the recipient for which they met disapproval, but only 7% or so feel that the family has been disapproving of them recently or that they have not been close to the patient. Thus, although a large subgroup may feel some compunction to make up for past wrongs, only a few could really be called "black sheep" in the more extreme meaning of the phrase.

One such incidence of a true black sheep donor is illustrated by the following case:

Brother donating to sister (Two days prior to transplant.)

INTERVIEWER. What might make you decide to donate?

DONOR. Well, I gotta say. . .someday I may need my folks. If I don't donate I know I can just forget I ever had any relatives.

INTERVIEWER. What do you mean?

DONOR. Just that. That's it. I can forget about ever coming home. . .that I ever had any family. Hell, someday I may need them to bury me. They don't give a damn about me now, but if I don't go through with this they won't even bury me. Dad never did think I'd do it.

INTERVIEWER. How do you know that?

DONOR. Mom told me.

INTERVIEWER. Why do you think he thought that?

DONOR. Oh you know. . .once a bum. He thinks I'm still just a bum. He don't think I'm worth anything. . .and I guess he just thought I wouldn't. He may not be wrong yet.

INTERVIEWER. About not ever having anything to do with your family again if you don't donate. . .of them not having anything to do with you. . .what about Joan? How does she fit in here then? Are there bad family feelings toward her. [Note: His sister Joan refused to donate to her sister.]

DONOR. No. They wouldn't anyway because she's not me.

INTERVIEWER. What do you mean?

DONOR. She's different than me. She lives an acceptable life.

In another case the father was the black sheep donor, and his wife hoped that his strong desire to donate to their daughter symbolized a change in his attitude to marriage and the family:

INTERVIEWER. How does your husband feel about donating?

DONOR'S WIFE. He was bound and determined he was going to be the donor right away. He hasn't spent time with his children. The 13-year-old needs his father. He has been a real problem. He's been

> counseled for it and they said his antics were to get his father's attention. My husband's gone a lot of the time and would rather drink beer with his friends than play with his kids. I think he would like to make it up. It's not been a good marriage. Hasn't been for some time. I hope this [illness] brings it back.

In addition to guilt deriving from their past behavior, some donors volunteer because of the guilt they expect to feel if they do not help their dying relative. According to the coding of the qualitative material, when asked why they were donating, 14% of the donors indicate that they will feel guilty if they do not donate, and 5% more claimed that either parents or other family members expected it. Of course other donors who are less self-perceptive or less verbal may also be motivated by a desire to avoid guilt.*

Family Obligation. The family clearly has the power to make members feel compelled to aid one another. This power stems in great part from internally felt obligation to help one's relatives. Individuals believe part of their role as family members is to make great sacrifices for other persons in their family—sacrifices they would prefer not to have to make but that they expect others would make for them if the situation were reversed. Seventy-three percent of the donors agree with the statement that it is the family's responsibility to find a donor; 50% of potential donors "agree a lot" and 17% "agree a little" that it fulfills a parent's role to donate to his child; 79% of the donors "agree a lot" that the transplant patient would donate to them if the situation was reversed. In the words of two of the donors:

Donor 1 (mother donating to her son.)

INTERVIEWER. Well, now that you're in for the tests. . . .How do you feel about the idea of donating yourself?

DONOR. It's the least I can do. Like my husband said, and I agree, we've done our part for our family. But our responsiblity doesn't end there for our children.

INTERVIEWER. What did you consider in making the decision?

DONOR. I think it is as involuntary as if you saw one of your kids slip off a curb. . .you would do what you could to help him.

* See the latter part of this chapter for a discussion of negative and positive feelings of "black sheep donors."

Donor 2 (son donating to mother)

DONOR. In that respect I don't like the idea of having to give up part of my body. I'm apprehensive. To be honest, I have to say I don't want to do it. But I have to. It's something that has to be done, and I'm not afraid. There are many things in life you have to do. No one likes to pay taxes, but you have to.

INTERVIEWER. People sometimes use the term "have to," but they mean different things by it. What exactly do you mean by it?

DONOR. As my responsibility as a family member and my responsibility to my mother, I have to do it.

Donors who perceive donation as a family obligation are less likely than others to have ambivalent feelings about the sacrifice. One might presume that a clear sense of moral obligation may make the decision an easier one to resolve. To risk one's life for a friend may be more difficult than to risk one's life for a parent, a sibling, or child to whom one feels socially approved obligation. The fact that parents are the most likely relatives to volunteer to donate (see Chapter 7) and among the least ambivalent donors reflects the normative obligation felt by parents in our society.

One feels comfortable criticizing the more blatant unwelcome types of family pressure that occur in 12% of the cases. However, to these authors, it seems naive to jump to a conclusion of inevitable family blackmail from our findings that situational pressures, guilt, perceived family expectations, a desire to remedy past wrongs, and felt family obligations are operative in motivating the donor. Furthermore, to assert that family donation should be minimized or disallowed on this evidence would appear unwarranted. When a dying patient's chance for life can be significantly improved, family members feel and accept as legitimate an obligation to make significant sacrifices for their close kin. Despite its difficulty for individuals involved, this is a dilemma that cannot be legislated away. Yet more careful psychological screening might help eliminate the minority of donors who suffer extreme ambivalence and doubt. The factors that predispose a donor to ambivalence are considered in a later section of this chapter.

POSTTRANSPLANT COSTS

Feelings of ambivalence and perceived family pressure do occur as significant difficulties for a minority of donors pretransplant. The persistence of negative feelings in the posttransplant period could represent major long-term as well as short-term costs for the donor.

Short-Term Costs

Posttransplant the donors experience a great deal of pain and discomfort, and they now carry a scar that runs from mid-abdomen to their back. When we administered the questionnaire five days posttransplant shortly before donors were discharged from the hospital, 96% of the donors said they were still feeling sore, and 28% indicated they were very sore.

In addition, there have been other medical problems related to the operation. In a review of 287 donors at the University of Minnesota Spanos et al. (1974) reported a 28.2% complication rate. The vast majority of these were minor complications—minor wound infections, mild urinary tract infections, transient pulmonary (lung) problems. No deaths occurred. However, four major complications were encountered (a rate of 1.4%). In three of these cases the donors later developed the same disease that had previously affected the recipient—in two cases glomerulonephritis, in another hemolytic-uremic syndrome. Although two of these donors show normal kidney function, one needed dialysis for two months and still shows some impaired kidney function. Whether donation itself jeopardized these three donors is unclear, because in each case it is possible that the disease would have affected both of the donor's kidneys had no donation taken place. Two other serious complications were more clearly related to the operation—a pulmonary embolus and a case of deep thrombophlebitus; in both cases the patients responded well to anticoagulation therapy with no subsequent recurrence.

This experience with donor complications is similar to that reported by Smith et al. (1972), Penn et al. (1970), Farrell et al. (1973), Bennett and Harrison (1974), and Bergan (1972). The death rate in a survey of 11 centers conducted by Bergan (1972) was 1,565 donor operations (0.06%).

In terms of the psychological effects of the operation, Kemph (1967) has reported frequent temporary postoperative depression in his series of donors. To determine the extent of letdown or depression in our data, we asked the donor:

> Some people report they feel depressed, or let down and unhappy, after surgery. Would you say you've been
>
> very depressed
> somewhat depressed
> a little depressed, or
> not at all depressed

> Many donors report the operation is an emotional experience for them—and they feel like crying more often after the transplant. Would you say this has been true for you or not?

Thirty-one percent of the donors report feeling at least a little depressed in the postsurgical period, and 19% say they feel more like crying. When asked in an in-depth interview about this depression, they indicate that the major sources of the problem from their point of view are the pain, worry about the recipient, or concern about their own present or future health.

Kemph and associates (1969) and others have speculated that after the operation the donor is neglected by the family, as everyone concentrates on the recipient, and that such neglect might lead to depression. Only three donors specifically attribute their depression to loneliness. However, five depressed donors complained of lack of care from nurses and doctors.

Donors expect the hospital as well as the family to be grateful for their donation. Yet the nurses on the donor service have little personal reason to feel grateful, and furthermore they do not have much time to give special attention and praise to the donors. This particular hospital housed the donors on a surgical service separate from that of the crowded recipient ward. The donors were on a crisis service where they were the healthiest postsurgical patients. Like many academic hospitals, unusual serious surgery is more frequent than is routine surgery on healthy patients—that is, than appendectomies or gall bladder operations. Thus the donor is bound to be among the healthiest in the surgical census and the least needy of attention. Partly as a result of our ongoing research, a special "donor doctor" was appointed to the transplant team whose sole responsibility was to the donors both living and cadaveric. This increased the physician attention to the donors but did not solve the lesser attention by nurses. In the words of two donors:

DONOR. Most of the staff on this station are way over worked and they don't have the time to give the patients. Like I had to get out of bed this morning to go to the bathroom and I couldn't get anyone to help me.

. . .

DONOR. You should have been here this morning. You would have seen a real crying scene.

INTERVIEWER. Why was that?

DONOR. They have been calling me fat ever since the transplant. After the transplant, after they had taken out two ribs and had cut from here to here they wanted me to turn over on that side so that they could get those bottles to run in. . . .I said that the bed was too small and the nurse said for normal people it isn't, you're just a big person. I know I'm fat, but if they felt it would be such a risk, why didn't they say so before the transplant. . . .Now that they have the kidney, they tell me I'm fat. . .four or five times they have told me that now. They take the kidney out and then you can make it on your own. . . .

Fear of discharge when they were not feeling fully recovered and capable of caring for themselves and a realization of the length of the scar were also identified as factors engendering depression in a small number of cases. The presence of very sick patients in the ward where they are housed also is depressing for some donors. When a mother gives new life, she is surrounded by other joyous patients. When a donor gives life, he is surrounded in this hospital by the dying and seriously ill. One might expect less depression in centers in which the postoperative environment of the donor is more benign.

In addition to depression, do donors experience negative feelings toward *donation itself* shortly after the transplant? A *small proportion* (5% or less) have very negative attitudes at this point, while a slightly larger group show some worries and concerns. At five days posttransplant, in answer to multiple-choice questions, 2% (three donors) say they are unhappy about having donated (in contrast to the 92% who say they are very happy about donation); 1% say they would discourage a potential donor in another case; 4% indicate they disapprove "a lot" of transplantation; 6% "agree a lot" that they have given up something that is part of them for nothing in return; and 2% (two donors) indicate they are not sure they would donate if they had to do it again. In addition, 14% of the donors say they are at least a "little worried" about their own health; 16% agree that donors are less attractive sexually; 26% agree that the size of the scar bothers them at least a little.

Obviously, to be able to predict which donors would experience such negative feelings posttransplant would be valuable, and in a subsequent section of this chapter the correlates of negative attitude are discussed. At this point the existence of a very small group of negative donors has been documented.

In cases in which the donor is depressed or not feeling well, the recipient is generally alert to this problem. Thirty-two percent of the recipients and 31% of the donors characterize the donors as depressed or lacking great cheer shortly after the transplant. Thus, in calculating the cost of donation, one should take into account whatever increase in the recipient's feelings of guilt and indebtedness occurs when he becomes aware of donor depression.

Long-Term Costs

Because donors were interviewed only if the transplant was successful and the patient reached a year posttransplant with a functioning kidney, we have to assume that we are underestimating long-term negative donor feelings. Eisendrath (1969) has indicated that donors whose kidneys are rejected feel less positive about the experience than successful donors. For 24 (18%) of the donors in our cohort, the kidneys were rejected or the recipient died. Our point here is not to argue that the unsuccessful kidney transplant is without cost; we recognize that the stress of a rejected kidney is severe, particularly for the patient, but also for his entire family and the donor. For example, one donor to whom we did talk several months after her brother had rejected her kidney reported the following:

INTERVIEWER. Let's go back now. He lost the kidney. How did you feel about that?

DONOR. That was awful. I really went into hysterics. I don't remember ever losing control like that. I screamed and cried and was really hysterical. My recovery was slow. I wasn't feeling well. That didn't help. I was really hysterical. I don't ever remember being out of control like that before. I felt a real sense of loss.

INTERVIEWER. What in particular were you upset about? I realize the whole thing was upsetting.

DONOR. That it didn't work.

INTERVIEWER. Was it fear for Clyde or a feeling that it was all for nothing? Or what?

DONOR. Both. What a waste for me and what a horrible thing for him.

What we wish to discover, however, is whether a successful transplant is also too costly for the donor, since it is the gains of the successful transplant that are used on the ethical balance sheet.

In the cohort of 111 donors who answered questionnaires at a year following a successful transplant, 59% say they were back to full activity in two months or less. However, 8% report it took more than six months to return to all daily activities, and 3% (3 donors) more claim that they never were able to "recover and resume all normal activities." For all three, the major complaint involves numbness around the scar tissue. The first is a woman who also reports a current bladder infection but is quite pleased to have donated: "I just feel happy to have been able to help someone. . .I just feel delighted everytime I think about it." The second is a 47-year-old man who complains that he could no longer manage the heavy lifting involved in farm work: "If I try to lift, it grabs." However, he also indicates he is quite happy with his donation. On the other hand, the third donor is very negative and believes that worry about his sole remaining kidney is contributing to the development of stomach pain and distress.

Thirty-four percent (38 out of 111) of the donors say they do not feel "completely" normal at a year posttransplant. However, for all but 17 of this group, they are referring to minor problems primarily regarding the numbness of the site or loss of muscle tone in the area of the scar.

Other more serious complaints involve the two donors who had developed glomerulonephritis in the remaining kidney posttransplant,* two donors who report weakness in lifting, two with urinary tract problems including a bladder infection and a kidney infection, and 11 donors who report they still tire more easily than before they donated. Most of those who complain about tiredness see it as a minor problem and often are not certain it is attributable to the donation. For four female donors, the tiredness is seen as more severe and debilitating. However, two of these women had another unrelated major operation the same year and believe they are still recovering from the combination of surgeries, and a third woman had been ill with hepititus three to four months after the donation.

For donors who are working, 12% returned to work within two weeks of the transplant, 51% within the first month, and 78% by two months. However, 4% (three donors) took more than six months to return. One was a woman who had been laid off a few months before the transplant for reasons unrelated to donation and returned as soon as she was called back; another was a male student who missed his final exams at school because of the donation and did not have enough money to return to school so finally sought a job; the third was a married woman with children who felt fine at a year but had delayed return to work. In general, heavy laborers were instructed to wait three months before resuming work. Although most donors were rehabilitated fairly quickly, the time

* The other donor who developed the same disease as the recipient was no longer in this cohort, because the donated kidney had been immunologically rejected.

lost from work as well as the financial cost sometimes involved must be considered significant sacrifices.

Regret at Donation. Significant psychological long-term costs seem to affect only a very small number of the donors. In answer to a multiple-choice question at a year after a successful transplant, only one donor (1%) says she does not know if she would decide to donate again if she had the choice. All others say they would donate again. Another two donors (2%) indicate they are "unhappy" about having donated, and 5% agree they have given up part of themselves for nothing in return.

The two most negative donors, according to the above measures, were also among the most ambivalent prior to the donation. When the first was asked if she would again decide to donate a kidney if she had the choice to make:

> I can't answer that. . . .Fortunately it turned out well. . . .If circumstances were the same, I'd go through the same process I'm sure. I'd have to be dragged, clawing all the way to get me here. . . .The patient has done exceptionally well. He's 100% o.k. . . .Before the transplant, it changed my mental makeup. . . .It was just a terrible strain. . . .After it was just such a relief.

Her feelings even now are ambivalent. In answer to another multiple-choice question, she rates herself as "very happy" she's donated. Her survival of the operation was quite a relief.

The second negative donor says:

> Like it's caused me to worry. This dumb thing has turned me into a hypochondriac. Now everytime I get sick I worry: "Why am I getting sick?" Maybe my kidney is flipping out.

Yet there is still ambivalence: When asked how "happy" or "unhappy" he is he donated, he indicates he is happy for the recipient but very unhappy with everything else. And when queried if he would donate again, he indicates he would.

The other donor who indicates he is "a little unhappy" with the donation is primarily concerned whether the transplant was the right choice for his teen-ager who had rejected an earlier kidney and had not grown since nine years of age. The father indicated he would have donated again if the choice were available.

Difficulty in Relationship with the Recipient. Cramond (1967) has noted that in some cases the long-term relationship between the donor and the recipient can become difficult. The recipient may be overwhelmed by feelings of indebtedness—a debt he can never repay. In turn, the donor may expect more gratitude than he has received. Or the donor may become overprotective—he may pressure the recipient to take better care of himself or to reduce his activity to protect the new kidney.

Bernstein has shown that some of these problems do affect the child as recipient and parent as donor (see Chapter 5).

In our total cohort only 7% of the recipients and 6% of the donors in answer to a multiple-choice question indicate that their relationship has become difficult because of the transplant, although 19% of the donors wish their recipients felt closer to them. In terms of problems of gratitude and indebtedness, the majority of donors report that the recipient and the family have expressed direct gratitude to them (56% and 64% respectively). Depending on the item we use to measure this aspect, somewhere between 5% and 10% of the donors report receiving too little appreciation from the patient or the family. Eight percent of the recipients indicate that the donor expects more gratitude than he has received at a year.

Nevertheless, in answer to a specific question, about 20% of the recipients tell us that they feel uncomfortable that they cannot pay the donor back. Guilt then appears to be more of a problem than the actual expression of gratitude on the part of the recipient. Thirty-six percent of the recipients indicate they feel some guilt at "having taken a kidney from a relative," although only 4% report a lot of guilt. It is worth noting however, that feelings of guilt were even more intense prior to the transplant, when 60% of the recipients said they felt some guilt "at asking a relative to donate" and 28% reported a lot of guilt.

Overprotectiveness on the part of the donor appears to be only a minor problem, although it seems to have some effects in approximately 20% of the cases. Fourteen percent of the recipients agree the donor tries to tell him what to do too often; 21% report the donor sometimes acts like he does not take good enough care of himself; 19% of the donors agree that they feel angry at the recipient for not taking care of himself. Many of the recipients, however, appear to enjoy rather than resent the extra solicitation of the donor and of other family members. They speak of the overprotectiveness with affectionate humor, interpreting it as evidence of the donor's caring for them rather than as an indication of their own indebtedness.

We asked both donors and recipients what jokes they had together about the kidney; clearly some frequent jokes of donors have barbs.

> I have told her that if she doesn't follow her doctor's orders that I will take my kidney back [an adult brother to his sister].

> Once in awhile I kid. A car yesterday almost hit us [the donor and recipient] when a friend was driving. I said "Watch it. That's the side my [remaining] kidney's on."

Using the humor as an outlet, the donor reminds the recipient that the gift can be regretted and that it has placed the donor in jeopardy.

Although extreme problems of indebtedness appear to disturb only a few of the donor-recipient pairs, when such problems occur they are quite interesting from a social-psychological viewpoint. When the donor does not receive enough gratitude for his gift, his reaction is not simply that of an angry creditor who resents taking a loss without receiving some tangible benefit in return. Rather he feels like he is being taken for granted, as if he is a "sucker." His very dignity is attacked.

Brother donating to a sister. (Pretransplant)

INTERVIEWER. What do you think about. . .you say you've been doing a lot of thinking?

DONOR. About the fact of. . .is it important enough to the recipient. I think of this. It's really important to me to know how important it is to the recipient. . . .

INTERVIEWER. Do you feel that your sister shows enough gratitude to you for this, or not enough?

DONOR. Basically, that's what I'm trying to say. I think she takes it for granted once the decision is made. Not just her, everybody but my wife and children.

INTERVIEWER. You feel your wife doesn't take this for granted?

DONOR. No, she doesn't think it's so easy. I think if I could start all over again today and if I asked my wife if I should go through with it, I think she would say no. . . .

INTERVIEWER. Does your sister or your folks know how you feel about this?

DONOR. They do now. I decided to have it out. I didn't like the way it was going. I felt there was too much being taken for granted. They just assumed everything was go. There was no red lights. Just go lights. When my folks were back here the last time, I had to get it out. I had to get if off my chest. So I did. I shook the whole family. My mother got so shook she had to go to the hospital. It was nerves. [It was a lot] of stress for her. But I had to get out what I

> thought. It was too much to hold back. I don't know if it was normal, but I had to let them know what was really going on. It was too much to hold back. . .I've never heard the feelings of my sister.*

Some recipients find expression of gratitude very difficult even though the donor clearly would appreciate such a gesture. The overwhelming value of a gift they cannot repay threatens their dignity. From one donor's point of view recalling the year after the transplant:

> I would say for 3 months [the recipient] tried to avoid me. I was never so crushed. I would call him up and he would be as cold as ice. I was destroyed. To this day I don't mention the kidney in front of him. Whenever I do, it turns him off. He has never come out and said "Thank you."
>
> I think he appreciates it. He's done everything but verbally thank me. My brother's a proud person. He doesn't take anything from anyone. . . .I couldn't accept one [a kidney] from somebody. It would probably bother me in the same way it bothered him.

A particularly interesting reaction also seems to occur when the donor demands "too much" gratitude or recompense. Then the reaction of the recipient may be to belittle the entire gift. Somehow the donor who is most demanding of recognition is the one who is least likely therefore to receive it. The demand is perceived as inappropriate and compromises or taints the entire gift. In the case of a daughter who asked her recipient mother to buy her an expensive coat prior to the transplant if she was going to donate, the mother's reaction to this donor even at a year post-transplant was the following:

RECIPIENT. She's a very selfish girl and not very mature in many ways. . . .She's not used to doing things for people. She didn't think her life should be constricted in any way. . . .She wanted a fur coat. It really shook me up. It was unnerving. . . .She was reluctant and unenthusiastic. . . .She's very calculating.

INTERVIEWER. [Multiple-choice question later in the same interview.] Some people say that if a family member donated a kidney they would feel uncomfortable as if they never could pay the donor back. Other people say this is not a problem. [Which do you feel?]

RECIPIENT. I'm not uncomfortable. I've put up so much. . .then she turns around and kicks us in the teeth.

* For a similar example see page 191 of this chapter.

In another case a brother comments about his sister who he knows was an ambivalent donor and who at a year is complaining of neglect.

> She feels slighted. . .jealous that I get all the attention. You have to understand though, my sister's a very jealous person.

The donor who demonstrates clear ambivalence prior to donation is likely to find the recipient reacting with hostility rather than gratitude for the gift. The reluctant gift may be accepted, but the donor loses more than the gift in exchange. Further analysis of this aspect of the gift relationship is presented in the final chapters.

Summary

The psychological costs for the donor appear to be most severe prior to the transplant and even there affect only a minority of donors. While one-quarter demonstrate pretransplant ambivalence, less than 5% retain highly negative attitudes about donation at a year after a *successful* transplant.* Only a small percentage of relationships between donors and recipients are significantly strained. Physical complications are rare, yet not so rare that the act of donation can be dismissed as without risk.

The highly dramatic instances of donor difficulty do occur, but we should not be blinded to the larger scene by their flare. More careful attempts to screen donors pretransplant might help to eliminate the few donors who will end up feeling very negative toward the donation even when it is successful.

BENEFITS OF DONATION

The ethical balance sheet is incomplete if we look only to see whether the negative aspects of related donation are too severe. In many cases successful donation may bring with it rewards for the donor. Obviously the greatest reward is the restored life and health of the recipient and the

* Hirvas et al. in psychiatric studies from Finland seem to find more trauma among their donors than do our studies. However, when the transplant was successful only 1 out of 38 of their donors exhibited what they characterize as "moderate to severe trauma" whereas 5 out of 20 of the donors in unsuccessful cases showed moderate to severe trauma. In fact, the majority of their successful cases demonstrated *no* discernable trauma (21/38) but there is a subgroup (16/38) whom they classify as showing *mild* trauma based on psychiatric interview. Whether the difference between the studies is a difference of measurement techniques, of investigator emphasis on positive vs. negative statements, or a real disparity between the centers is unclear.

meaning of that life to his immediate and larger family. Are there other benefits for the donor?

Psychological Gains for the Donor

Pretransplant Motives. The reasons the donors give for donating are instructive in terms of the gains they expect to receive. We have explored the more negative aspects of donor's motivational schema—family pressures, obligations, and expectations. Yet there are many other reasons the donor feels the sacrifice is important. The primary reason is to help save the recipient's life. For many relatives the recipient is a central person in their life, whose loss would be a major tragedy. Ninety-three percent of the donors "agree a lot" that they are "thankful I'm able to help by donating;" 83% offer this as their reason when asked in an open-ended way why they were donating. In fact two donors wished to save the person's life so badly that they hid their own prior medical problems from the doctors. The following comment illustrates this type of strong motivation: "The doctor said there would be a lot of pain. I can take a lot of pain for something like this. That makes no difference when you really love someone."

Some view donation as a chance to do something worthwhile in life. In fact 78% agree that "donation will make their whole life more worthwhile." Other donors see the act as a religious or moral one, as fulfilling God's will (9%). A few donors (7%) want to donate themselves to protect another family member: A parent does not want her other child to donate; a sibling senses reticence on the part of a sister and wishes to protect her as well as the recipient.

Another motive becomes important to adolescents: They want to prove to themselves and their parents that they are mature rather than childish. A key task of adolescence is to prove that one can successfully operate as an adult, that one will be able to leave the status of adolescent. Donation, for 6 out of 26 adolescents, promises to aid in this task:

> I would feel more grown-up if I were accepted [for donation]. My mother would not sign for me for a car [before]. If I donated maybe she would think twice of me and be convinced I could handle the car.

> Now when a crisis comes up I think I can handle it better. I was always told I act older. Now it seems I can really prove to myself I can go through with things. It's a test of growing up [see Bernstein and Simmons, 1974].

Some volunteers (23%) seemed to be extraordinarily eager to donate, hoping they would be the family member chosen rather than someone else. To these persons the chance to donate could very well benefit their self-picture:

> When I found out the [blood] tests were all over, I wrote to the doctor here and said if my brother and I were both equal I wanted to be first donating.

> The decision for me to do it was really very easy. There was really no choice. I think a person often feels "if only I had the power to save someone's life," and you wish for that power. This opportunity to be a donor kind of fulfills that wish.

Sadler et al. (1971) report similar motivations on the part of living unrelated donors who had responded to a mass media campaign. One such donor from their series discussed her motivation in a panel discussion: "You always dream of running into a burning building to save someone. But that opportunity doesn't come to everyone."

The desire to be a hero, to save another's life, appears to be a motivation in at least a small number of cases. Most of the donors, however, seem to be attempting primarily to avoid the loss of a loved one.

Posttransplant Self-Image Gains. Fellner and Marshall (1970), Eisendrath (1969), and Sadler et al. (1971) have found in their psychiatric studies of donors that the self-picture appeared to be improved by donation. We have attempted in this larger series of donors to measure more precisely the extent to which this is so and for whom it is so. Table 6-2 shows that in response to several items, some 30 to 60% of the donors at a year posttransplant agree they feel like a better and more worthwhile person after having donated, that donation is a high point in life making their entire life more meaningful. These feelings are present by five days posttransplant and persist or increase by a year posttransplant.* In addition, about one-fifth of the donors agree that the act is a heroic one. In the words of the donors themselves at a year after the transplant:

INTERVIEWER. Why would you encourage someone to donate?

DONOR. (donated to sister). To save a person's life makes you feel like a better person. There are rewards.

. . .

DONOR. (donated to sister). I think I see myself as a little more human and patient. Just the fact of giving part of my body. . .and

* These items were buried among many other items testing agreement with negative and positive attitudes toward the transplant.

TABLE 6-2 POSITIVE SELF-ASSESSMENT BY DONORS POSTTRANSPLANT

	5 days post-transplant ($N = 128$)	1 year post-transplant ($N = 111$)
I'd like you to tell me if you agree a lot, agree a little, disagree a little, disagree a lot, with these ideas:		
AGREE		
Donating was really a high point in my life making everything seem more meaningful.	60%	70%
Donating an organ makes one feel he is a bigger and more worthwhile person.	44%	61%
A person willing to donate a kidney is almost a hero.	14%	22%
Do you somehow feel like a better person after having donated a kidney?		
YES	45%	42%
Since the transplant, do you think more highly of yourself, that you're a better person than you were before the transplant; do you think less highly of yourself; or is there no change in the way you think of yourself?		
BETTER PERSON	16%	32%
I'm going to read you a list of ways some donors feel and I'd like you to tell me if you've felt this way very much, a little, or not at all recently when you think about the transplant.[a]		
FEELING THIS WAY "VERY MUCH"		
Worthwhile	63%	69%
Proud	40%	36%
Brave	16%	15%
Thrilled and excited	18%	21%
Generous	15%	14%
FEELING THIS WAY "VERY MUCH" OR "A LITTLE"		
Heroic	25%	32%

[a] These were interspersed with negative adjectives. The other items in this table were scattered through the questionnaire.

donating to someone who's going to live because of it. . .I guess I consider it one of the more worthwhile experiences of my life.

. . .

DONOR. (father donated to his 8-year-old daughter). For a parent, it gives you an awful deep satisfaction in fulfilling your vocation as a parent. . . .I really feel good about it, especially when you knew Susie before and knew her after. . . .Physically she wasn't within 25% of her capacity physically before. Her school marks are much better. She thinks and reacts—she does everything better. In physical education at school there are very few who can keep up with her. . . .I think it's made a better group of people out of us. I think it's given all of us a better belief. It's made us closer to each other. . . .[It's given us] a better belief in God.

. . .

INTERVIEWER. How do you generally feel now about having donated?

DONOR. (donated to mother). Great! It's fantastic to see. When I lived with her she was [always] sick. It's great to see how healthy she is now and to see her happy! And grateful!

. . .

INTERVIEWER. What words would you use to describe a living relative who donates a kidney?

DONOR. (donated to sister). It's a wonderful feeling, that's all.

When the donor is asked about the effect of the donation, he sees it then as increasing his self-esteem. But is this improvement evident when donation is not made so salient? Among other psychological measures, a global self-esteem scale was administered to the donors at the time of their original work-up before they knew they would be acceptable as donors and again at five days and a year posttransplant. This is the same self-esteem scale used to measure changes in recipients over time (see Chapter 3 and Appendix A). The happiness scale described earlier was also administered to donors pre- and posttransplant.

Tables 6-3 through 6-5 show that, like the recipients, the donors experience a significant boost in self-esteem and happiness after the transplant. Only 38% of the donors score high in self-esteem pretransplant, in comparison to 54% at five days posttransplant and 50% at a year. Only 57% demonstrate high scores in happiness pretransplant, in contrast to 72% at a year after the donation (Table 6-3). If we compare the donor's scores a year after the transplant to his own ratings pretransplant, we see that two to three times as many donors show improvement in self-esteem and happiness after the donation as demonstrate erosion in these areas (Table

TABLE 6-3 SELF-ESTEEM AND HAPPINESS FOR DONORS PRE- AND POSTTRANSPLANT

	Donors		
	Pretransplant	5 days posttransplant	1 year posttransplant
Low self-esteem[a]	36%	18%	21%
Medium self-esteem	27%	28%	29%
High self-esteem	38%	54%	50%
	100% (124)	100% (118)	100% (109)
Low happiness[a]	5%	3%	6%
Medium happiness	38%	23%	21%
High happiness	57%	74%	72%
	100% (120)	100% (119)	100% (108)

[a] For findings in this table, according to a chi-square test, $p < .02$.

TABLE 6-4 COMPARISON OF INDIVIDUAL DONOR'S SCORES ON SELF-ESTEEM AND HAPPINESS OVER TIME

Comparison of	Donor's score becomes worse over time	Donor's score stays the same	Donor's score improves over time	Total
Self-esteem pretransplant and 5 days posttransplant	17%	24%	59%	100% (111)
Self-esteem pretransplant and 1 year posttransplant	26%	21%	53%	100% (96)
Happiness pretransplant and 5 days posttransplant	17%	35%	48%	100% (109)
Happiness pretransplant and 1 year posttransplant	24%	32%	44%	100% (93)

6-4). In fact 53% end up with higher self-esteem than they had when they started. The long-term exhilaration and improvement in the self-picture demonstrated by the recipient appears to extend to the donor in many cases. The pair together have surmounted a momentous crisis, due to the donor's impressive sacrifice.

Yet perhaps the difference in the donor pre- and posttransplant does not reflect a positive gain from donation. Perhaps instead the pre-transplant score reflects an unusually depressed state due to the patient's illness and fear of the impending operation for himself. Posttransplant the donor may be simply reverting to his usual positive state. Comparisons with other control groups presented in Table 6-5 tend to belie this alternate explanation. Pretransplant the donors' scores and their distribution on the Bradburn happiness item are equivalent or better than those of national and local control groups, as well as nondonors in their own family. Posttransplant the donors' scores are considerably higher than that of control groups. Sixty percent of donors say they are "very happy" a year after the donation, compared to only 34% of the donors pretransplant and 26 to 37% of the control groups. Without a measure prior to the time when donation was raised, one cannot be certain the change over time is a positive outcome of the donation experience. Yet certainly the evidence points in this direction. Altruistic acts as significant as this one can represent a peak life-experience with far-reaching benefits for the donor's self-picture and overall level of happiness.

Donor Gains in Relationships with Others. Not only is a major altruistic act intrinsically rewarding, it is likely to be positively reinforced by those who are significant to the donor. The donors report receiving much praise and gratitude. When given a list of comments that might or might not have been made by others to them, 75% of the donors indicate that people have said they are proud of them; 65% have heard others say their donation is "great"; 56% that it's heroic.

DONOR. There are different things. I try to think about it. I knew this was happening. My primary feelings were, first, fear. And second, pride.

INTERVIEWER. Pride? How is that?

DONOR. Well, it is, in a way, an ethical choice or something. I mean, it makes you look like a good guy. It sounds so terrible to say.

INTERVIEWER. No. . .

TABLE 6-5 HAPPINESS OF DONORS AND CONTROL GROUPS

	Donor			Controls, Twin City[a]		National control[b]		
	Pretransplant	One year Posttransplant	Nondonors	Control 1	Control 2	1963	1963	1965
Taken all together how would you say things are these days? Would you say you are:								
Very happy[c]	34%	60%	26%	37%	37%	36%	32%	30%
Pretty happy	58%	35%	68%	54%	56%	55%	51%	53%
Not too happy	8%	5%	5%	9%	6%	9%	16%	17%
	100% (134)	100% (111)	100% (174)	100% (75)	100% (75)	100% (2460)	100% (1501)	100% (1469)
In general how satisfying do you find the way you're spending your life these days? Would you call it:								
Completely satisfying[d]	26%	37%	19%					
Pretty satisfying	64%	59%	71%					
Not satisfying	10%	4%	10%					
	100% (133)	100% (111)	100% (174)					

[a] The entire study in which these samples were used is reported in Simmons et al., 1974.
[b] Bradburn, 1969, p. 40.
[c] According to a chi-square analysis of the difference among the two donor groups and nondonors, $p < .001$.
[d] According to a chi-square analysis of the differences among the two donor groups and the nondonors, $p < .01$.

DONOR. Well, it's true. . .it makes you look that way. I mean, like I have friends over, and they ask how my sister is, and I tell them. . . .I mean, I get this feedback, and it says I'm a good person.

Donors also report that the family feels closer to them now. At a year posttransplant almost 25% of the donors see the rest of the family as closer to them now. In particular, the relationship to the recipient is significantly improved. Whereas 59% of the donors rate themselves "very close" to the recipient pretransplant, at five days posttransplant, 77% of the donors feel this close. Similarly, pretransplant 55% of the recipients see themselves as "very close" to the donor, but by three weeks posttransplant 86% feel themselves this close. This increased closeness that occurs almost immediately posttransplant persists at a year posttransplant, with 71% of the donors and 77% of the recipients describing themselves as "very close" to the other.

Furthermore, when asked to make the time comparison themselves, 53% of the donors at a year say they feel closer to the recipient since the transplant. Was this increased closeness produced by the act of donation or simply by the shared family crisis? Because only 26% of the nondonors report increased closeness to the recipient after the transplant, we must assume that the act of donation itself plays a major part in improving the relationship. This increased closeness plus the marked improvement in the recipient's health and personality is rewarding for the donor. As one exhilarated 20-year-old boy stated at a year posttransplant:

> Right after the transplant she thanked me a lot. Since then [she says] "Thanks big brother." She is growing now. She credits it to me. . . .[Before] she'd just come home and do her homework. Now she's out and around. . . .I got a lot in return. Like she's having a lot more fun now. She's a lot closer to me.

A Typical Case. The following case report is typical of the positive attitudes with which many donors and recipients face this potentially stressful event.

The patient is a 15-year-old high school student, whose malfunctioning kidneys were discovered at a routine physical exam. He was referred to an area hospital for further testing where he remained for 11 days. At some point during this hospitalization the possibility of total kidney failure and treatment by transplantation was mentioned to the patient and the family. When his kidney functioning did not show improvement, he was transferred to the University for further work-up. Very soon after arrival here, he was told that irreversible kidney failure was imminent and that transplantation would be the treatment of choice. The family was informed by the medical staff of the statistical probabilities of transplantation and of various types of donors and specifically that a sibling donor would probably be the closest match and therefore the best donor.

The family consists of the patient, a 19-year-old sister, a 12-year-old brother and two natural parents. After being told of the blood testing procedure to determine matches, both parents and the 19-year-old sister were tested together the next day. The parents were at the University and available for testing. The daughter was called the night the family found out about testing, was asked to come the next day, and did, traveling about 300 miles to be tested with her parents. All three were found to be acceptable donors, but the sibling was found to be a closer match. Because all three had indicated prior to the blood tests that they would be willing donors, the sibling volunteer entered the hospital first for the donor work-up. She was found to be healthy and acceptable physically as a donor, and the transplant was scheduled and performed within three weeks of the blood testing. The transplant was successful; the donor was discharged without complication on the sixth postoperative day; the patient was discharged without complication on the twelfth postoperative day.

Regarding feelings about donation, the donor had this to say:

INTERVIEWER. How did you first find out about the possibility of a transplant?

DONOR. He went into the hospital and that night he called me. Tommy and I are real close. We are like that [crosses fingers]. There is a four-year difference, but we are very close. He told me that he had kidney disease and was in the hospital. Transplantation was mentioned as a remote possibility. But we have been very open about discussing the possibility. After talking with Tommy, I called my parents and found out from them more of what happened. As soon as I found out about the possibility of a transplant, I told him I would be willing to do it. We are very close to each other. I would prefer that I did it more than my folks. I have a brother who is too young. But even if he could, I would prefer if I did it because I wouldn't have to be that active [in sports].

INTERVIEWER. How do you feel about the possibility of donating?

DONOR. I just don't want a big ugly scar. I am very willing to do it. I don't like to sit around and think about it, but if it happens it happens. . . .

INTERVIEWER. Did you know right away you would definitely do it, or did you think it over?

DONOR. I knew right away.

INTERVIEWER. Sometimes even though a person knows right away, there are thoughts that run through their mind about donation. . . .

DONOR. My only consideration was about childbirth, whether it would be natural after. . . .But Dr— answered all the questions about that.

INTERVIEWER. How does your fiancé feel about the possibility of your donating?

DONOR. He knows that I would do it and there has been no question really. He understands how close we are. He has just accepted it.

She further says about her fiancé later:

DONOR. He and Tommy are just about as close as I am. He knows it was the only natural thing to do. He's more calm than I am about it. He just accepted it. We were both concerned about the childbirth, but we both talked to Dr. —though.

INTERVIEWER. What were you told or what did you find about the risks of donation to yourself?

DONOR. That they'd never lost a donor, and it shouldn't have any bearing on having a child.

This donor had to take time off from college in order to donate, causing her to get behind a quarter in her college work and postponing her graduation a quarter—[which she says she doesn't mind]. Her younger brother "thinks it's great I'm doing it." Her friends "strongly approve." She mentions no one who disapproved. She indicates both pre- and posttransplant that she doesn't feel the transplant brought the family any closer, because they were close to begin with.

INTERVIEWER. Would you agree or disagree: Any family member who donates a kidney could be considered something like a hero?

DONOR. That really bothers me. I don't think there should be any glory. There was a news article back home that played it up. It's no big deal!

The recipient, who indicates no problems with accepting the kidney says the following, concerning the time when he was told about transplantation.

INTERVIEWER. Was anyone with you?

RECIPIENT. Yes, my parents.

INTERVIEWER. What did they say at that time?

RECIPIENT. If they matched up they would be glad to donate a kidney. Both them and Sally said they would. They all matched, but Sally is the best match.

INTERVIEWER. How do your folks feel about the transplant?

RECIPIENT. It is necessary. They're all for it. They're happy I could have it. Ten years ago nothing could have been done.

INTERVIEWER. How does Sally feel about the transplant and donating?

RECIPIENT. I don't think she minds. She wants to give. She is worried about the scar. She really wants to, but doesn't want to have a scar when she wears her bikini.

INTERVIEWER. How do you feel?

RECIPIENT. If you got to have it, you got to have it. It is scary. I've never really been sick before. I've never had major surgery before.

5 days posttransplant

INTERVIEWER. How do you generally feel now about having donated?

DONOR. I'm very happy I did it.

INTERVIEWER. What does Tommy say about your donating?

DONOR He's called me several times to tell me how great it is that I did it. He is thrilled with it.

INTERVIEWER. Looking back, why do you think you decided to donate in the first place?

DONOR. Because I love my brother.

A year post transplant

She says it took two weeks to resume all her normal activities.

INTERVIEWER. What do you think Tommy feels about your donating?

DONOR. He shows a lot of gratitude, but not in a direct way.

INTERVIEWER. How, can you give me an example?

DONOR. We were just always super close. Probably we're just closer now.

INTERVIEWER. How do you generally feel now about having donated?

DONOR. Really no different than I felt then. It was just something that had to be done.

INTERVIEWER. Do you think your family has been changed in any way by the transplant experience?

DONOR. Somewhat.

INTERVIEWER. How has it changed?

DONOR. In that you now value the everyday things of life more.

The donor, like the recipient, sees the transplant as illuminating basic life values, as increasing the fundamental appreciation of life (see Fellner and Marshall, 1970; for similar case reports).

WHICH DONORS BENEFIT MOST

Two pictures have emerged in the course of this chapter: the first of an ambivalent pressured donor embroiled in family conflict and maintaining negative feelings and difficult family relationships at a year post-transplant; the second of a donor eager to rescue the loved recipient and demonstrating long-term elation, boosts in the self-picture, and increased closeness to the recipient. The fact that the second type of donor is found much more frequently than the first alleviates some ethical concerns about the use of related donors in general. Yet these concerns would be further attenuated if psychological screening could weed out the more negative donors.

Therefore, we have investigated the correlates of negative and positive feelings toward donation. Several scales were created from multiple-choice items to aid in this analysis: a scale of pretransplant ambivalence (see Table 6-1), of negative feelings and regret about donation at five days and at a year posttransplant,* and a scale measuring the extent to which the donor feels he is a better and more worthwhile person and more heroic because he has donated—the "better person" scale (see Table 6-2).

* Although only a few donors have *extremely* negative feelings, donors do differ in the degree of positiveness or negativeness they feel, and these scales attempt to capture such differences.

The exact scales and their coefficients of reliability are presented in the appendix.

Five major factors appear to be related to the donor's response to this experience: (1) his background and family statuses; (2) his interpersonal relationships within the family; (3) his personality pretransplant, (4) his pretransplant attitude toward donation, and (5) his concerns about the patient's prognosis.

Family Statuses

Sex-Roles. The male donor's reaction to donation is very different from the female donor's reaction. Prior to the transplant the male is more likely to be ambivalent than is the female ($r = .23, p = .007$). Mothers are more likely to be free of ambivalence than fathers (58% vs. 29%) and sisters more likely than brothers (56% vs. 28%); sons are more likely to score high in ambivalence than are daughters (27% vs. 11%). Posttransplant males persist in having more negative feelings toward donation both at five days ($r = .22, p = .008$) and a year after the event ($r = .20, p = .02$).

However, not all males react to donation negatively, and those who do not are more likely than are females to rate themselves as better persons after the transplant. At five days posttransplant 23% of males versus 8% of females score high in the "better person" scale ($p = .03$), and this difference persists to a year posttransplant (40% vs. 26%).

What these results suggest is that donation is a more momentous event for the male. He is more likely to question whether he wishes to make this sacrifice. If he does make the sacrifice, he reacts more dramatically—either with regret or with a great boost in the self-picture. The female appears to take donation more for granted, neither reacting as negatively nor as likely to perceive the act to be an extraordinary one on her part, as an act that proves her greater worth as a person.

Perhaps donation seems to the female to be a simple extension of her usual family obligations, while for the male it is an unusual type of gift. In our society the traditional female role is one in which altruism and sacrifice within the family is expected; the female is the customary family nurse and caretaker in times of illness and need (Litman, 1974).

In fact, entering a hospital and suffering pain and body manipulation to give life to another is ordinarily a major part of her role and purpose in life. Giving birth to an infant is congruent psychologically with the act of giving a body-part so a loved one can be reborn, so he can have a "second chance at life." The imagery of rebirth, of helping a person to be reborn, occurs frequently in conversations with transplant families, as Rapaport noted in *A Second Look at Life* (1973). In the words of one mother, who felt guilty that her daughter had inherited diabetes:

> I would rather donate [than have my son donate] because Betty's my daughter and I want to help her. I kind of failed at it the first time, and I'd like to do what I can for her. . . .I would like to give her a second chance. She's had a rough life since she was little—since she was 8. She's been in and out of hospitals so many times. . . .I just think I should be the one [Her eyes fill with tears as she talks of the illness.]

Because in her mind she "failed" in the first giving of life, she would like to be the one responsible for a more successful second opportunity.

From a male's point of view, there is no life experience or expectation like childbirth that prepares him for this act of donation. Thus he may have stronger ambivalences and doubts even after the transplant. In any case, whether his feelings are positive or negative, he is more likely to feel he has performed an exceptional act. If his feelings are positive, as the majority of men's are, he is more likely to reap self-image benefits from this extraordinary gift.

Other Family Statuses. Donation is an extreme example of family help-giving behavior. The question arises as to the strength of the ties among blood relatives in the American family. In terms of cultural definition, the expectation that *parents* will aid and sacrifice for their children is indeed a strong one. The obligation of adult siblings to one another or of adult children to their parents would appear much less clear.

Parents are less ambivalent than other family donors ($r = -.21, p = .01$) and have less negative feelings about donation immediately after the transplant ($r = -.15, p = .06$), although this difference disappears a year later. Overall, brothers and sons are more negative than other relatives. In terms of a perceived boost in the self-picture, parents do not differ consistently from other donors in their scores on the "better person" scale.*

In the case where siblings and children are used as donors, more than one family unit is likely to be involved. The donors, if married, are members both of their family of origin and their family of procreation. Some donors feel caught between obligations to these two families, between obligations to the recipient and to the spouse and children who are dependent upon their continued health (see Chapters 7 to 9 for further discussion of this conflict). The power of this conflict is reflected in a

* If anything, at a year posttransplant parents are slightly less likely to credit donation with rendering them a better person ($r = -.09$).

comparison of the feelings of married and unmarried donors. Siblings and children, if married, are more likely than their unmarried counterparts to be ambivalent donors ($r = .19, p = .06$), and to report negative feelings at a year posttransplant ($r = .35, p = .002$). Other data indicate that siblings and children who are married also perceive themselves to be less close to the recipient than do the unmarried donors.

One other characteristic of a person's status in the family involves the presence or absence of other potential donors. If an individual believes he is the only possible donor in the family, the obligation he feels to donate might be stronger. Does such a donor require additional protection from the medical staff to prevent him from donating under duress? Although such donors are slightly more likely to be ambivalent pretransplant ($r = .12$) and at five days posttransplant ($r = .10$), they are no more likely than others to demonstrate negative feelings at a year after the transplant. In fact donors who are the only possible donors are more likely than others to believe that donation has improved their worthiness as individuals. They are more likely to score high on the "better person" scale at five days ($r = .27, p = .002$) and slightly more likely a year posttransplant ($r = .10$). Thus these data would not support any *a priori* exclusion of such donors, although in any screening process they are slightly more likely to appear among those initially more ambivalent and requiring consideration.

Interpersonal Family Relationships

The most obvious hypothesis is that persons who feel closer to the patient pretransplant will be particularly desirous of donating and will maintain the most positive attitudes over the long run. In truth the data support this reasoning, although the correlations are not large. The correlation between closeness to the patient and ambivalence is $-.14$ ($p = .08$), between closeness and short-term negative feelings $-.18$ ($p = .02$) and for long-term negative attitudes $-.20$ ($p = .03$). Because parents and females are closer to the patient than others, the question arises whether closeness to the patient remains an important correlate of later adjustment if we control for these factors. Above and beyond parenthood and being a female relative, closeness still matters, but to a smaller extent. Donors who report they are closer to the patient are still less likely to show negative feelings at any time after the transplant ($r = .12, p = .09$ for five days; $r = .16$ for negative feelings at one year). Prior closeness to the patient appears to have no effect upon the donor's perception of himself as a more worthy person.

Moving from the donor's emotional relationship with the recipient to his interpersonal role within the entire family, we are led to examine the impact of the donation on the "black sheep" donor. There are few true "black sheep," but there are many donors whose past included a major act that met family disapproval. Here the broad conception of "black sheep" motivation is used, and both those who presently are subject to family disapproval and those whose past led to problems are included. (For the exact scale, see Appendix C.)

"Black sheep," though not clearly more ambivalent prior to the transplant, do end up with slightly more negative feelings posttransplant ($r = .13, p = .08$ at five days; and $r = .16, p = .07$ at a year).* Although right after the transplant, "black sheep" donors are slightly less likely than others to perceive themselves as better persons due to the donation ($r = -.11$),* this difference disappears by a year.

Thus in the long-run the "black sheep" donor is somewhat more likely than other relatives of his type and sex to react negatively. In some cases the desire to compensate for past wrongs and to reinstate their position in the family appears to be frustrated. The complexity of this reaction is seen in the following case report of an adult "black sheep" donor who had donated to his sister. Prior to the transplant he indicated that his parents did not approve of his lifestyle. In the postsurgical recovery period the medical staff observed him being fed by his mother. However, this increased closeness appeared short-lived. At a year posttransplant he made the following comments in reaction to a conflict over money with his parents in which he felt he had been wronged:

> DONOR. They asked me to do it [donate] and I did it, and then they turned around and ripped me off. The only time they want me around is when they need something. . . .[I told my mother I'm in financial trouble] She could care! . . .The falseness of people. . .they're real nice to you when they need you.
>
> INTERVIEWER. What words would you use to describe a donor?
>
> DONOR. A fool. . .I feel like an idiot. . . .I'd still do it for Janey, I'm glad I donated for Janey's sake. I wish I could have told the rest of them—in not such pleasant words.

The tendency to perceive oneself as a better person after donation appears to be more a response to one's family position *after* the transplant than prior to it. That is, those donors who report receiving more *explicit*

* This partial correlation between "black sheep" status and attitude toward donation holds constant whether or not the donor was the recipient's parent and the donor's sex. This control is necessary because males and nonparents are more likely to be "black sheep."

gratitude from patient and family are more likely to indicate that donation has rendered them a better person. The correlations between the score on the better person scale and reported expression of gratitude from the family are .11 at five days and .30 ($p = .001$) a year later. Gratitude from the recipient is also somewhat important for the donor's self-image—the correlations are .10 and .12 respectively. At a year posttransplant the donor is also less likely to have negative feelings about donation if the family has explicitly thanked him since the transplant ($r = -.22$, $p = .01$), and if the recipient has done likewise ($r = -.18$, $p = .03$).*

Personality

As indicated earlier, the donor's self-esteem and general level of life-happiness was measured when he or she first entered the hospital for a work-up. These pretransplant measures do not correlate with ambivalence to donation before the transplant, but they are significantly associated with the donor's posttransplant reaction, although many of the correlations are not large. Patients who appear to be less *happy* in general prior to the transplant have more negative feelings to donation a year later ($r = .27, p = .005$). They are also slightly less likely to report a boost in the self-picture at five days ($r = .11$), although this difference disappears by a year. Also, initially *low self-esteem* is associated with negative feelings immediately after the transplant ($r = .14, p = .07$), but this difference does not persist. Persons with low self-esteem prior to donation are slightly less likely to report that the donation has made them better persons at both points in time ($r = .10$ and .08).

Thus persons most in need of improvement in the self-picture are not the ones most likely to perceive the donation as having this particular effect. In fact a negative attitude toward one's life during the pretransplant period appears to generalize to the specific posttransplant attitude toward donation. A generally negative self-attitude pretransplant places one at somewhat greater risk in terms of reaction to the donation event.

Prior Attitude to Donation

Another predictor of negative attitudes posttransplant is the donor's *specific attitude to donation* pretransplant. The correlations between pretransplant ambivalence and negative feelings at five days is .15 ($p = .06$), and between ambivalence and negative feelings at a year is .31

* Explicit gratitude does not mollify negative feelings shortly after the transplant, however.

($p = .001$)* Long-term improvements in the self-picture, as measured by the better-person scale, are not affected, however, by pretransplant ambivalence. Ambivalent donors are not less likely than others to experience this benefit of donation.

While ambivalence prior to the transplant may alert one to more vulnerable donors, the lack of a *very* high correlation indicates that many persons who are ambivalent pretransplant react positively after the operation is over.

Concerns About the Patient's Prognosis

One type of donor—the A-match family member—presents particular ethical problems. A transplant with an A-match kidney almost always is successful, with better than 90% of patients showing long-term kidney survival. If the patient surmounts early infection problems in the first year and if there are no technical difficulties, the physicians expect almost indefinite kidney function. Thus the A-match donor, who is almost always a sibling, is likely to be under particular pressure to donate. Does such a patient require particular protection psychologically? Contrary to expectation, A-match donors are *less* likely than others to indicate ambivalence ($r = -.17$, $p = .07$, controlling for type of relative). In addition, after the transplant the A-match donor reacts much like the individual who perceives himself to be the only possible donor. Both types of donors may feel more obligated than others to donate, and the evidence shows that both types react more positively posttransplant than do others who were less obligated. At a year after the transplant, the A-match donor is less likely than others to demonstrate negative feelings ($r = -.16$, $p = .05$, controlling for type of relative).

The greater expectation of success on the part of the A-match donor is probably largely responsible for their lower ambivalence and fewer negative feelings. In worrying about the protection of donors who are under special obligation to donate (the A-match donor and the only possible donor) one ought not to discount the possibility that a strong obligation may lessen the likelihood that the donor will have second thoughts. The donor may more easily regard his sacrifice positively if he believes his duty was strong. If other relatives would have been as adequate a donor as he, the fact that he voluntarily placed himself in jeopardy may cause some psychological discomfort.

For all donors, not only A-match donors, the patient's level of health at a year after the transplant is important. We asked the donor at a year

* If sex and type of relative are controlled, the correlations are reduced to .09 and .29 ($p = .004$).

In recent months would you say the transplant patient has been

Very healthy
Somewhat healthy
A little healthy, or
Not at all healthy

Donors who perceive the patient as more healthy tend to have slightly less negative attitudes toward the transplant ($r = -.12$). The sacrifice has not been in vain.

Before summarizing this section, we should examine the effect of one additional factor upon the donor's response to donation—that is, his age. Ethical questions have been raised about the use of minors as donors. Are they truly capable of informed consent? The use of older donors, aged 50 and above, has also been questioned because they are likely to be greater surgical risks (see Chapter 2). In our previous work (Bernstein and Simmons, 1974; Spanos et al., 1973) we have demonstrated that these two groups are likely to have very positive attitudes toward donation, both before and after the transplant. In the cohort described here, 23 donors aged 16 to 21 have been used as have 25 donors aged 50 and above. Although age differences do not show consistent patterns, the youngest and oldest donors are surely no more likely than others to have negative attitudes toward donation. In fact, if anything, the ones with the most negative attitudes appear to be those in their later 20s or 30s, the life-cycle stages of childbearing and nurturing. The youngest and oldest donors are usually free from obligation to care for young children. The donation and the threat to their health does not place their own family at the same level of risk.

The youngest donors complain much less of soreness right after the transplant than does any other group, even those in their mid and late 20s. In a review of 26 adolescents worked-up for donation, 18 of whom were used, Bernstein and Simmons (1974) also indicate that the majority of adolescents appeared to be under no blatant family pressure to donate. Seventy-three percent of the potential donors in the series (21 out of 26) and 89% of the actual donors (16 out of 18) were subject to no undue pressure. In many cases, in fact, parents tended to protect the adolescent from the surgical process and either hesitated to ask about donating or were opposed to donation until convinced by the adolescent himself. Of the five potential donors classified as experiencing some pressure, only three experienced more than mild pressure. The first case involved a retarded schizophrenic teen-ager who was excluded by the staff on psychiatric grounds. The second was also not used as a donor but had been pressured in favor of donation by one parent, while the other was opposed to her donation. The third case was a "black sheep" donor who felt rejected by the parents who wished him to donate.

Six adolescents (23%) could have been classified as "black sheep." This rate is comparable to the 29% in the entire sample of donors of all ages who reported doing "something major in their life which met family disapproval." The behavior of the six "black sheep" teen-agers that brought censure included drug problems, living in a commune, holding nonconformist philosophies, delinquency, and reckless driving resulting in the death of a passenger.

Out of all the adolescent donors, only one indicated long-term emotional difficulty. This was a donor who pretransplant had agreed to talk to the sociologists only after being assured that his ambivalence would not be reported to the medical staff who might then prevent his donation to his sister. Subsequent to the donation he indicated fear of developing kidney disease and required short-term therapy for a depressive reaction about a month after the transplant. At a year this fear still remained, as did some turmoil with his family.

More typical adolescent reactions at a year after the donation are the following:

Donor 1

> The kids at school said I had guts [and] they don't. My parents said it was thoughtful and there was a lot of hugging that never happened before. They didn't think I could do it because of my age.

Donor 2

INTERVIEWER. How do you generally feel now about having donated?

DONOR. I feel real good. Proud. Happy.

INTERVIEWER. [later in questionnaire]: Since the transplant, would you say you think more highly of yourself. . ., less highly of yourself, or would you say there is no change.

DONOR. There's been a little change. . . .I saved someone's life!

Summary

In this analysis the types of donors who are more likely to react negatively have been identified. Males appear more likely than females to treat the donation as a momentous occurrence; they show more extreme negative *and* positive reactions. Relatives other than parents, particularly brothers and sons, are more likely to respond negatively, especially if they are married and have obligations to a family of their own. Holding constant the nature of the blood-relationship to the patient (that is, whether or not the donor is the recipient's parent), the following types of donors are less likely to respond positively: donors who pretransplant are emotionally less close to the patient, "black sheep" donors, individuals who do not receive explicit gratitude from the family after the transplant, persons who show low happiness and low self-esteem on pretransplant personality measures, donors who demonstrate marked ambivalence before the operation. Donors who believe the patient is not doing well at a year also have more negative feelings about the donation. In addition, certain other donors are more likely to react well to the experience: relatives who are more obligated to donate because they are an A-match or the only possible donor. Neither the donors' education nor income predict their adjustment to donation.

Although many factors help to predict the donor's posttransplant reaction, none of the associations are high enough to warrant automatic exclusion of any one type of donor. If we consider all the above discussed factors together, using multiple correlation statistics, we find we have explained the following percentages of variance:

1. 12% of the variance in donor ambivalence ($R = .35$, $p = .04$)
2. 15% of the variance in negative feelings five days posttransplant ($R = .39$, $p = .09$)
3. 36% of the variance in negative feelings at a year posttransplant ($R = .60$, $p = .01$)
4. 15% of the variance in the better person scale—five days posttransplant ($R = .38$, $p = .06$)
5. 7% of the variance in the better person scale at a year posttransplant ($R = .26$)

In comparison to many other sociological studies, the proportion of variance that is explained is respectable. Yet more is left unexplained and unpredictable. Even the donors who appear to be most vulnerable frequently react positively to the experience, and some donors have negative reactions that could not be foreseen. The fact that extremely negative reactions are rare and positive ones frequent must be taken into account in any attempt to exclude donors on psychological grounds.

CONCLUSION

The donor and recipient share intimately the experience of a major life crisis, and they most often emerge with intensely forged ties of closeness and with a long-term exhilaration and life-appreciation greater than that seen in the ordinary population. The typical donor feels little or no ambivalence related to the basic decision to donate but does have concerns about the surgery. His main motive for donating appears to be an intense desire to save the life of a person who holds high value for him. While unwelcome direct family pressure is not a problem for the majority of donors, more subtle pressures appear to be inevitable. The donor frequently learns of the need for a kidney directly from the ill and needy recipient or in a situation in which other family members are volunteering. Volunteering at such an instant in such a group situation must seem highly desirable, especially to a donor who would be positively oriented in this direction in any case. Feelings of family obligation are common and in fact may make the decision an easy one. Parents almost always feel that their role requires them to make this sacrifice, as well as many other sacrifices, for their child.

Immediately posttransplant the typical donor is in quite a bit of pain and discomfort but generally has no regrets about donating. He feels closer to the patient, an emotion that is well-reciprocated; he receives a great deal of praise and gratitude from the family; and he frequently views himself and his life as more worthwhile because of the donation. This increased closeness to the patient and family, the positive feelings toward donation and the self, persist in the successful cases at a year posttransplant. Elation at the restored good health of the recipient is frequent. Although recipients do feel some guilt about the gift they cannot reciprocate, most recipients and donors report there are not major problems in their relationship at a year posttransplant.

Among others, Katz and Capron (1975) have suggested societal policy curtailing the use of related donors in transplantation because of relatives' basic ambivalence and the possibility the donation will have negative psychological effects. These results suggest that such a policy would be premature in terms of most related donors.

Despite the benign picture for the majority of donors, however, at all points in time there appear to be a small group of donors (5%) who are extremely ambivalent or regretful of their decision. In this chapter we have attempted to isolate factors that correlate with a less positive reaction to donation. No one factor is predictive enough to establish a policy automatically excluding a particular type of donor. However, more effort aimed at eliminating the extremely ambivalent donors would be advisable, as would counselling help for other relatives who wish to donate despite normal fears.

7

THE NONDONOR: MOTIVES AND CHARACTERISTICS

ROBERTA G. SIMMONS,
DIANE BUSH,
SUSAN KLEIN

The recipient and the donor are not the only family members significantly affected by the transplant. All blood relatives are faced with a question of whether to offer a kidney. The nondonor has been defined as the relative who never offers the gift of a kidney; he never makes the commitment of having his blood tested. The question arises as to what factors distinguish a nondonor from a donor, what differentiates a family member who is willing to make such a major sacrifice from another who is unwilling. Specifying the differences between them should help illuminate the nature of the bonds within the extended family as well as add to knowledge about altruistic behavior in general.

Our task in this chapter, then, is to explore the differences between donors and nondonors. Later in Chapter 9 we focus on the stress to which the nondonor and other family members are subject. The experience of the nondonor should be entered into the calculus of the social-psychological costs and gains of this new technology.

METHOD

The goal of this aspect of the study was to collect information on all nondonors in the 205 families that were followed in depth from October 1970 to September 1972.* Information about the nondonors was gathered prior to the transplant throughout the donor search from the qualitative interviews with them or other family members. Also basic data were collected concerning each of the 1187 potential donors in these families, allowing us to compare nondonors to donors and to volunteers who were not used and to relatives who received medical excuses.

In addition, questionnaires were administered to 186 nondonors approximately one month after the transplant. These interviews at a month posttransplant were to capture the opinions of these relatives at a standard point in time after a transplant that was to this point still successful.

In some cases we were also able to interview nondonors pretransplant when they visited the patient during one of his many pretransplant hospital admissions or during dialysis. However, given the fact that these were persons who chose not to volunteer a kidney, they were less likely to visit the patient and therefore less likely than other family members to be interviewed by us pretransplant. Altogether, we interviewed 206 nondonors either before or after the transplant or both.

In general the refusal rate for the questionnaires was relatively low (8% of all nondonors approached). However, our questionnaire and interviews tended to be confined to nondonors whose relatives had a successful posttransplant course for at least a month, excluding nondonors (N = 77) whose relatives either were never transplanted or did not survive the early postoperative period. For nondonors who were not interviewed, substantial information about them was collected from other family members.†

* Among these 205 families were 184 cases in which the recipient was actually transplanted.

† In actuality there were 357 nondonors in these families. In addition to the 77 who were not interviewed because the recipients did not reach one month posttransplant and in addition to the 18 refusals, 10 nondonors were excluded because their recipients received transplants long after our interviewing of nondonors had ceased, and six could not be reached. In addition, early in the data-collection process, we confined our nondonor interviews to siblings, parents, and children and only later included aunts, uncles, cousins, and so on,

Before the findings are presented, our technical definitions of a relative's donor status should be made clear:

1. *A donor.* A family member whose kidney was actually implanted in the recipient.
2. *A volunteer.* A family member who had his blood tested and who explicitly indicated willingness to donate or allowed the family to assume that the blood test carried this connotation. His offer must not have been contingent on all others still eligible trying to go first. A volunteer could later be found medically ineligible for donation.
3. *A verbal offer.* A member of the larger family (e.g., aunt, uncle) who said he or she would donate if no one in the closer family was eligible. In these cases the person never had to go for a blood test because a closer relative was able to donate.
4. *A nondonor.* *(a)* A sibling, parent, or child who refused to donate, failed to have his blood tested, or indicated he would donate *only* if all others still eligible were first ruled out medically.
   (b) A member of the larger family who was approached for donation and did not offer to donate or if he did offer verbally did not proceed to the blood test once all closer relatives proved ineligible.
5. *A relative ineligible from the start.* A relative under 16 or over 65. A relative with a well-recognized medical problem that would exclude him from consideration according to the transplant physicians (e.g., diabetes, cancer). These latter relatives were never considered for donation because of their health.
6. *A person with a medical or age excuse.* A relative between 16 and 20 or 60 and 65 whose family never considered them eligible or whom the physicians declared ineligible because of age. A relative for whom donation was considered, but who was found to have a legitimate medical problem precluding donation, according to the transplant physicians. The medical excuse occurred before the family member volunteered or refused to donate.

---

who were asked to be donors but did not volunteer. Thus 25 of such nondonors failed to receive questionnaires. Finally, there were 14 nondonors whose status was recognized by the coders only after the appropriate time had passed for the interview. Primarily they were persons not fully recognized as nondonors by the family. They were defined to us as ineligible from the start because of age or a medical excuse, or in a few cases they were termed volunteers. However, upon carefully rereading the material it was clear that at some time before excuses were given, these family members had been considered as possible donors and they all had failed to have their blood tested, although there was ample time to be tested. Thus the nondonor interviews were more likely to be completed (1) in successful cases, (2) if the family recognized the nondonation as such, and (3) if the nondonor was a sibling or parent or child of the recipient.

When we speak of the *potential donors* in the family, all siblings, parents, and children between 16 and 65 except those defined as ineligible from the start are included. Relatives from the larger family (aunts, uncles, etc.) are included only if they were approached as possible donors by the family or staff.

Finally, to facilitate comparison among donors and nondonors for certain analyses we utilized only one nondonor per family. Because there is only one donor per family, we did not want differences between donors and nondonors to be artifacts of the peculiarities of the few families that happened to have larger numbers of nondonors. Thus where we had questionnaires from more than one nondonor in a family, a random nondonor was designated to be used in these particular analyses. We term the resultant group of 124 as the "random nondonors" and specify when they are being used instead of the total sample.

THE EXTENT OF NONDONATION

Is the altruistic gesture within families a rare or common phenomenon? Is the recipient who requires such a major sacrifice likely to find it forthcoming, or is he instead likely to discover himself isolated because of the exorbitant request? The strength of kinship bonds and the generosity of human nature receive an unparalleled test in the kidney donation situation. If the patient is liable to be refused or ignored when asking for a related donor, a case could be made against putting him in an unnecessarily stressful and unrewarding situation.

Table 7-1 shows that most extended families have at least one member who volunteered to donate a kidney to the recipient. Out of the 184 transplanted patients in this cohort, 61% actually received a kidney from a related source. In addition, for the majority of patients who received cadaver kidneys, there *were* family volunteers who, for reasons of health or blood type, proved ineligible (21% of all recipients were in this situation). These figures mean that 82% of recipients found at least one family member who was willing to donate a kidney to them and who went as far as having a blood test. In another 4% of the families, there could be no donor search because there were no eligible relatives to be approached. This leaves only 14% of the recipients who were faced with extended families in which *none* of the eligible members volunteered.

However, looked at from another angle, in 59% of the families, there was at least one nondonor in the close family (Table 7-2). In fact, three-quarters of all recipients who received cadaver transplants had at least one sibling, parent, or child who could have been tested for donation but

TABLE 7-1 VOLUNTEERING FOR DONATION AMONG RELATIVES OF 184 TRANSPLANT PATIENTS

Recipient received kidney from related donor(s)		61% (112)
Recipient received kidney from cadaver donor(s) only		
Recipients who had at least one relative volunteer to donate a kidney (although such relative later found ineligible)	21% (38)	
Recipients who never had any eligible relatives (there was no donor search)	4% (8)	39% (72)
Recipients who had eligible relative(s), but no one volunteered to donate	14% (26)	
Total transplant patients		100% (184)

TABLE 7-2 FAMILY VOLUNTEERING BY TYPE OF DONOR WITHIN FAMILY OF ORIGIN AND PROCREATION[a]

	Patient received kidney from			
Family volunteering	Related donor(s)	Cadaver donors	Both related and cadaver	Total
Everyone possible volunteered or had a legitimate medical excuse	51% (53)	14% (9)	(3)	36% (65)
One or more nondonors in the family	49% (51)	74% (49)	(7)	59% (107)
No donor search in the family—no eligible relatives	—	12% (8)	—	4% (8)
	100% (104)	100% (66)	100% (10)	100% (180)

[a] In this table only siblings, parents, and children are considered. In four families there were potential donors whose status was unclear and so could not be classified.

did not do so. Thus volunteers and nondonors are common in these families, and the individual recipient is likely to be exposed to both.

A surprisingly large percentage of all persons who could have volunteered to donate a kidney actually did offer to do so. Table 7-3 shows that in total, 57% of all eligible relatives actually donated a kidney or volunteered to make this extraordinary gift.

In other transplant centers where less emphasis is placed by the physicians on the need and advantage of related donors, the extent of volunteering would be expected to be less. However, where the need is stressed, the majority of family members are willing to make this major sacrifice to save the life of their dying relative.

DIFFERENCES BETWEEN NONDONORS AND DONORS

Status Differences

Type of Relative. Which relatives are the most likely to volunteer to donate? If one of the key elements in donation is the commitment to the norm that one is obligated to help family members, we would expect a

TABLE 7-3 VOLUNTEERING TO DONATE BY RELATIONSHIP OF ELIGIBLE DONOR TO PATIENT[a]

	Relationship of eligible donors							
	Mother	Father	Daughter	Son	Sister	Brother	Other relatives who were approached	Total
Donated or volunteered	86%	86%	66%	66%	48%	46%	50%	57%
Did not volunteer, nondonor	14%	14%	33%	34%	52%	54%	50%	43%
	100% (74)	100% (70)	100% (54)	100% (66)	100% (217)	100% (27)	100% (97)	100% (815)

[a] Relatives who received medical or age excuses without volunteering or refusing are not included in this table. Only relatives who needed to reach a decision are presented.

higher proportion of volunteers among occupants of family roles in which helping and responsibility are most clearly institutionalized. In American society, therefore, we would expect parents to be more willing to make this sacrifice than other eligible relatives, and indeed they are. Table 7-3 shows that 86% of eligible fathers and mothers either volunteered to donate an organ or actually donated, in contrast to two-thirds of the children and slightly less than half of the siblings. According to this test, the bond of obligation between parents and children appears stronger than the tie among siblings.

The lesser willingness of siblings is more striking, given the unwillingness of recipients to consider their own children as donors and the emphasis physicians place on sibling donors. At this center the physicians usually encourage the recipients to search among their siblings, because genetic laws indicate that 25% of siblings will be perfect tissue matches, protecting the donated kidney from immunological rejection. No other relative is anywhere near as likely to be a perfect match to the recipient.

Although siblings volunteer less frequently, they are still more likely than any other type of relative to end up as donors, both because there is a larger pool of them to start with in many families (if we look at members of eligible age) and because siblings who volunteer are likely to be better matches than the parent or child volunteers. Out of all the related donors in this cohort, 48% were siblings, 32% parents, 16% children, and 3% were from the larger family.

In other societies the particular family members who are most obligated to help and those members most deserving of help may be very different than in the United States. We would expect differences in the relative obligation of parents and children to one another, of male and female family members, of youngest and eldest siblings. Suggestive of such variation is the comment by a Moslem man who came from Lebanon to donate a kidney to his eldest brother:

INTERVIEWER. Why do you think you decided to donate in the first place?

DONOR. My eldest brother is considered a leading person in our family. Since my father died he has been a leader to us.

Age, Sex, and Class. The absolute age of the potential donors appears to affect their likelihood of volunteering. When the blood relationship to the recipient is controlled for, donors and other volunteers are likely to be younger than nondonors. Among the recipient's children for example,

87% of the donors and 91% of the other volunteers are under 30, in contrast to only 74% of the nondonors. Among the siblings 46 to 47% of the donors and volunteers are this young, in comparison to only 28% of the nondonors. The few parental nondonors appear to originate from the oldest age group: 71% of them are over 50, in contrast to 35% of the donors and 54% of the other volunteers. Thus, as a whole, volunteers are a younger group than nondonors.* Younger family members are undoubtedly more optimistic about their own health and their ability to withstand operative risks. We would expect a person's consciousness of his own mortality to increase with age, as members of his generation die with greater frequency. The fact that one is taking a risk with his life may appear more real to the older individual than to the younger one. To the young, death is something that happens to someone else. Among the donors, for example, those under 21 are the least likely to indicate they are frightened of surgery. In answer to a multiple-choice question posed pretransplant, only 27% of this youngest group agreed they were frightened, compared to 37% to 63% of other age groupings.

Absolute age is not the only factor at issue. Among sisters and brothers, age relative to the recipient is also important. Donors are much more apt than nondonors to be *close in age* to the recipient. While 42% of the sibling donors are within two years of the recipient's age, only 16% of the random nondonor siblings are this close. At the other extreme, for 21% of the random nondonor siblings, there is a discrepancy of 10 years or more between their ages and those of the recipients, while only 7% of the donors are this far removed from the recipient in age.

For example, one nondonor sister who was 20 years older than her recipient brother indicated she was a lot less close to the recipient than to a sister much closer in age:

> You kind of stick to your family that you're closest to. I was already married when Henry [recipient] was born. . . .We weren't brought up to play together. I was already gone when he was a baby. I am 20 years older than him. I did not even know what kind of a baby he was.

Does the sex of the potential donor also affect his likelihood of volunteering? In fact, although males who actually donated a kidney were more likely to be ambivalent than were female donors (Chapter 6), Table 7-3 shows no sex difference in the proportions volunteering to donate in the first place. However, while the *actual sex* of the donor doesn't affect

* The age-difference between donors and nondonors persists in general when the potential donor's marital status is controlled.

the likelihood of volunteering, sex *relative* to the recipient does matter. Once again, the lines of cleavage or bonding among siblings in a family appear to be based on similarity of sex as well as age. Among the siblings, 60% of the donors are the same sex as the recipients, while only 40% of the random nondonors are of the same sex. No such pattern emerges between the generations (parents donating to children and vice versa). Thus siblings who actually donate are more likely to be of the same sex and age as the recipient than are those who do not volunteer.

Social-class position might also be expected to distinguish the donor from the nondonor. Many studies (see Chapter 2) indicate that more educated persons have more favorable attitudes toward modern medicine, transplantation, and cadaver donation. These favorable attitudes are part of an entire *weltanschauung* (i.e., configuration) of pro-science, secular, and less traditional life views. Our data do indicate that donors are more likely to hold higher social-class positions than non-donors, controlling for age. Thirty-six percent of donors aged 21 and above have attended at least some college, in contrast to only 21% of nondonors.* Donors are also more likely to be in middle-class jobs rather than in working or lower-class occupations. Among males, fully 52% of the donors and other volunteers hold middle-class jobs above the clerical and sales level, in comparison to only 25% of all the nondonors and 35% of the random nondonors. In addition to possible subcultural differences between the classes in attitude toward medicine, these differences may reflect the fact that donation is often perceived as more of a sacrifice when income is less. Time out of work and travel to the hospital may be more difficult to absorb financially in blue-collar homes, particularly because heavy laborers are advised not to return to work for three months. Eight percent of the nondonors to whom we spoke were heavy laborers who specifically mentioned that the three months away from their job was too great a burden to assume. The exact level of sacrifice depends on the sick-leave policies and insurance coverage affecting each potential donor.

Racial background might also affect one's tendency to donate. However, our population has too few non-whites to test out racial differences. It is certainly possible that other centers treating more families of lower socio-economic status and more non-whites might find lower proportions willing to volunteer for donation.

* Because we did not administer quantitative questionnaires to volunteers who did not donate, we do not have as much information about them as we do for the actual donors and nondonors. This chapter concentrates therefore on the differences between donors and nondonors. Information about other volunteers is included if possible, however, and is clearly identified as such.

Family Relationships

Closeness to Recipient. A potential donor can be close to a recipient in two ways: literally—that is, he can live nearer to the patient—and symbolically or emotionally. One could certainly predict a closer emotional relationship between the donor and recipient than between the nondonor and recipient, and our data support this prediction. However, most of the quantitative data from recipient and donor have been collected after the identity of the donor was known. Thus we cannot be certain that the greater closeness between recipient and donor preceded the donor search.

Prior to the transplant all potential donors were listed by name and the recipients were asked how they felt toward each. Were they very close, somewhat close, a little close, or not at all close to that particular relative? Recipients indicated they felt very close to 63% of the donors, 65% of the other volunteers, 59% of those excused, but only to 42% of the nondonors. Similarly, Table 7-4 indicates that for every type of relative, donors felt closer to the recipients than did nondonors.

Some indication that this difference in closeness may have predated the donor decision is found when the donors and nondonors are asked how frequently they visited, telephoned, or wrote to the recipient prior to his illness. Exluding cases in which the potential donor lived in the same

TABLE 7-4 EMOTIONAL CLOSENESS TO RECIPIENT BY DONOR STATUS

	Parent		Sibling		Child	
	Nondonor	Donor (pre-transplant)	Nondonor	Donor (pre-transplant)	Nondonor	Donor (pre-transplant)
Perceived closeness to recipient						
Very close	60%	82%	34%	47%	48%	50%
Pretty close	30%	16%	49%	44%	30%	46%
Not close	10%	2%	16%	10%	22%	5%
	100%	100%	100%	100%	100%	100%
	(10)	(45)	(122)	(62)	(23)	(22)

household as the recipient, 63% of the donors visited as often as once a month in contrast to 52% of the nondonors; in cases where the potential donor lived in a different town, 28% of donors wrote every month or more, as opposed to 13% of the nondonors. These differences persist when geographical distance between the two homes is controlled.

The difference in feelings of emotional closeness extends beyond the dyadic relationship between potential donor and recipient. The nondonor appears to view the emotional relationships within the family quite differently from the donor. When asked in a multiple-choice question to rate the closeness of the family they share with the recipient, 61% of the donors describe the family as very close in contrast to only 47% of all nondonors and 46% of the random nondonors. These differences hold whether one examines siblings, parents, or children as potential donors.

Thus the nondonor perceives not only himself but the entire family as less emotionally close than does the donor. In some cases the donor and nondonor are still part of the same nuclear family. In other cases the family of which donor, recipient, and nondonor are a part is not one unit. The members (parents, siblings, children), originally part of the same immediate family as the recipient, now have established families of their own which may have settled quite far apart. The donor and nondonor may never have been part of each other's household, as in the case in which one is a sibling, the other a child of the adult recipient. The family segment salient to one potential donor may be quite different from the segment salient to another. Thus the level of family cohesion may appear quite different to one potential donor than to another.

What role does geography play in these relationships? Surprisingly little. Excluding potential donors who share a household with the recipient, nondonors are no more likely than donors to live far from the recipient. Instead, the key factor appears to be whether the relatives are still part of the same immediate family as the recipient. For all types of relatives, those who live in a different home from the recipient are more likely to be nondonors than those who share the same household—for example, among siblings, 40% of those in a different home are nondonors, in contrast to only 22% of those who live with the recipient; the relevant figures for children are 32% versus 11%; for parents 15% versus 8%. However, once the relatives have left the original common home, geographical distance does not seem to impair the giving of this extraordinary gift. The emotional bonds forged in a family appear to be able to withstand the challenges of widespread geographical mobility so typical of our society, at least in cases where the need is as extreme as that experienced by the dying recipient.

Despite the importance of emotional closeness to the recipient in differentiating donors from nondonors, only five nondonors admit a lack of closeness as a motive against donation, although 26 (13%) of those to whom we talked imply it.

INTERVIEWER. Generally, why do you think someone living would decide to donate a kidney to a relative?

NONDONOR BROTHER. I figure there are three reasons. You love the person, or you feel obligated, or there's no other choice. Like if my wife needed a transplant I wouldn't hesitate a minute. And like the girl who was giving to her father. She loved him and she probably felt obligated since she was his only child.

Few were as direct as the following nondonor daughter:

> My father is almost a total stranger. He's not warm [when I see him]. We do not have a good relationship. . . .My husband thought he was out of order in asking.

Informal Family Roles. As noted above, donation as a type of helping behavior within the family appears to be influenced by formal statuses and roles—by age and sex-roles, by the type of relative involved (parent, child, or sibling). Informal patterns and roles also develop within families. Our question is whether informal patterns predating the donation situation affect the likelihood of a particular relative volunteering his kidney. Most relevant would be the tendency of a family member to assume responsibility within the family unit. To investigate whether donors were persons who always played a more responsible part in the family, we asked both donors and nondonors

Would you say generally

1. You've always taken a lot of responsibility in your family
2. You've had no more responsibility than anyone else
3. That you've taken less responsibility than the others

Would you generally say you're a person whom the family depends upon

1. More than upon others in the family
2. Less than upon others in the family
3. About the same as they depend upon others in the family

Certainly according to their own perceptions, the donor and nondonor appear to be enacting roles to which they have become accustomed.

Sixty-seven percent of donors say the family depends upon them more than on other relatives, in contrast to only 27% of nondonors. Only 4% of donors report they have had less family responsibility than others, in contrast to 12% of nondonors. (These findings persist when the type of blood-relationship to the recipient is controlled.)

In the words of one donor when queried about several of his nondonor siblings:

> It seems like I always had to do everything. No one else takes any responsibility much. Even at home, I always was the one who mowed the lawn or put up the storms. . . .It seems like they don't care. I know they do. It's just that I'm an activist. . . .I have to make an effort for Bobby. No one else is.

Yet the nondonor is as likely as the donor to report that he has aided the ill recipient in ways *less demanding* than the sacrifice of a kidney, such as driving, babysitting, financial aid, and household help.

In addition to the degree of family responsibility held by the potential donor, the general level of esteem in which he is held would appear important to investigate. As indicated in Chapter 6, several investigators have posited that family "black sheep" are likely to donate in the hope of making restitution and assuring a warmer place for themselves in the family's regard. The experimental literature on altruism emphasizes the importance of guilt in engendering helping behavior (Freedman, 1970). Yet, although such cases were identified in our cohort of donors (Chapter 6), there is little evidence in our data to indicate that "black sheep" are more likely to volunteer than they are to become nondonors. In cases in which the donor was the patient's sibling or child, he was asked which child in his family was thought to be particularly difficult for his parents to handle. If we classify the donor status of all relatives so identified, we find virtually no difference in the proportion of donors, volunteers, and nondonors who were labelled difficult children (15% of donors, 19% of other volunteers, and 15% of nondonors). Furthermore, when we asked the recipients who were their father and mother's favorite child, donors were more, rather than less likely to be mentioned as the father's favorite (18% of donors vs. 9% of nondonors), and there is no difference in terms of the mother.

The informal role of the *recipient* within the family would also appear important to engendering willingness to donate. The issue is whether this informal role is perceived differently by donors and nondonors. Of particular relevance is the esteem the recipient is perceived to hold and the extent to which he has fulfilled his past family obligations to the potential donor.

If equity processes are operative, one would predict that if the recipient is seen as well-respected and satisfying kinship obligations to the potential donor, relatives will be more likely to reciprocate by coming to his aid. In fact, in answer to a multiple-choice question,* 63% of the donors see the recipient as commanding high respect in the general community, in contrast to only 46% of the nondonors. In addition, 61% of the donors, but only 25% of the nondonors, rate the recipient as "a lot better than average" in fulfilling kinship obligations to them.†

Opposition from the Nondonor's Immediate Family. The essence of the donor decision-making process is that it involves more than one family. It pits one's family of origin against one's family of procreation—the family one grew up with against the family one has chosen to establish. The health and continued well-being of the potential donor is of great importance to his own immediate family; whatever sacrifice he makes in health, money, or time out of work is a sacrifice for them as well. The anxiety and worry engendered by the operative risk to his life is also a cost for the potential donor's family. In many cases the spouse is opposed to the donation, placing the potential donor in a role conflict between the discrepant expectations of his two families. A nondonor sister discussed her dilemma:

> I guess Mary wrote and asked me to do it [donate to her]. . . .I told my fiancé about the letter Mary sent and he said, "No, wait until she calls you." Before I

* Generally, how much respect to you think people who know (the transplant patient) have for him? Would you say that (he, she) is generally respected

- More than the average person
- About the same as the average person, or
- Less than the average person

In your opinion, over the years, how good a (father, son, mother, daughter, brother, sister, etc.) has (the transplant patient) been? Would you say (he, she) has been

- A lot better than average
- A little better than average
- About average
- A little worse than average, or
- A lot worse than average

† Of course, in all of these analyses we are speculating as to the most likely causal sequence to explain the relationship between variables. Because we did not measure these individuals prior to the donor search, however, we cannot be certain of the causal direction. In this case donors or nondonors may have altered their perceptions of the recipients after they made their decision to donate or not donate, in order to make their attitude consistent with their behavior. However, it seems more likely that the attitude toward the recipient preceded and, in part, determined the choice of whether to donate.

> heard about the letter I had decided no. My fiancé didn't want me to. When I told him about the letter. . .he said, "No." He was at the state if I did it, forget everything. It was really a mess. If I didn't do it I felt like everybody would be against me. Finally Don [fiancé] said, "OK but don't think you're changing my idea of it."

This nondonor later received a false medical excuse after discussing her feelings with the physician.

In fact, spouses of nondonors are more likely than those of donors to express opposition to the donation (78% vs. 16%). Whether this opposition is the cause or consequence of the nondonor's own doubts is impossible to determine. The spouses may be reacting to subtle negative cues emitted by the nondonors and may be attempting to protect them. In comparison to blood relatives, the spouses of the potential donors appear free to play more "selfish" roles without meeting family or community disapproval. In some cases the opposing spouses may be serving as the potential donor's excuse. Unable to admit their own indecision or unwillingness, they may place the blame on their marital partners, who are not expected to feel as great an obligation toward the recipient. For the spouse, the recipient is only an in-law, not a close blood relative, and the expectations for sacrifice are considerably different. Whatever the exact dynamics, the spouse and the nondonor appear to reinforce each other in their negative decision, while the donor and his spouse are likely to reinforce a positive choice.

In the nondonor interviews we asked:

> What kinds of concerns and doubts do you think people have about donating? Or what kinds of reasons make people think they shouldn't donate?

> You mentioned that you thought about donating. What things did you worry about? What sorts of things seemed to weigh against your donating?

Seventy-two percent of the nondonors on whom we had information and who had their own families (116 nondonors) indicated that they perceived the donation as a conflict between the recipient and their own family (spouse and children), and 103 of these same nondonors felt their own family must take precedence. In contrast, only 39% of the donors who had separate families of their own mentioned this role conflict. Most of these nondonors saw donation as a threat to their health which would jeopardize the welfare of their own family, or they mentioned their spouse's opposition.

Given this tendency of nondonors to define donation as a conflict between the interest of their two families, it is not surprising to find that they are more likely than donors to be married. That is, they are more likely to be in a position to experience this type of conflict. Seventy-seven percent of the nondonors, but only 66% of the donors, were married. This difference persists when the type of blood relationship to the recipient is controlled—for example, among the siblings 78% of the nondonors, but only 57% of the donors, were married. It also persists when age is controlled.

Furthermore, among the married relatives, nondonors are more likely than donors to have children (93% vs. 75%) and in specific to have children under age 18 (74% vs. 64%). Married donors in contrast are more likely to have an empty nest. Moreover, the nondonor *with* children is more likely to mention the conflict between his obligations to the recipient and to his own family, if some of these children are still in the nest, that is if his youngest is under age 18 (52% vs. 71%).

Societies would be expected to differ in the norms that define the obligations to one's family of origin as opposed to one's spouse and children. One family from India, for example, excluded a brother as a potential donor because he had been recently married and the arranged-marriage agreement with the bride's family was based on the assumption that the groom was in perfect health (rather than missing one kidney).

Although primary opposition to donation appears to come from the donor's own family of procreation, some pressure against the sacrifice could originate from the family of origin as well. Interestingly, the nondonors are more likely than the donors to report that their parents had negative feelings toward donation—34% of the nondonors whose parents were alive indicated that one or both parents were opposed, in contrast to only 8% of the donors.

Thus in not volunteering a kidney the nondonor is likely to receive support from key family figures. In fact, 17% of the nondonors felt particular justification in their choice because an authoritative family member clearly did not wish to consider them as possible donors. In 30 cases, for example, the recipient and his or her spouse indicated they did not wish their own children to donate (49% of all cases in which children were eligible donors). In our society it is extremely difficult for parents to accept a child's maiming himself for their sake. While parents are expected to make unlimited sacrifices for their children, the reverse is not the case.

CASE Mother needs transplant

HUSBAND OF RECIPIENT. We found out in June [that she needed a transplant] and decided then that our own children were not eligible. My wife says she'd rather die than use one of them.

SON OF RECIPIENT. I thought about it. But my mother got hysterical everytime anybody mentioned it. She'd scream "You can't touch my children. . . .I won't let you."

In some families such opposition to their donation was accepted, and the nondonors assumed they were not in the donor pool. In other families, the potential donors proceeded to be blood-tested despite family opposition. One daughter went in secret for the test in order not to arouse her recipient father's anxiety prematurely.

CASE 20-year-old daughter volunteering to donate to father (at time of blood test)

Dad didn't want me to come. He didn't want me here. And I don't think he wants me to donate. . . .He doesn't know I'm here. . . .I always said to him if he needed a kidney he could take mine. . .he always said, "No, I don't want yours."

Thus if there is opposition within the family to a particular member donating, that opposition may lead him to interpret the situation as one in which he does not have to make a choice because he is unacceptable as a donor. He may not define himself as a nondonor, even though persons in other families in the same situation proceeded to volunteer.

Attitudinal factors

In addition to differences in status attributes and family relationships, nondonors and donors would be expected to be distinguishable from one another in terms of their attitudes toward medical procedures in general and transplantation and donation in particular.

Attitude to Transplantation and Donation. As expected, nondonors hold less favorable attitudes toward transplantation and donation than do the donors. In a series of multiple-choice questions, we asked donors and nondonors how willing they would be to donate a kidney to each of several types of relatives (see Table 7-5). We had also asked these same questions of a random sample of persons in the Twin Cities who had signed organ donor cards (volunteering their organs for transplantation upon their death) and a control group of their neighbors who had not signed such cards. Table 7-5 shows that the nondonors report themselves less willing than the donors or the donor-card signers to donate to all types of relatives (even when educational background is controlled). In fact, they are even less willing to donate to their siblings, fathers, nieces, or nephews than are the control group of neighbors. However, the vast majority in all of these groups say they are willing to donate to their own

TABLE 7-5 WILLINGNESS TO DONATE TO VARIOUS RELATIVES AMONG DONORS, NONDONORS, AND CONTROLS

I'd like you to tell me if you think you would be definitely willing, probably willing, or definitely unwilling to donate a kidney to the following:

	Definitely Willing Among			
Kind of relative to whom would donate	Donors pre-transplant (*N* = 142)	Nondonors (*N* = 177)	Donor-card volunteers (*N* = 80)	Neighbor controls (*N* = 80)
Aunt or uncle	14% (124)	7% (164)	13% (70)	10% (69)
Sister or brother	72% (142)	42% (172)	59% (76)	56% (70)
Mother	88% (106)	60% (131)	67% (69)	59% (56)
Father	85% (93)	52% (115)	66% (58)	61% (51)
Son or daughter	96% (99)	88% (136)	96% (51)	86% (58)
Niece or nephew	28% (116)	15% (171)	32% (71)	28% (67)

children. Parental obligation clearly outweighs all other family responsibilities. On the one hand, how much obligation an adult has to his various relatives is unclear—unclear enough to produce sizeable differences among groups in their willingness to aid any one type of relative. There are no clear norms defining the situation. On the other hand, however, there appears to be considerable consensus concerning which types of relatives can legitimately expect greater sacrifces on their behalf. While the absolute proportions vary from group to group, the rank-order of relatives remains the same. Donors, nondonors, donor-card volunteers, and controls concur in their willingness to aid their children first, their parents second, then their siblings, nieces and nephews, and finally their aunts and uncles. These attitudes are a perfect reflection of the behavioral choices reported earlier—that is, parents of ill children are the most likely to volunteer to donate, followed by children donating to parents, with siblings the least likely of the close relatives to offer.

In fact, in explaining their failure to volunteer, 9% of the nondonors indicate that the particular recipient at issue is not a close enough type of relative to warrant donation. Whereas there would be no hesitation in donating to one's own child, donating to a brother is problematic.

INTERVIEWER. How do you generally feel about a living related person donating a kidney for transplantation?

NONDONOR BROTHER. I told my brother before I'd give up one they'd have to try one if not two of someone else. . . .If something happened to my kid's kidney. . .I'd be more apt to give to my own kids. I told him they could try a cadaver. . .and they'd they'd have to before I'd do it.

Several aunts, uncles, and cousins and five nondonor half-siblings also explained that the recipient was not a close enough relative. The half-siblings saw their own full-siblings as closer emotionally and a more legitimate responsibility, as is clear in the following two cases:

HALF-BROTHER. It was a shock to me because we're not that close because I don't hardly know her. . . .Since I've been born, she's been married. I've only seen her on casual visits. . . .It seems weird because we aren't that close, but we have the same father and were checked for that reason. If it was Susy [his full sister] it would be different because I lived with her all my life and I would be more willing to give her one.

* * *

INTERVIEWER. Did you or anyone else in the family ever consider donating [to half-brother]?

HALF-BROTHER. I have to my own family or to my [whole] sisters, but other than that I wouldn't. . . .If my wife or kids needed me, I sure would.

In further exploring differences between the attitudes of donors and nondonors, we asked if the following types of relatives should be considered as donors: a young unmarried person, a relative who is in his 50s, a mother of young children, a father of young children, a woman of childbearing age, and a relative who is in his early 60s. In all cases nondonors are less likely than donors to think such people should be definitely considered as donors. In addition, in answer to other multiple-choice questions, nondonors are less likely to agree that the family should be the first place to turn in the search for a donor (77% vs. 95%); and nondonors indicate less favorable attitudes than donors toward kidney transplantation in general (71% vs. 92%).

Of course we cannot conclude with certainty that these attitudinal differences existed prior to the donor choice being made, because the measurement occurred after that point.

Perceptions of Risk and Benefit. One explanation for the less favorable attitudes could be that people perceive the statistics and risks differently. The nondonors are less likely to believe that a sacrifice of their own kidneys would help the patient more than would the use of a cadaver organ. In terms of benefit to the recipient, 37% of the nondonors agree with a statement indicating there is no difference between the success rates of cadaver and related transplants; only 5% of donors and 20% of recipients see no benefit to related vs. cadaver donation.

Moreover, in terms of risk to themselves, the nondonors, in response to in-depth questioning were much more likely than the donors to mention worry about their long-term chances with one kidney and concern about their future (48% vs. 17%; 72% vs. 34%). Similarly, 32% of nondonors "agree a lot" with the multiple-choice statement, "The thought of surgery really frightens me," in comparison to 21% of the donors.

This fear of medical procedures may predate the entire issue of transplantation and contribute to the nondonation.However, instead nondonors might have begun to emphasize the negative aspects of donation only after making their choice, in order to justify their behavior. Or donors may be repressing their anxieties; or their initial fear may have been alleviated by the contact they all have with a transplant physician. Only 26% of nondonors have talked with a doctor about the issue, and only 16% have spoken with a transplant or kidney specialist.

Furthermore, when nondonors do consult a local physician (a physician who is not a kidney specialist), that physician frequently expresses disapproval. Of those nondonors who spoke with one or more physicians, 49% report that at least one doctor was opposed to the donation. Persons who become donors also report that the local physicians were opposed, although less frequently: 32% of donors who consulted a local physician prior to their decision report receiving negative feedback. Thus nondonors are less likely than donors to have their anxieties alleviated by consultation with a transplant physician; instead, their fears are liable to be reinforced by their local private practitioners. When asked about their feelings toward donation, 78% of the nondonors who had consulted local physicians expressed worry over a donor's long-term life-chances with one kidney, compared to 58% of these who saw no doctor and 36% of those who talked with a transplant physician or other kidney specialist.

Whether these physicians are opposed to donation in reality or whether they are responding to cues emitted by the ambivalent nondonor is not clear. In some cases the local doctor may be attempting to protect the obviously fearful relative by suggesting he should not donate. However, the doctor's opposition may have a more generic origin. If the physician is responsible only for the potential donor and has had no contact with the recipient, he would appear to be under subtle pressure to oppose donation. Although the risk to the donor is small (a fact of which the doctor may not be aware), the doctor is exposing himself to possible censure if complications do arise and he has recommended the procedure, particularly because the procedure is of no benefit to the donor. The safest and most conservative course for the relative would be to avoid donation, and the local doctor is likely to recommend this option, especially if he senses any fear or reluctance.

Not only are nondonors likely to show a somewhat higher level of fear of the surgical procedure in a quantitative sense, but in some cases the difference is almost qualitative in nature. That is, among the nondonors there are 21 persons who have had a long-standing well-recognized fear of the hospital and medical techniques. No donor resembled these persons in level of anxiety.

CASE Family members were asked about the possibility of one son donating to his father

INTERVIEWER. What about the possiblity of Henry donating?

SISTER. He would give it, should Jane and I not be able to. But he's very bad—he's unbelievable hospitals, needles, everything. Our doctor doesn't think he should do it [given his fears].

* * *

INTERVIEWER. How did your children feel about donating?

MOTHER. Two of them were OK, but Henry can't take it. Hospitals and doctors and all that gets to him. Once when he was a kid there was a dead chicken on the road and I told him to take it and put it on the spreader. He said he wouldn't do it. I threw the chicken toward him and told him to do it right now. When I got over to him he was white as that lab coat you're wearing. I realized then how he felt. I apologized and sent him to the house. He didn't come out of the house the whole day.

* * *

INTERVIEWER. What about Henry?

FATHER. He was hesitant. . . .When they came down he would have liked to have come. He said, "I'd like to come down and see what they have to say. Even if I don't donate. . . ." He's so frightened. He can't stand the sight of blood. It just frightened him to walk into a sick room. . . .We tease him all the time. When he came to visit me in the hospital he kept saying, "Let's go. . .let's go. . . .Let's go" He just doesn't want to visit very long.

In addition to a general fear of related donation, the nondonors are likely to define themselves at *particular* risk. In discussing why they did not volunteer, 30% of nondonors claim they are ineligible or less eligible than others because of past or present health problems. In reality none of these health problems was severe enough to automatically preclude consideration for donation, although upon more rigorous medical examination some of these nondonors may have been ruled out.

In the potential donor's calculation of risk versus benefit, one would expect him to weigh the alternative of other relatives volunteering instead of him. According to Schwartz's (1970a, b) theory of altruistic decisions, the more likely a potential helper is to ascribe responsibility to himself rather than to others, the higher the probability he will act in accordance with the moral norm to help. Altruism experiments (Latané and Darley, 1970) show that a person is more likely to help a stranger if he is the only one available to do so. In this case we would expect to find a higher percentage of volunteers among relatives who are the only possible donors than among those who perceive others as also eligible. After family members with medical or age excuses are eliminated, relatives can be classified as the only possible donor or as one of several possible donors among children, siblings, or parents. In fact, as predicted, our data show that 77% (17 out of 22) of all relatives who found themselves the only possible donor in the close family volunteered to donate in contrast to 57% (394 out of 689) of potential donors who were in families where there were other eligible donors ($p < .10$).

In the five families where the only possible donor did not volunteer, two involved children from a recipient's first marriage. Neither of these children had seen their parent for years and both resented the lack of warmth and attention they had received after the divorce. The donation situation highlights the discrepancies between biological and emotional ties in the family. The weakening of emotional linkages that occurs in broken families is made quite clear to all parties when the issue of this major family sacrifice is raised.

The other three only possible nondonors did not volunteer for idiosyncratic reasons. One sibling was frightened and offered to build his recipient sister a house instead, perhaps out of guilt. A parent decided not to donate when his wife became ill with cancer. He was afraid to take any risk with his health which could leave his large family parentless.

Thus, with a few exceptions, the only possible donor is particularly likely to volunteer help. Furthermore, these data may be underestimating the number of donors affected by this feeling of being the only person who can help. According to the above classification, 7 out of 120 (6%) of the parents, siblings, and children who actually donated were the only possible donors early in the donor search. However, in families where there appear to be several possible donors, the numbers may become reduced as time goes on. Many of the volunteers turn out either to be the wrong blood or tissue type or to have a medical problem, leaving fewer possible donors in the family. In fact, by the time of the transplant 40% of all actual donors "agree a lot" with the statement, "I am really the only family member who could donate."

Ironically, smaller families with fewer eligible potential donors are more likely to produce a volunteer. Table 7-6 shows that among families with eligible siblings, those with only one eligible sibling were the most likely to find that at least one sibling volunteered (51%). Moreover, at the other extreme, in the five families with 10 or 11 siblings, no sibling offered his kidney. To have several siblings is advantageous to a recipient because of the likelihood that there will be a perfect tissue match among them. However, the more siblings he has, the less likely any one of them will feel the responsibility to volunteer.

In addition to determining whether he is the only possible donor, a relative may calculate his suitability against that of other family members before deciding whether to volunteer. In fact, 18% of nondonors to whom

TABLE 7-6 NUMBER OF ELIGIBLE SIBLINGS AND PRESENCE OF SIBLING VOLUNTEER

Is there a sibling volunteer or donor?	1 Sibling	2–3 Siblings	4–6 Siblings	7–9 Siblings	10–11 Siblings
Yes	51%	34%	37%	27%	0%
No	49%	66%	63%	73%	100%
	100%	100%	100%	100%	100%
	(37)	(62)	(57)	(15)	(5)

we talked said they did not volunteer because donation appeared to be less costly for another relative in terms of money, time, their own family needs, or some other factor (see Chapter 8). Twelve percent did not offer because another relative seemed to be more highly motivated.

In summary, the gift of a kidney entails considerable inconvenience, pain, and cost for a donor and his family. To some family members the cost is perceived as too great and the benefit too unsure. The alternative of another relative or a cadaver donor may seem more wise. The level of obligation one owes to various relatives is ambiguous, and family members do not agree in their definitions of obligation. These differences in attitude and perceptions appear to be correlated with family members' donor status—that is, with their tendency to have volunteered or become nondonors.

Personality Differences

The question of whether donors and nondonors differ fundamentally in personality-type is one to which we can give only peripheral answers. Given the tremendous amount of material we wished to cover with nondonors and our concern that they would be unwilling to devote more than one hour to an interview, extensive personality measures were not included. Cleveland's study (1975) of 30 persons who had signed donor cards willing their organs in the event of their death and an equal number of control individuals opposed to cadaver organ donation indicated that donor-card volunteers were more likely to be "internalizers," that is they were more independent, autonomous, resistive to outside influence, reliant on internalized goals, and more likely to express hostility intropunitively with attendant feelings of guilt and depression. While we did not use measures that could determine whether our donors were more likely than our nondonors to be internalizers, we did measure the level of self-esteem and happiness of both groups.

Two alternative hypotheses could be advanced concerning the self-esteem and happiness of both groups:

Hypothesis 1. (*a*) *Persons with particularly low self-esteem are more likely to volunteer to donate because of a personality need to think better of themselves.*

(*b*) *Similarly, persons who are less happy will volunteer to donate to improve internal feelings of well-being—they will attempt to help another person feel happier themselves.*

These motivational forces will probably not be conscious ones.

In their series of living unrelated donors, Sadler and associates (1971) note that some individuals with low self-esteem do seem to exhibit this type of motivation. By saving the life of another, they hope to give meaning to their own unsatisfactory life and to demonstrate their own worth as individuals. In addition, Cialdini and associates (1973) present some experimental evidence in support of their hypothesis that one of the motivational forces behind altruistic behavior is the desire to counteract unhappy feelings, whatever their source. The theory is that altruism and the good it produces will alleviate feelings of unhappiness, even when the origin of such feelings is unrelated to the altruistic act. In Chapter 6 we noted that the self-esteem and happiness of donors does appear to improve after the donation of a kidney. However, while the consequences of altruism may be beneficial to the individual's feelings of well-being, the premise that those who select the altruistic act are more in need than others of such an improvement does not necessarily follow.

The alternative hypothesis is the following:

Hypothesis 2. Optimistic, happier individuals with high self-esteem will regard the risk of donation with more sanguinity and will be more willing to take the chance and donate a kidney.

Cleveland's (1975) study cited above would support this hypothesis associating donation with initially high rather than low self-esteem. There is evidence that his measures of internalization are correlated with indicators of high self-esteem. [See Isen (1970) for evidence of greater charity among individuals who are made to feel successful in an experiment. Also see Trimakas and Nicolay, (1974).]

Our data show little difference between the donors pretransplant and the nondonors in terms of happiness or self-esteem (e.g., see Tables 3-5, 6-5). However, if anything, the nondonors appear slightly less happy than the donors and the controls. These data, though limited in the number of dimensions measured, do not point to a fundamental difference in the self-picture or level of happiness of donors and nondonors.

Our study of MMPIs of donors at the time of their physical work-up also does not indicate great personality differences between donors and normal controls (see Figure 3-1). On most scales there is no difference, although donors do score a little higher on defensiveness (K-scale), psychopathic orientation (Scale 4), and alienation (Scale 8).

However, one additional life-attitude that we measured did distinguish nondonors from donors—that is, faith in people. A scale designed by Rosenberg (1965) was used to differentiate individuals with a high trust in others from those with low faith in other people.* The reasonable prediction is that the altruistic individual would demonstrate higher faith in people than those unwilling to make major sacrifices for others. In fact, 74% of donors and 71% of recipients score high in faith in people, in contrast to only 43% of nondonors. These results must be interpreted with caution because the measurement occurred after, rather than before, the donor decision was completed, and the subject's view of others may have been affected by the presence or absence of his own generosity. Yet, in our view, the probability is that the causal direction is as originally formulated—that a person's view of others as trustworthy and generous will facilitate his own tendency to help those others.

Other types of altruistic behavior might relate to personality-type differently than does the organ-donor situation. Many types of altruistic acts involve helping a stranger or groups of strangers at relatively low cost and low benefit to the self, in comparison to this act. Blood donation, small gifts of money, going to the aid of a person in trouble, returning a lost wallet, helping to make telephone calls, signing an organ-donor card are all examples of the type of altruistic behavior that has been investigated (Macaulay and Berkowitz, 1970; Titmuss, 1971; for an exception, see Schwartz, 1970b). Although such acts could trigger considerable cost (if a stranger being helped was not trustworthy or if medical complications occurred during blood donation), the expectation is that the cost will be minimal; whereas the sacrifice for a kidney donor of undergoing a painful operation and having an organ removed is a significant one even if all proceeds smoothly. More important, the benefit to the self of saving the life of a loved one is also significant, while many altruistic acts have no obvious benefit to the individual providing help. The individual who chooses to go out of his way to help someone when there is little intrinsic reward for him may be different in personality from other persons (although the personality variables that have been tested have not been very good predictors in these types of helping studies). In the related donor situation, however, many other variables may be more powerful

* Would you (1) agree or (2) disagree with this? If you don't watch yourself, people will take advantage of you.

Would you say most people are more inclined to (1) help others, or more inclined (2) to look out for themselves?

Some people say that most people can be trusted. Others say you can't be too careful in your dealings with people. Do you feel (1) most people can be trusted or (2) that you can't be too careful?

Human nature is really cooperative. Do you (1) agree or (2) disagree?

No one is going to care much what happens to you, when you get right down to it. Do you (1) agree or (2) disagree?

motivators—closeness to the recipient, feelings of obligation to both of one's families—so that personality-type becomes less important.

However, there are several dimensions of personality that should be measured before such a conclusion is accepted; for example, propensity to risk-taking behavior (see Kogan and Wallach, 1967), tendency to ascribe moral responsibility to the self and to delineate consequences of one's act (see Schwartz, 1970 a, b), and tendency to internalize or to externalize (Cleveland, 1975). London (1970) finds that Christians who aided Jews to escape from Nazi Germany had demonstrated a particularly great level of adventurousness and risk-taking behavior earlier in their lives.

Situational Factors

In studies of *minor* levels of altruistic behavior, situational factors appear to be important. Darley and Latané (1970), for example, show that the individual's likelihood of offering help to a stranger seeking directions is influenced by the details of the situation in which help is being asked. However, the importance of situational factors in *major* decision-making has probably been underestimated. The more traditional approach is to explore, as we have just done, the impact of background statuses, interpersonal relationships, attitudinal, and personality variables upon important life-choices. There would appear to be few decisions as major as the one to donate a kidney. Yet there are several indications that the character of the situation in which one is told about the need for a kidney in itself influences the outcome. Just as in our discussion of situational factors in Chapter 6, however, this analysis must be regarded as tentative. Despite careful coding of multiple stories of the same event, such reconstruction is difficult. Cases where independent coders could not agree are excluded from analysis.

First of all, the donor is more likely to have been informed of the donor need *in person* than is the random nondonor (80% vs. 58%); the nondonor is more likely to have been informed by telephone or letter. This difference is still evident when we control for nature of the blood relationship between the recipient and potential donor and for the geographical distance between their homes. Among those who live more than 100 miles away, donors are *more* likely than random nondonors to have learned of the need by telephone or in person than by letter. Clearly the pressure to respond would seem greater when the potential donor is face to face with a family member asking for help. The letter would appear to be the least powerful means of communicating the patient's urgent need, and the nondonor is the family member who receives these weaker calls for help.

If we conceive of a two-stage information flow—from the recipient, recipient's spokesman, or doctor to certain potential donors and then from the latter to the rest of the family—the relatives who become nondonors are the ones who are part of the second rather than the first stage of communication. In fact, while 44% of the donors and 26% of the other volunteers were the first family members to be notified of the donor need, only 10% of those who became nondonors learned about the problem first.

We could argue that the dying patient, his spokesman (usually mother or spouse), and the expert physician are more persuasive communicators than are the other relatives. Thus those who hear of the problem from the former are more likely to volunteer to help. However, because there is definite evidence that the person the recipient approaches first is the relative to whom he feels closest and the relative who lives nearest, the question arises whether these situational factors have any power in their own right or whether they are mere reflections of the patterns of emotional and geographical closeness in the family. When we control for the closeness of the relationship between potential donor and recipient, we still find that those who become nondonors have been (1) informed later than donors about the patient's need; (2) have been informed in a less personal face-to-face manner; and (3) were less likely to be notified directly by the patient, their own mother, or the physician. For example, among the potential donors to whom the recipient felt "very close" emotionally, 43% of the individuals who became donors and 44% of the other volunteers were the first family members to be notified of the donor need, in contrast to only 11% of those who became nondonors. Among those rated less close, 22% of the donors, 24% of the other volunteers, but only 8% of the nondonors were told before other family members. Regardless of emotional closeness, those who became volunteers apparently were more likely to have been part of the early communication process than those who became nondonors.

Controlling for the geographical distance between the homes of the recipient and potential donors does not modify these results either. Both among those who live in the same household as the recipient and among those who live farther away, the future donors and volunteers were more likely to have been notified early and more personally than were the future nondonors.

Thus the structure of communication is different for those to whom the recipient feels close and those to whom he is less close. But above and beyond the emotional feelings of closeness, the situation under which the potential donor hears of the need for a kidney appears to exert an influence on his final decision.

Although the structure of communication between the patient and the donor is different than that between the patient and the nondonor, the content of the initial message appears to be similar. In Chapter 6 we noted that a greater pressure is put on the potential donor if he is ordered to donate or asked directly than if he is informed of the need without an immediate answer being required. The donors do not appear to be exposed to any more direct a message originally than the nondonors, although they may have been over time (see Chapter 9). Furthermore, the donors are no more likely than the nondonors to be subject to undue family pressure. Two independent coders agree that 32 *nondonors* (16%) were clearly subject to family pressure to donate. Approximately the same percentage of *donors* (11%) were also subject to family pressure. Pressure to donate was more likely to result in *major* family stress for nondonors than donors. In the 11 families out of 205 (5%) where pressure was classified as a major stress, eight involved pressure toward nondonors, two toward donors, and one toward other volunteers. Stated differently, in these families 21 nondonors found pressure a major stress, compared to two donors and one volunteer.

The Situation and Perception of Oneself as a Nondonor. Another important aspect of the situation is whether it allows a relative to avoid perceiving himself as a nondonor. Ten percent of the nondonors indicate that they did not consider donation because they were not asked to do so. Given the difficulties in clear communication when asking for such a major favor, it is not surprising that many family members do not believe they received a clear request (see Chapter 9). The recipient is often more likely to hint than to ask clearly for such a substantial sacrifice. Yet the indirect request may be so unclear that the potential donor either does not hear it or is able consciously or unconsciously to avoid it.

Many nondonors claim their health precludes donation, although their health problems were not major. In some cases the medical excuse appears to have been mentioned for the first time in the interview with the sociologists, and the family has never heard about it; in other cases the family accepts the excuse as legitimate, even though in other families similar persons have volunteered; and in some families the excuse is not accepted.

SISTER. (donor) One of the reasons my husband said he was against it was because he didn't see any of the others popping up to volunteer. . .and he's right about that. . . .Why didn't the others come? They have families. . .and other things they hide behind!

INTERVIEWER. Do you feel they should have offered?

SISTER. I can't understand why they don't. They should. . . .My brother. . .I told you about him before. . .

INTERVIEWER. Yes.

SISTER. Well, I found out that yellow jaundice has nothing to do with this. That's with the liver.

INTERVIEWER. Do you think your brother knows that?

SISTER. Oh yes. . .he's hiding behind that just like the rest are hiding behind their families. He said he wanted to do it, but if he really did he'd check it out. I bet he knows it has nothing to do with it.

Still other nondonors (15%) define themselves as ineligible because another potential family donor has already volunteered, although this fact does not in reality eliminate the usefulness of their being tissue-typed and matched also. As Schwartz (1970a) notes, one way to evade altruistic behavior is to deny one's own responsibility for giving help. Although by using such excuses many nondonors avoid perceiving themselves as unwilling, other family members note their failure to volunteer and define the situation quite differently (see Chapter 8).

These discrepancies in perception could be predicted by attribution theory (Jones and Nisbett, 1971). Frequently the actor in a situation, in this case the nondonor, will perceive his action or nonaction to have been attributable to the characteristics of the situation rather than to any basic personality trait or motivation in himself. The observer, in this case the recipient and the family, will label the act as consistent with underlying traits of the actor and attributable to his true motivations. The actor is aware of the great variety of situational stimuli affecting him and of his own confusing battery of emotions. The observer is primarily aware of whether the actor proceeds in one direction or not, and to produce cognitive clarity he places a structure of consistency and meaning on that behavior. In this case the nondonor will perceive his lack of volunteering as a function of the particular way events structured themselves; and the recipient or family will perceive the nondonation as an indicator of motivational state, in this case as a lack of love or as selfishness. While some nondonors' excuses appear to be rationalizations to protect their own self-picture or conscious attempts to impress the outsider, others seem to represent legitimate differences in perceptions of events. In other instances the family over time comes to support rather than contradict the nondonor's view of himself (see Chapter 9).

CONCLUSION

Altruistic behavior presents social-psychological theory and the skeptical layman with a puzzle to resolve. According to reinforcement theory and exchange theory, individuals give to others to achieve certain rewards for themselves (Darley and Latané, 1970). If the gift is given without expectation of any external reward, as in the case of most altruistic behavior that has been studied (voluntary blood donation, help to a stranger), theories arise to identify the rewarding aspects of the situation. If the organ donor risks his own life "merely" to save that of a relative, the skeptic regards this extraordinary gift as the outcome of an ethically dubious situation.* According to Fellner and Schwartz (1971), altruism has fallen into "disrepute." The organ donor must be operating to assuage guilt (the "black sheep" donor), to alleviate feelings of low self-esteem and unhappiness or in response to high levels of family pressure.

Our study (Chapter 6) has identified some donors who do appear to be responding to internal guilt and external family pressure. Yet the comparison of nondonors and donors shows no difference between the two groups in the proportions who seem to be "black sheep," no difference in the percentage subject to undue family pressure, and little difference in underlying self-esteem and happiness. Insofar as we have evidence, nondonors were as likely as donors to be family "black sheep," to be pressured by their families to donate, and to suffer from a low self-picture in need of a boost. These factors, which if operative could raise ethical questions, do not appear to be the overriding motivations for organ donors.

There *are* differences, however, between individuals who volunteer to donate a kidney and those who do not. These findings seem to indicate that in truth the anticipated "reward" for the donor lies in saving the life of a loved one and in fulfilling the family obligations that appear most important to him.

The fact that donors are so much closer emotionally to recipients than are nondonors is one indication that the major reward for the donor lies in preventing the loss of an emotionally significant person. The donors'

* Macaulay and Berkowitz (1970) define altruism as "behavior carried out to benefit another without anticipation of external reward" (p. 3). If one considers the continuation of an important relative's life an external reward, a definitional problem emerges—even when the motivations are relatively "pure" ones, can organ donation be defined as altruism if the donor is dependent upon the transplant recipient emotionally or physically? The major issue discussed above, however, is not a definitional one, but whether individuals are capable of making major sacrifices to help another person simply because of a wish to help or because of the desire to remove that person from distress. Or do major sacrifices of that type stem from less "positive" emotional sources?

perceptions of their own motivations agree with this conclusion, as indicated in Chapter 6.

Figure 7-1 summarizes the variables that are important in distinguishing donors from nondonors. Each of the variables represented is correlated with the fact of donation or nondonation. In the diagram these variables are arranged in the causal sequence that seems most likely. According to this proposed schema, several intervening attitudes and emotions predispose a family member toward volunteering to donate an organ, and certain structural variables enhance the likelihood that these attitudes will be present. The key intervening attitudes include a high degree of emotional closeness between recipient and potential donors, a positive view of the risks and chances for benefit of the medical procedures, a strong feeling of family obligation to help, and a failure to define the choice as a conflict between the recipient and one's own family of procreation.

Several of these intervening variables can be linked to *subjective utility theory*. According to subjective utility theory, the likelihood that an individual will make a risky decision is a function of his various perceptions: (1) the apparent chances of success if the risk is taken (in this case the individual's perception that a related transplant will be successful); (2) the value he places on the successful outcome (the value the recipient's life has for the potential donor as measured by the closeness between them); (3) the perceived chances of failure (the donor's perception and fear of the risks to himself); and (4) the cost of failure to him (Kogan and Wallach, 1967).

Unfortunately because those intervening attitudinal variables were measured after the donor choice became known, we cannot be certain that these differences preceded the donor search. Thus the causal ordering in Figure 7-1 is hypothetical; it is consistent with our data but still remains to be tested conclusively. The structural variables, however, in almost all cases did precede the decision to donate; and where arrows are drawn, these variables are correlated in the indicated direction with the relevant intervening variables. Thus, first of all, one of the most important structural variables appears to be the nature of the blood relationship between the potential donor and the recipient: Within the family of origin, the recipient's parents are by far the most likely to volunteer an organ, with children the next most likely, and siblings the least likely to volunteer. A reasonable hypothesis is that this difference is due to the fact that parents experience greater feelings of obligation and closeness to the patient than do other relatives because of the role-expectations and norms governing parenthood.

Second, the lines of cleavage, bonding, and obligation in a family are

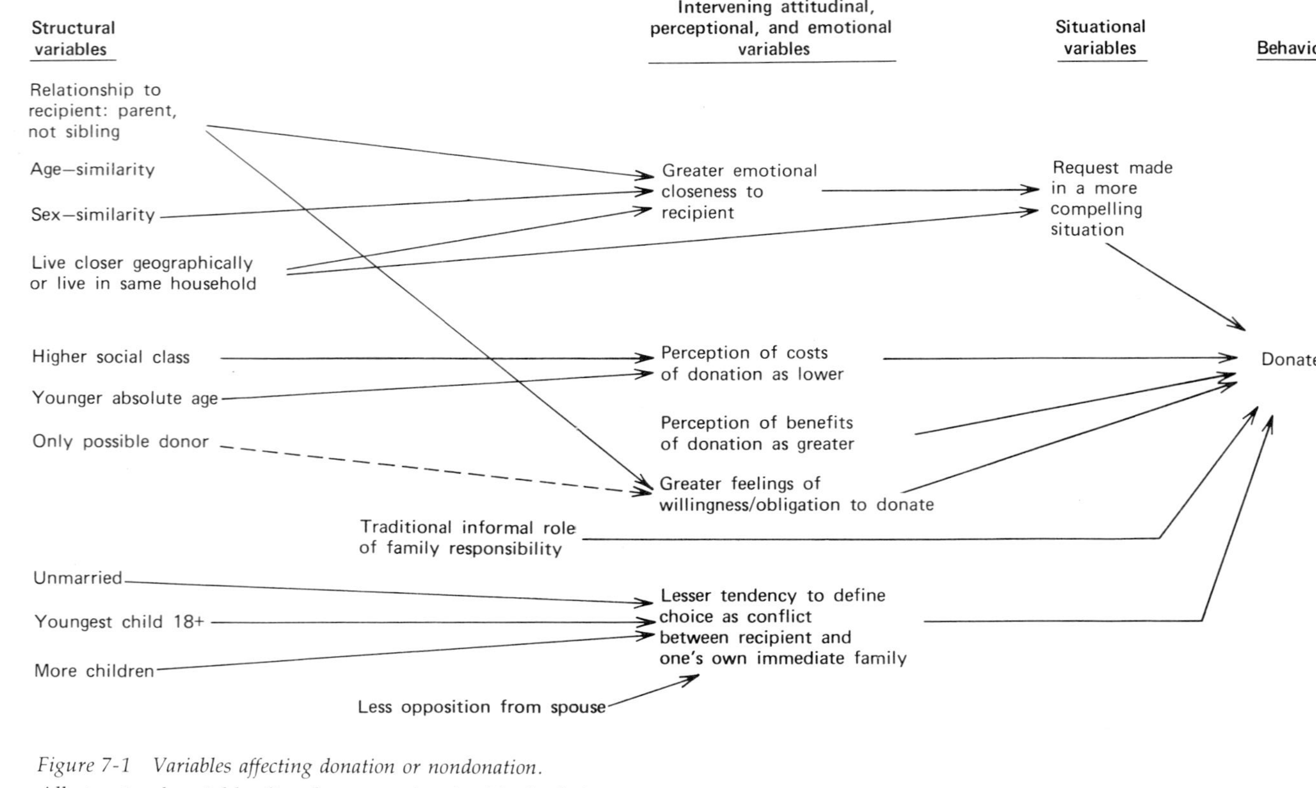

Figure 7-1 Variables affecting donation or nondonation.

All structural variables listed are correlated with the behavior of donation/nondonation. The dotted arrow indicates presumed causal link, although no adequate test of hypothesis is possible with data.

further explicated when we look at the potential donor's age, sex, and residence. Relatives still sharing the same household and siblings closer in age to the recipient and of the same sex are more likely to volunteer to donate. We hypothesize that these findings are reflections of the greater emotional closeness of these relatives to the recipient. The closest bonds among siblings in the family thus appear to be among those similar in age and sex who have not yet left home.

Third, certain absolute status characteristics render family members more likely to volunteer a kidney—a higher education and occupational status and a younger age. All three characteristics are related to a more positive view of the risks and benefits of donation and are probably indicative of a different life-outlook in various socioeconomic groups and age cohorts. With higher education comes a greater faith in modern science, medicine, and technology. With advancing age may come a greater awareness of one's own mortality; among the young, the possibility of death may seem unreal. In addition, the financial costs of donation may appear less great for relatives in middle-class occupations than for those holding blue-collar jobs.

Fourth, certain aspects of the family constellation and its organization of informal roles appear to be important. The member who is the only possible donor in the family of origin and the members who have always taken greater family responsibility than others are more likely to volunteer. Feelings of obligation seem to be more intense among only possible donors.

Fifth, the role of the situation in which the request for help is made appears to be significant. Family members who are closer emotionally to the patient and who live nearer are more likely to be informed of the need in a compelling situation. They are among the first told of the donor need, are most likely to be informed in person rather than, for example, by letter. Even when emotional and geographical closeness are held constant, those informed in these more compelling situations are more likely to be donors than nondonors.

Finally, individuals who appear to have greater obligations to their own family of procreation are less likely to donate. Siblings and children who are married, who have more children, who have children too young to leave the "nest," and whose spouses are opposed to their donation are more likely to be nondonors. Persons in these situations are more likely to define the situation as a conflict between their normative obligations to their families of origin and their duty to their own immediate families, a conflict they feel must be resolved in favor of their own families.

To what extent do these factors explain the difference between donors and nondonors? The structural variables in the first column of Figure 7-1 account for 38% ($p < .001$) of the variance in the decision to donate or not donate. If we add the intervening variables, 53% of the variance is explained ($p < .001$).

In general, according to this analysis, the key factors differentiating donors from nondonors involve their formal and informal roles and relationships within their two families—the family they share with the recipient and the family they have founded themselves. The donor-decision situation thus sets in relief some of the bonds of closeness within the "larger" family. In addition, the study of this decision contributes to the literature on altruism by adding a case in which the consequences of the help-giving act are major rather than minor, in which the level of self-sacrifice and the potential for gain literally involve issues of life and death. In a situation where there are such large stakes involved, a surprisingly high proportion of family members volunteer to sacrifice one of their own kidneys to save the life of their dying relative: 57% of eligible family members volunteer and take the definite preliminary step of having their blood tested. Nothing in the results reported in this chapter comparing donors to nondonors points to a need to restrict the *right* of individuals to give this extraordinary type of help.

8

THE DECISION TO BE A DONOR

The field of medicine provides the sociologist with a rich research site for the study of individual and family decision-making processes. Physicians, patients, and patient's families are faced with decisions and choices whose impact and urgency certainly cannot be overestimated (Farber, 1960; Fox, 1959; Rosenstock, 1961). In areas of new medical technology, where decisions are less likely to be routinized, the study of decision-making processes is particularly fruitful.

To the outsider few decisions in the life-course would appear as major and as crisisbound as that confronting the potential kidney donor. Clear norms to guide this decision-maker are absent. What are the procedures used by family members as they decide who, if anyone, will take the risk of donation and make the necessary sacrifices?

Although decision-making has been extensively studied in the laboratory situation and in larger-scale organizations, there have been few studies of the real life processes that occur as individuals in a family attempt to make major, highly stressful, and risky decisions (Aldous et al., 1971; Kogan and Wallach, 1967). Our purpose in this analysis is to use the transplant experience to enhance our knowledge, to help develop the theories of the ways major life-decisions are made. Therefore this particular chapter may be of more interest to a behavioral scientist than to the general reader. (In the summary the main findings are delineated and their policy relevance is indicated.)

Most of the chapter is focused on the *individual* family member's perception of his own decision-making process (see Simmons et al., 1973), although the processes that take place in the *family* are examined briefly toward the end of the discussion. In Chapter 7 we attempted to identify factors that help to predict whether a person will donate or not. In the first part of this chapter we concentrate instead on the individual's perception of his decision-making.

SOURCES OF INFORMATION

There are three sources of information for this chapter, the first two of which have been discussed in detail earlier: (1) the quantitative questionnaire material for recipients, donors, and nondonors; (2) the in-depth qualitative case material collected over time for 205 families, 114 donors, and 357 nondonors (235 about whom we have clear enough information to use in the analysis); and (3) 52 intensive qualitative interviews with family members at the time they were being blood-tested and typed for donation.*

The second source, the long-term case studies, involved repeated interviews with recipients, spouses, and as many members of the extended family as possible (including all potential donors, spouses, and even sometimes in-laws) through the donor search to allow us to reconstruct decision-making and commitment events.†

* For a relative to be accepted as a donor he must follow certain procedures. He has to have his blood typed to make certain it is compatable. Although some potential donors already know their blood type or obtain this information outside the University, all must be tissue-typed and crossed-matched through the University Hospital to eliminate cases in which the recipient has developed antibodies against the donor's tissue. Most donors are tested for both blood type and tissue type at the same time at the University. If there are several possible family donors, these laboratory tests may identify the person whose tissue type most closely resembles that of the recipient. Once potential donors successfully pass these initial screening procedures, one such family member is admitted into the hospital for three days of extensive testing. Through this work-up the staff determines whether his health and kidneys are adequate for donation.

† For the donors, one in-depth interview always took place at the time the donor was being physically worked-up, before he or she was definitely approved as a donor; although many donors had been interviewed prior to this point also. However, the main questionnaire interviews of the *nondonors* took place approximately a month posttransplant. Although the memory of nondonors on the questionnaires at a month posttransplant might be expected to

Because the blood-testing event occurs relatively early in the sequence of events leading to donation, we felt it would be useful to explore the extent of decision-making and commitment at that time through a definitely scheduled interview. Many blood-tested relatives do not go on to become donors, either because they are the wrong type or have physical problems or because another family member is used. In addition, some of them become nondonors after this point. From July 1972 to February 1973 we interviewed all persons blood-tested at the University prior to their learning the results of the tests. The 52 individuals interviewed at that time were from 27 families.

Two independent coders were asked to classify the decision process of each donor, nondonor, and blood-tested relative according to three basic models of decision-making: the classical model of rational deliberation, the instantaneous-decision model, and the postponement model (see below). Their classification was based on information from the qualitative interviews and from the open-ended material in the questionnaires. Judgements of family processes were made similarly. Reliability was generally satisfactory and will be discussed below.

THE INDIVIDUAL DECISION

In discussing the ways in which donors and nondonors arrive at their choices, the focus is on the *perceived process* of decision-making—the extent of deliberation, the perception that a decision was reached, and the speed with which it was reached.

In the light of prior work in this area, several decision-making models are advanced, and we analyze the extent to which the cases fit these models.

Obviously the way people act to resolve the donor decision would not be expected to be generalized to all human decisions. The congruence would be expected to be greater for similar types of decisions, however, and therefore it is useful to classify the donor problem (see Brim et al., 1962; Tallman, 1970, for classifications of problems). First, we are defining a decision as a set of actions and cognitions related to and including the choice of one alternative rather than another (see Backrach and Baratz, 1970; Dahl, 1960). The number of alternatives possible is one key charac-

---

be somewhat distorted, the repeated qualitative interviews of many family members prior to the transplant allow us to identify and analyze some of this bias. See Olson and Rabunsky (1972), and Janis and Mann (in press) for a discussion of the limitations of self-report measures in decision-making studies.

teristic of a decision. In this case a potential donor who is informed of the need for related donors either volunteers to donate or he does not. It is a decision with *two basic alternatives* for the individual (see Brim et al., 1962), although some donors choose a third road and make offers conditional on the ineligibility of all other family members. At the family level, however, several alternatives (several donors) are often possible.

More important in terms of decision characteristics, this is a *major life decision* with *high stakes*. After being implemented, the decision is *irreversible*. It is not a decision where the outcome is assured, but it falls into the category of a decision made under *risk* where the *probabilities* of success and failure are *known* (see Tallman, 1970; Taylor, 1965). That is, the probabilities are known to experts, but not all potential donors seek out this expert knowledge and not all perceive the probabilities accurately.

It is a decision made in a *crisis situation* usually with an implicit though not clear-cut *time deadline*. The time lead between knowledge of the need for a donor and the patient's readiness for a transplant varies from case to case with some urgency present in a high frequency of situations. Given the availability of the dialysis machine to keep the patient alive, delay is possible. When other family members volunteer to donate or the recipient places himself on the list for a cadaver kidney, a time boundary is set on the decision-making process.

The decision is *nonrepetitive* rather than customary, and the *norms* to aid in its resolution are relatively *unclear*.

Finally, the *family context* of the decision is important. This is a decision affecting the individual's central and intimate *interpersonal* relationships. Unlike a simple gambling situation, for example, where an individual's decision to bet on a horse does not involve a negotiated conflict of interest with other individual gamblers, the donor decision is embedded in a *potential bargaining* or *strategy* situation (Tallman, 1970; Turner, 1970). The donor's narrow interest is in some conflict with the recipient's as well as with other potential donors'—if one family member donates, another does not have to.

Unlike other family or group decisions, however, the solution is not dependent on the concerted action of all members or even of a large subgroup. If a wife wishes the family to move to another home, agreement of some other family members is usually necessary. If a group member wishes to devote group resources to the development of a costly program at the expense of other activities, some member agreement is likely to be required. But if the potential donor is of age, he may volunteer to donate without consent of other potential donors; and if he is found medically eligible, the recipient's and the family's problem is resolved.

The decision-maker has the power to resolve the problem *as an individual*, although bargaining and strategy may assume importance.

The potential impact of these decision characteristics upon the model of decision-making used is discussed below as relevant. The issue to be discussed here is not how the individual should make decisions, but how he does make them—in what processes he perceives himself engaging.

The view of the actor as an "economic man" motivated to increase reward and decrease cost has historically led to an emphasis on the rationality and deliberativeness of his decision-making behavior (Pollard and Mitchell, 1971; Simon, 1957; Taylor, 1965). The model of the decision-making or problem-solving widely used and emerging from such a tradition has been presented by Hill (1970) and Brim et al. (1962) among others. It includes the following stages: (1) identification of the problem, (2) collection of relevant information, (3) production of action alternatives, (4) evaluation of the expected outcomes of each alternative, (5) a deliberate selection of one alternative, (6) implementation of the decision, and (7) evaluation of the actual outcomes. As will be evident later, the key elements of this model in our view involve the period of *conscious deliberation* and evaluation of alternatives and the equally *conscious choice* of one alternative. We term this classical rational model the "model of deliberation."* (See Figure 8-1)

In its original form the model was an *optimizing* or *maximizing* one (see Glueck, 1974; Janis and Mann, in press; Taylor, 1965)—that is, it is based on the assumption that the decision-maker weighed the positive and negative outcomes of *all* possible alternatives accurately and made the optimal choice. More recently, especially in organizational theory, this view of the rational *decision-making* process has been widely attacked (Katona, 1953; Simon, 1957; Taylor, 1965), particularly on the grounds of the incompleteness of information available to the actor, the subjective values attached to alternative outcomes, and the fact that all possible alternatives and outcomes are unlikely to be considered. According to Simon (1957), man's rationality is "bounded," not complete. The actor necessarily has a simpler and more uncertain map of the domain relevant to his decision than is likely to be optimal. Because his information search may be limited, the actual probabilities of various outcomes will be less important to his choice than the perhaps inaccurate probabilities he perceives. An objective value cannot be placed on all the consequences of

* In earlier work (Simmons et al., 1973a) we termed this simply the "rational model." However, to avoid fruitless arguments over whether other cognitive processes of arriving at choice are ultimately "rational," we have renamed this model to emphasize its major characteristic—the presence of deliberation.

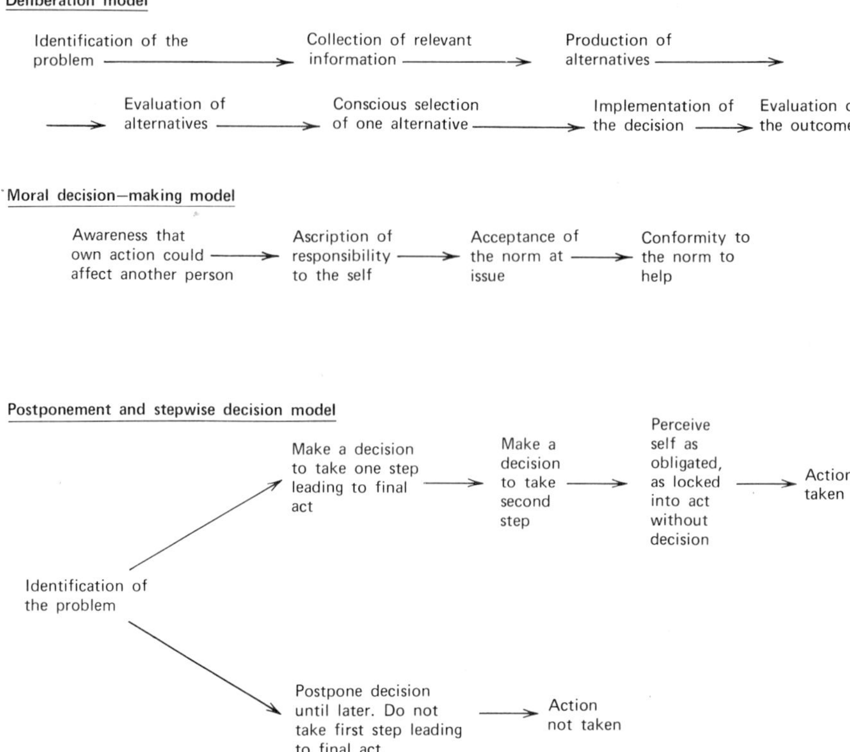

Figure 8-1 Initial decision-making models.

his choice, so his own subjective values (utilities) are used.* Instead of considering all alternatives, an individual may look at only one or two and decide if their outcomes are satisfactory.

In fact, because of this last characteristic, noted by Simon (1957), a major distinction has been drawn in the literature between "optimizing" decision models and "satisficing" models (see Glueck, 1974; Janis and Mann, in press; Taylor, 1965). That is, does the individual, limited as he is, still *attempt to weigh the outcomes of many possible alternatives* to make the optimal choice, or does he choose the first alternative that "satisfices"—the first alternative that is "good enough" and meets minimal standards. In either case, the process as originally described by Simon (1957) and Taylor (1965) still appears compatible with the main stages in

* See Kogan and Wallach (1967) for summaries of models of Expected Value, Subjective Expected Utility, etc. as applied to decisions of risk.

the classical "model of deliberation" outlined above (see Rados, 1972). Each stage, from information search through evaluation of alternatives, may be curtailed in comparison to that ideally *required by "economic man."* Yet the organizational theorists still describe a *period of deliberation* in which the outcomes of at least one alternative are weighed against desired ends, and they still emphasize a *conscious decision*. Even the "satisficer" spends some time deliberating to see if an alternative meets minimum standards (Cyert et al., 1956).

While a model of deliberation, either in its "satisficing" or "optimizing" form, may be appropriate for administrative problem-solving within complex organizations, alternate models may far better fit major life-decisions or choices made in an expressive context like that of the family. This analysis is an attempt to answer the question of whether the individual decision-maker—the donor, the nondonor, and the blood-tested volunteer—perceives his process as one of *deliberation* and *rational weighing of outcomes followed by a clear decision* or whether some other process seems to fit his perceptions better.*

MORAL DECISION-MAKING MODEL: A SATISFICING MODEL OF INSTANTANEOUS CHOICE

Schwartz (1970a, b) posits a model that stands in opposition to the classical model of deliberation—that is, in opposition to a pattern of deliberation and conscious weighing of costs and gains. He terms this model "moral decision-making." Fellner and Marshall (1968, 1970) and Fellner and Schwartz (1971), in their studies of a smaller sample of kidney donors, have seen donation as an example of this type of decision. According to this theory, three steps are necessary if the person is to decide to make the "moral" choice to help another person (see Figure 8-1). *First* the person must become aware that his particular actions have consequences for the welfare of the other person. This is the equivalent of the first stage in the deliberative decision-making model—that is, the identification of the problem, plus the knowledge of the advantages of one of the decision choices. Thus this step *per se* does not distinguish between the models. In this case the donor would have to be aware that donation of an organ by a relative would help to save the life of the recipient. *Second*, the person would have to ascribe some responsibility to

* Some theorists (White, 1970) have distinguished between the term *choice* and the term *decision*, and reserved the term *decision* for just those choices that are made after rational deliberation. Although we do not follow this lead, the question would remain: What life choices fit a classical model of "deliberation" and which better fit some other model?

himself rather than to other potential actors or to chance. The potential donor would have to see himself, not simply other relatives, as having some responsibility. *Third,* he would have to accept the moral norm at issue. In this case he would have to perceive donation as an act of virtue or an obligation.

Fellner and Marshall (1968, 1970) point to the speed with which their donors committed themselves to donation, as an indication that one is dealing with a moral rather than a deliberative decision-making process. Their donors generally perceive that they've made no decision at all—that they knew at once upon hearing of the need that they would be willing to donate. *They report no process of deliberation before volunteering*. The instantaneous character of the decision choice is what strikes us as very different from the classical model of deliberation. Although Schwartz's model is designed to apply to any decision involving help-giving behavior, the *instantaneous* choice is what interests *us* at this point (see Schwartz, 1975).*

The reader should be reminded that our concern here is the actor's *perception* of his decision process, or his *conscious* cognitive work. We are not claiming that a person whose decision-making approximates an instantaneous model is unaffected by the expected costs and gains of his act, by the subjective or actual utilities. The process, not the ultimate rationality of the choice, is at issue—the fact that the actor does not consciously take time to weigh these utilities.

In response to Schwartz's work (1970a, b), to our own earlier published material in this area, and to other literature, Janis and Mann (in press) characterize instantaneous moral decision-making as one type of "satisficing decision." If a person is using an *optimizing* strategy, he *must* deliberate and explore the consequences of a variety of alternatives. However, with a *satisficing* strategy one simply refers to a minimal decision criterion or criteria. Although an individual who is following a satisficing strategy may take time to seek information and deliberate whether a particular alternative meets these minimal standards, he may instead make such a rapid calculation that the effect seems instantaneous to the decision-maker and observers alike. In a normative area the minimum decision rules may simply be "Is this problem my moral responsibility?" "Is this the morally right thing to do?" In fact if the norm is strong enough, as it might be in a family context, the person may feel that it would be immoral for him to deliberate or consider other options open to him.†

* See Simmons et al., 1973a for a discussion of the "impulse model," as an alternative model to deal with instantaneous choice.

† Janis and Mann note that there is a continuum between optimizing and satisficing models with many types of decisions falling between. One type of decision we would characterize

The Decision of the Donor: The Instantaneous Choice

Do the actual donors in our large sample tend to report this speedy type of decision, this immediate choice without any deliberation or further information-seeking? Kogan and Wallach (1967, p. 128), as well as Ferber (1971) have predicted the opposite: They hypothesize that the more grave the situation or costly the choice, the more information will be sought by the decision-maker. Yet many have noted that in times of crisis and stress, there is a narrowing of the cognitive organization of the moment, fewer alternatives are perceived, and decision-making becomes more rigid (Holsti, 1971) and presumably less deliberative.

We are concerned here with the donor's decision to volunteer to donate if eligible. (In families where there are several eligible donors, another family decision has to be made to choose one of these persons. This decision is discussed in Part II of this chapter.)

Table 8-1, based on multiple-choice questionnaire responses, shows that 88% of donors report that they considered donating as soon as they found out about the need; 78% said that they knew right away they would donate—they did not think it over. Over 70% either say that the decision was "not at all hard" for them or spontaneously tell the interviewer that it was no decision at all. Thus there is indication that the majority of donors perceive themselves as making a very rapid and easy choice.

In addition, coding of the qualitative material from donors and other family members indicates that 61% of the donors would be classified as making an immediate choice, according to the judgment of two independent coders (see Table 8-2). That is, according to the donor and usually several family members, the majority of donors *volunteer immediately upon hearing of the need* without any time delay or any period of deliberation, and they themselves regard their choice as no decision at all. The donor describes his choice as instantaneous, and in most of these cases we have verified with several family members the fact that the donor volunteered *as soon as* he heard of the need.

Table 8-2 also lists subcategories of this immediate decision, according to the hardness of our evidence and the "pureness" of the case. For 38% of the donors the case is "pure" and the evidence is well verified by other family members. In a few cases other key family members were unavailable and family verification of the donor's story of immediate volunteering was not secured, or the donor was unable to volunteer abso-

as deliberation, but that is a hybrid type is the "validating decision" described by Glueck (1974) and Soelberg (1967) in which the individual has a strong bias toward his first satisfactory opportunity, but creates a second alternative that does not survive the comparative evaluation because of motivated distortion.

TABLE 8-1 SPEED OF DONOR'S DECISION (QUESTIONNAIRE RESPONSE)

When did you first consider donating?	
As soon as you found out about the need	88%
Sometime after that	12%
	100%
	(117)
Did you	
Know right away you would definitely do it?	78%
Think it over?	22%
	100%
	(125)
How hard a decision was it for you to decide to donate?	
Very hard	4%
Somewhat hard	10%
A little hard	13%
Not at all hard	64%
(Spontaneous—"It was no decision.")	9%
	100%
	(135)
How difficult a decision was it for you to decide?	
Very difficult	5%
Somewhat difficult	10%
A little difficult	13%
Not at all difficult	59%
(Spontaneous—"It was no decision.")	12%
	100%
	(135)

lutely immediately because he received the request by letter and no family member was present. In two other cases the donors did not volunteer the first moment they heard of the need because the situation appeared inappropriate: That is, a local physician was informing them of the need for a transplant and the necessity to try and refer the patient to a transplant center. Although the probable need for a donor crossed these relatives' minds, it did not appear necessary to volunteer to a physician who would not be caring for the patient. In addition, two donors felt that their willingness to donate was obvious and expected, and that they needed to say nothing specific to volunteer at the initial encounter. In other cases the donor volunteered immediately when the need was advanced and reports an instantaneous choice; but there is some evidence that he may have considered the possibility earlier, as in the cases where the patient had been transplanted previously or where transplantation had been mentioned as a future possibility years before it was raised seriously. In two of the least pure cases, the donor who reports an instantaneous choice did not volunteer at the initial expression of need, although the situation would have been appropriate for him to do so.

As noted in Table 8-2, the coding reliability here was very high. The independent coders were asked to classify all the donors according to three basic patterns of decision-making, adding categories if necessary. The three patterns were: (1) this model under consideration of immediate choice, (2) the classical model of deliberation, and (3) a pattern of postponement to be discussed below. Once all the subtypes listed in Table 8-2 were added, there was agreement in all but six cases out of 114 (5%). Thus there appears to be little difficulty in identifying those donors who volunteer immediately without a time delay for deliberation.

The character of these instantaneous choices is demonstrated by the following typical comments:

CASE 1 *Donor (mother)*

Me? I never thought about it. . .I automatically thought I'd be the one. There was no decision to make or sides to weigh.

* * *

CASE 2 *Donor's wife*

You mean did he think about it and then decide? No—it was just spontaneous. The minute he knew. . .it was just natural. The first thing he thought of. He would donate.

* * *

TABLE 8-2 MODEL OF DONOR DECISION:

MORAL DECISION-MAKING MODEL: IMMEDIATE VOLUNTEER, NO DELIBERATION		
TOTAL		61% (71)
Subtype		
1. Donor and family agree the volunteering was immediate.	38% (44)	
2. Donor reports convincingly instantaneous decision and commitment, but we have no family verification or contradiction.	5% (6)	
3. Donor reports convincingly instantaneous decision but could not commit himself immediately (request was in a letter, situation inappropriate).	3% (3)	
4. Donor reports convincingly instantaneous decision but did not say anything because donation taken for granted.	2% (2)	
5. Donor and family agree the volunteering was immediate, but this is a second transplant.	4% (4)	
6. Donor reports volunteering immediately, but before he knew it was a possibility for *him*, some evidence he may have thought about it.	6% (7)	
7. Donor reports he knew instantaneously but did not say anything, although situation appropriate.	2% (2)	
8. Unreliable which subtype. Agree "immediate volunteer."	2% (2)	

CATEGORIZATION OF DONORS BY INDEPENDENT CODERS

MODEL OF DELIBERATION: PERIOD OF DELIBERATION AND A CONSCIOUS CHOICE		
TOTAL		25% (28)
Subtype		
9. Donor reports deliberation and conscious choice.	21% (24)	
10. Two decisions: first immediate volunteer, then reopened decision and deliberated.	4% (4)	
POSTPONEMENT AND STEPWISE DECISION-MAKING MODEL		5% (6)
11. No conscious choice. Donor reports postponing final decision while taking small steps that lock him into donation.		
Unreliable		5% (6)
Not enough information to code		4% (4)
TOTAL		100% (114)

CASE 3 Interview with donor's sister

INTERVIEWER. Who told you about the need for a donor?

DONOR. (sister). [The recipient]I came back from my vacation. She picked me up at the plane. I knew something was bothering her. After Dad went to bed I said "OK, what's bugging you?" The evening was fraught with emotion.

INTERVIEWER. What was your initial reaction?

DONOR. The initial reaction was, "Of course, I'll do it."

INTERVIEWER. What was so emotional for her and for you?

DONOR. To her the fact that I lost my husband and then had to go through this. To me the fact that she was so sick.

INTERVIEWER. [later] When did you make your final decision to donate a kidney?

DONOR. I don't think it was a decision. I really didn't consider much. I kept thinking "What was the decision?" My sister kept saying I had to make a decision? I kept thinking what was I supposed to be thinking about. As far as I was concerned. . .I would donate a kidney.

Interview with recipient about the first time she mentioned a transplant to her sister

INTERVIEWER. Do you remember what you said to her at the time?

RECIPIENT. I think I told her that I had a choice of going on the machine or having a transplant. I didn't have to say much because she [knows something about medicine] and. . .is just one of these gals, and said immediately that she would do it.

* * *

CASE 4 Interview with recipient

INTERVIEWER. Who first talked to the donor about the transplant?

RECIPIENT. My husband and I. She visited often. She came in when I was still crying right after the doctor told me. She said "Don't worry. You can have mine." I thought after she thought about it she might change her mind, but she didn't.

INTERVIEWER. How long did it take for the donor to decide to donate?

RECIPIENT. A couple of seconds when she found out about it.

When the donor in this case was asked the same question, she said:

DONOR. I didn't think about it. That's what I'm here for.

The power of the sense of normative obligation that is operating here to produce such a speedy decision is illustrated by the following typical comments.

MOTHER. (donor to adult son) I can't understand these people who stop and think when it's their children. My neighbors told me how wonderful I was. I said, "You'd do the same if it was your kid." They said, "I'm not so sure." I was shocked. I thought a person would do anything for their kid.

BROTHER. (donor) I guess I see it as my Christian duty. . .and brotherly love.

GRANDMOTHER. (donor) It kind of scares you but. . .we try to do whatever we can for her; after all, I'm her grandmother.

Blood-Tested Relatives: The Instantaneous Choice

When we widen our sample to include the relatives who submitted to the blood test as well as those who actually donated, the same speedy decision is evident. By the time of the blood test, the majority of persons (57%) had already definitely decided to donate and had informed the family of this fact. Of these, most report that their choice was instantaneous—48% of the *total* (Table 8-3). This percentage is reduced to 42% if we delete those relatives who, regardless of their internal process, did not immediately commit themselves, although the situation was appropriate.

Of course, despite our cross-examination on this issue, we cannot prove that no thoughts about donation crossed the donor's mind before the need within his own family was raised. The point at issue is that, despite the importance of the decision, there was no attempt to delay it until careful deliberation and investigation could occur. Once again, the high reliability between coders should be noted.

A comparison of Tables 8-2 and 8-3 indicates that a higher proportion of actual donors than blood-tested relatives fall into the category of immediate volunteer, although in both cases the proportion is sizeable. There are

TABLE 8-3 MODEL OF DONOR DECISION:

MORAL DECISION-MAKING MODEL: IMMEDIATE VOLUNTEER		
TOTAL		48% (25)
Subtype		
1. Immediate volunteer, family verification.	21% (11)	
2. Relative reports instantaneous choice but no verification or contradiction.	4% (2)	
3. Unreliability between subtypes 1 and 2.	2% (1)	
4. Relative reports instantaneous choice but he himself initiated concept of transplantation and donation.	4% (2)	
5. Relative reports instantaneous choice but could not volunteer immediately because of situation.	4% (2)	
6. Relative reports volunteering immediately but may have thought about it before knew possibility for him.	6% (3)	
7. Relative and family always took for granted for many years he would donate; he feels there was no moment of choice.	2% (1)	
8. Relative reports instantaneous decision but did not volunteer immediately though could have.	6% (3)	
MODEL OF DELIBERATION		
TOTAL		23% (12)
Subtype		
9. Deliberation and conscious choice made to donate.	10% (5)	
10. Deliberation but final choice not made yet.	11% (6)	
11. Two clear decisions. First immediate volunteer, then reopening of decision with deliberation.	2% (1)	

DECISION-MAKING OF BLOOD-TESTED RELATIVES

POSTPONEMENT MODEL		
TOTAL		4% (2)
Subtype		
12. Relative postponing decision. Says may not have to make decision if wrong blood type.	2% (1)	
13. Relative indicates postponement of deliberation and of decision, but does not explicitly say may not have to make decision if wrong blood type.	2% (1)	
UNCLEAR IF WILL BE POSTPONEMENT OR DELIBERATION MODEL		
TOTAL		17% (9)
Subtype		
14. Same as 12, but also says wants more information before making decision.	6% (3)	
15. Same as 13, but also says wants more information before making decision.	6% (3)	
16. Unreliable between 12 and 13.	2% (1)	
17. Relative indicates postponement of deliberation until family indicates time for blood test. May have decided to donate in process of coming for blood test.	4% (2)	
Not enough information to code		4% (2)
Unreliable		4% (2)
TOTAL		100% (52)

two explantations for this discrepancy between donors and those blood-tested. The first is that there is a basic difference in motivation between the two groups, because only some of the blood-tested volunteers become the actual donors. The family members actually proceeding to become *donors* may be the most eager of those originally blood-tested and the most likely to have been able to make an immediate choice.

An alternative explanation is that the report of the blood-tested volunteers, secured at an earlier point in time, is less likely to be distorted by memory than is the report of the actual donors. Once their decision is made, the actual donors may be motivated to report they did not deliberate on the issue of whether to help save a loved one's life. Thus a higher proportion of donors than blood-tested volunteers will appear to have made an immediate choice, although the difference is due to measurement inaccuracies.

Some factors are contradictory to this latter explanation, however. Many donors were also interviewed early in their decision-making process, and this analysis draws on the information gained at that time. Second, as indicated above, other family members independently verify the story of a high proportion of those donors who claim they volunteered immediately upon hearing of the need. Third, within the blood-tested group, those who later became donors can be compared to those who did not. Twelve of the 52 blood-tested relatives (23%) became actual donors. The question arises whether this subgroup is more likely to make an immediate choice than the other blood-tested subjects. Although the number of cases becomes too small to be more than suggestive, the persons who became donors would appear to be more likely to have been immediate volunteers originally than were the other blood-tested relatives (75% vs. 42%, $p < .05$). The difference in decision-making between donors and blood-tested volunteers is probably reflective of a real motivational difference rather than a measurement problem.

The Decision of the Nondonor

Two independent coders were asked to decide for the nondonors as well as for the donors and blood-tested volunteers whether the decision-making process best approximated a moral decision-making model, a deliberation model, or a postponement model. The nondonors therefore were classified into the following three groups (Table 8-4): relatives who report no deliberation, who from the beginning never considered donation; relatives who underwent a period of rational deliberation and made a decision not to donate; and relatives who postponed a decision until events made nondonation inevitable.

Table 8-3 shows that coding reliability is not so high for nondonors as for the donors and volunteers, although it is still within satisfactory limits. In the following discussions we use only the cases in which the independent coders were able to agree.

Immediate Decision-Making Among Nondonors. According to the coders, 21% of the *nondonors* either never considered themselves as *possible* donors (Table 8-4); or they knew immediately they would not donate. These nondonors are the direct counterpart of the *donors* who never deliberated on whether they would give but knew instantaneously that they would. This pattern thus fits the instantaneous, moral decision-making model (see Figure 8-1) as interpreted by Fellner and Marshall (1968).

In 14 of these cases, the need of the recipient was recognized but the obligation or responsibility to help him either was never attributed to the *self* or was rapidly denied. This attribution of responsibility to the self is a very important stage in the moral decision-making process (see Figure 8-1). The following quotation is an example of such a case. When asked about donation, the nondonor (the brother of a recipient in a family with many potential donors) talked about other members of the family but does not mention himself.

INTERVIEWER. In many families it is not easy to decide whether a patient will receive a cadaver or related kidney, and who will donate. How difficult do you think this was for your family to resolve?

NONDONOR. I'm talking third hand. I really can't say. It would be difficult. I don't know.

INTERVIEWER. Did you or anyone else in the family besides the donor ever consider donating?

NONDONOR. I'm not sure. I heard [some of *them*] were to be tested and then it was put off.

When asked if they or anyone else in the family considered donation, the nondonors in this subgroup either fail to mention themselves or directly tell us they did not consider the possibility of their own donation. The remainder of the interview and material from other family members support this picture.

Other immediate decision-makers among the nondonors do not fail to recognize the fact they are eligible to donate, but they report that they immediately realized they would not do so. They attribute the potential

TABLE 8-4 MODEL OF NONDONOR DECISION:

MORAL DECISION-MAKING MODEL: NO DELIBERATION		
TOTAL		21% (49)
Subtype		
1. No deliberation. Nondonor never appears to have considered himself as a donor.	6% (14)	
2. No deliberation. Nondonor refused at first hearing of donor need.	6% (15)	
3. No deliberation. Nondonor knew immediately he would not donate. Did not refuse openly.	3% (6)	
4. Unclear if 2 or 3.	4% (10)	
5. Unclear if 1 or 3.	2% (4)	
MODEL OF DELIBERATION		
TOTAL		31% (73)
Subtypes		
6. Deliberation and conscious choice.		

CATEGORIZATION OF NONDONOR BY INDEPENDENT CODERS

7. Two separate decisions made. One involved deliberation.	4% (9)	
8. Nondonor demonstrated overwhelming long-standing, well-recognized fear of hospitals. In addition, he deliberated.	.4% (1)	
POSTPONEMENT MODEL		24% (57)
9. Nondonor postponed decision until nondonation inevitable. No conscious final decision.		
Nondonor Perceives Self as Volunteer		6% (15)
Eligible Nondonor not considered by family and does not consider self as possible donor.		5% (12)
Unreliable		12% (29)
TOTAL		100% (235)

responsibility to themselves, but instantaneously reject the idea of donation. (Table 8-4, 2 or 3).

INTERVIEWER. When was it you first heard about the transplant?

NONDONOR SISTER. About five years ago. He [the recipient's husband] said, "Maybe one of you girls can donate."

INTERVIEWER. What did you say when her husband called?

NONDONOR SISTER. I was shocked [probe] I did say I cannot do that because I don't think my husband would allow me.

Of course we cannot classify this group of *nondonors* with as much certainty as we can the corresponding group of *donors* and volunteers who appear to have made an *immediate choice*. In the case of the *donors* we can validate each of their own reports with that of another family member who agrees the donor offered to donate immediately as soon as he knew of the need. But we cannot similarly validate the nondonor's perception that he never considered donation. Throughout the donor search, however, we did ask many key family members about their perceptions of the status of each potential donor, and in none of these cases did any relative indicate perceiving any deliberation or information-search on the part of this group of nondonors.

A lower proportion of nondonors fit into this category of immediate choice than do the donors or blood-tested relatives. To avoid normative responsibility or to decide immediately to act counter to an altruistic family norm may be more difficult than to decide to act in accordance with the norm. In addition, after-the-fact nondonors may tend to buttress a decision with clear reasons, when in fact there was no deliberation prior to the decision (see Janis and Mann, in press).

THE CLASSICAL MODEL OF DELIBERATION: A CONTINUUM FROM SATISFICING TO OPTIMIZING

The Decision of the Donors and Blood-Tested Relatives

Although the majority of donors thus do not appear to follow a pattern of deliberation and choice, there are certainly a sizeable subgroup who do so. Our data, like those of Katona and Mueller (1954), Hill (1970) and Brim (1962), show individual variation in the extent to which persons appear to use the deliberative mode. In our study, according to the judgments made by independent coders, 25% of the donors and 23% of the blood-tested relatives seem to have approximated a classical decision-making pattern. These donors and blood-tested relatives *did not volunteer immediately* upon hearing of the need but had done some *deliberating* and weighing of costs and gains.

As shown in Figure 8-1, in the deliberation model and the moral decision-making model the first step involves the identification of the problem. After this first step, the models diverge. According to the deliberation model, the individual then collects relevant information, identifies and evaluates alternatives, and finally makes and implements a decision. All of the individuals in our study obviously identified the problem. More to the point, at least 17 out of 28 of these donors (61%) and 25 out of 49 blood-tested relatives (51%) sought more information about donation than was provided by the transplant staff or the patient. Unlike the "immediate" volunteers, these donors consulted physicians for information prior to committing themselves. Forty-seven percent of the deliberative donors gathered information before the transplant from their own local doctor instead of, or in addition to, the transplant physicians.

Although a sizeable percentage of these "deliberators" did seek out information, a large proportion of both the donors and blood-tested relatives failed to do so. In fact a predilection to donate and key initial acts were taken based on very little new information other than that provided by the family. Only two or three deliberators in the blood-tested relative group had done any reading about donation between the time they found out about the need for a donor and the time of the blood test, and only two out of 12 had consulted a physician. The following case is typical:

CASE Interview with blood-tested volunteer immediately after blood drawn. She has not yet talked with any medical staff.

INTERVIEWER. Do you feel now you have made a final decision that you would want to donate a kidney, or are you waiting until after the blood test to make your final decision?

VOLUNTEER. No, I think I'm pretty sure of giving. . . .

INTERVIEWER. You feel you've decided?

VOLUNTEER. Yes.

INTERVIEWER. How much did you think it over, the reasons in favor and against?

VOLUNTEER. I thought quite a bit.

INTERVIEWER. What did you consider?

VOLUNTEER. Like being an invalid. If I would be able to run and do stuff. . . .

INTERVIEWER. Anything else you thought about?

VOLUNTEER. Just about how bad he needed it. The pros and cons. I guess other people have transplants and come out OK, I'm sure I'll be OK.

INTERVIEWER. Have you read anything about people who have transplants or donated kidneys?

VOLUNTEER. No. I didn't know there was such information. . .I've never seen anything. Of course, I haven't really looked.

INTERVIEWER. Have you heard anything about transplant patients or donors from people?

VOLUNTEER. No. I heard my aunt and [the recipient] say about a patient they met in the hospital. One of his brothers donated and he went home in a few days. I'm sure they must do thorough tests.

INTERVIEWER. Do you know anything else about what it means for the donor to donate a kidney—any effects or anything?

VOLUNTEER. No, that's why I want to talk to Justine [the nurse-administrator of the transplant program].

INTERVIEWER. Now. . .I have a question. You said you had decided that you will donate if [you are the right type]. You've also indicated that you still have questions you want to ask, which I think is understandable. Do you feel that you have made your decision now, or are you waiting until you have questions answered to make a final decision.

VOLUNTEER. No, I'm going to ask the questions, but if my blood is OK, I'll do it. I still want to talk to someone though, just to know more.

This blood-tested relative characterizes her future information-seeking as "bolstering," as an attempt to gather more data to reinforce and support a decision already made (see Janis and Mann, in press). The decision itself, however, was made on the basis of very little independent information; the only information secured was transmitted by her own family.

After the blood test most donors directed their information-seeking toward the transplant physicians rather than toward an outside source. As indicated above, only 47% of the deliberators had spoken with a physician outside of the University transplant staff before the three-day work-up, whereas 58% had spoken with the transplant physician. At the time of the three-day work-up the transplant staff explained and in many cases reexplained the risks and benefits to all donors. Yet by this time most deliberators had already arrived at a final decision to donate.

Despite this lack of extensive information-seeking, these donors and blood-tested relatives all satisfy Step 4 of the Model of Deliberation. All of these individuals spent some time evaluating alternatives—that is, they all indicated some weighing of pros and cons before volunteering. According to their own and other family reports, none of these individuals volunteered when they first heard of the need. In fact, for the donors of this type a range of one day to more than two years passed between the initial learning of the donor need and the final decision.

Finally, the perceptions of all of the donors in this group were congruent with the fifth step of the model—they all seemed to feel they had arrived at a conscious decision to donate and then proceeded with the work-up to implement the decision. However, as noted in Table 8-3, the information from the blood-tested relatives indicates that the final decision of many of these deliberators was not made until after the blood test.

Thus the presence of a period of conscious deliberation and the greater likelihood of seeking independent medical information before commitment differentiates these donors from the so-called immediate decision-makers. However, there are several characteristics they share with immediate, moral decision-makers. Normative and emotional elements frequently play a large role in the decision-process of these "deliberative" donors. Normative criteria enter into the very weighing of costs against gains, into the "utilities." Questions arise as to the nature of their moral obligations: Is this type of altruism morally prescribed? Is it *their* particular responsibility as opposed to someone else's? Seven of these donors consulted their ministers in the process of deciding. Eighteen percent emphasized the guilt they would feel if they did not donate and their relative died, and 29% stressed their family obligation to a relative of this type. In the words of one of these donors at the time of the three-day work-up:

> I felt a great deal of social pressure. It's possible social pressure makes the decision for you. . . .I think you just can't let something like this go by—especially if there's no risk to you. I think you'd feel like a bastard. . .You feel it's a good contribution to make and you feel good. . . .He [my father] is a person I love and he's worthwhile. . . .My self is completely in the hands of the hospital staff. They say there is no risk, and I simply have to believe them and with

> societal and personal pressures. . .they make my decision for me. . .not myself. I believe most people end up in situations like this due to circumstances, not because they have a list of good and a list of bad reasons, and one side outweighs the other. . . .You see I'm just not used to it. I'm used to weighing the facts. [About donor risk], I have to accept someone else's decision.

This donor was one who attempted to follow the classical deliberation model and found himself frustrated by having to weigh normative obligations against a risk to the self and by his lack of expert knowledge in evaluating the risk. One could interpret his remarks to indicate that his desire to save the life of his father, in itself, did not outweigh the presence of risk, but the normative pressure from others to fulfill his filial obligations and his need to maintain a favorable self-image tipped the hat. He became a donor without shedding all fear and ambivalence. All patients are told of the actual small donor risk, and his attempt to state there was "no risk" may reflect a tendency of decision-makers to attempt to buttress the choice they have already made by distorting the probabilities of success or failure (Janis and Mann, in press).

Deliberative Decision-Making Among Nondonors

According to Table 8-4, a sizeable minority (31%) of the nondonors perceive themselves as having deliberated about donation and having arrived at a conscious decision not to donate. In accordance with the deliberative model outlined in Figure 8-1, all of these nondonors have identified the problem of donation. In addition, the majority have sought information about donation (Step 2 of the deliberative model). Although only 23% of the *immediate* decision-makers among the nondonors have done some reading or spoken to a donor or an acquaintance of a donor or talked with a physician about donation prior to the transplant, 65% of the *deliberative* nondonors have sought such information—30% from their own local physician,* 20% from the University doctors only, and 15% from the literature. Once again it is obvious that even among those who deliberated about the donor-decision, a sizeable proportion (about one-third) have failed to seek any expert information.

In terms of the steps of the deliberative model subsequent to information-seeking (see Figure 8-1), all of this group of nondonors indicate they have engaged in some evaluation of the alternatives, in some deliberation (Step 4 of the deliberative model). Either in the qualitative material generally or in answer to questions, they all say they

* As indicated in Chapter 7, individuals who consulted their own physicians were likely to find their doctors were definitely opposed to donation.

thought about being donors: (Did you or anyone else in the family besides the donor consider donating? How hard a decision was it for you to decide whether to donate or not to donate? Did you know right away you definitely were not going to donate, or did you think it over?) Finally this group perceives themselves as having *arrived at a decision* not to donate, which they then acted upon.

Once again, normative considerations frequently played an important part in the deliberation. Although the overriding reasons against donation involved fear of the short- and long-term health risks of the operation (see Chapter 7), the deliberative nondonor frequently indicates that he did not perceive the decision as a weighing of costs against benefits. Instead, as discussed in Chapter 7, he regarded the choice in terms of a role conflict between his *normative obligations* to his family of procreation and his *obligations* to the recipient, and he concluded that his obligations to his spouse and children must take priority. Fifty-nine percent of this type of nondonor fit into this category.

In some of these cases the decision was an easy one, but in others the role conflict engendered some feelings of guilt. The following quotations exemplify the role conflict:

NONDONOR SISTER. [My husband] is against me doing it. Taking a chance with my health. We have three young children who are my first responsibility. I didn't know what was more important—to give to my sister or to keep my health for my own family where my most responsibility was.

NONDONOR SISTER. You get hung up between your own husband and kids (we have two girls) and your sister. Who do you owe your loyalties to? You'd like to help your sister, but then [if something happened] who would take care of your family. . .or if our own needed a kidney [I] couldn't give.

For four deliberative nondonors, a minister rather than a physician was consulted as part of thc information-seeking.

The major distinction we have been making here is between the immediate and deliberative decision, between a clearly satisficing decision and one that attempts to optimize. However, in the donor selection instance, both are set in the context of strong normative pressures and felt family obligations. Both demonstrate characteristics of the moral decision-making model. Also, even among those classified as deliberators, the decision-making process falls far short of optimization in many cases, because a high proportion of these individuals fail to seek out expert information.

POSTPONEMENT AND STEPWISE DECISION: A MODEL OF INCREMENTALISM AND EVASION OF DECISION

The Decision of the Donors

During the qualitative interviewing with actual donors a pattern of decision-making that we had not predicted came to light, and therefore we asked our coders to code for this pattern in addition to the moral and deliberative patterns. According to this coding, in a small number of cases—that is, six cases—the donor *never* felt he had decided to donate a kidney, or he felt that he had only made that decision at the last minute. Instead he had made a series of small exploratory steps and then found himself locked into donation. He agreed to take the less difficult early tests: to have his blood drawn and tested and then his tissue tested to see if he were eligible for donation, while postponing any final choice until later. Upon hearing that he was eligible, he then agreed to have the three days of extensive testing to see if he were physically healthy enough, again, in his own mind, postponing any final decision. With each step taken, however, more and more of the relevant actors—the patient, the other relatives, the physicians and nurses—assumed he had already made the decision to donate. With each step taken, withdrawal became more difficult because of these building expectations of others. Soon he felt locked into donation without ever having decided to give (see Figure 8-1 for a diagramatic presentation of this pattern). Ambivalence in some but not all of these cases was extreme.*

The immediate donors make an instantaneous choice; the deliberative donors delay decision but come to a conscious and considered choice; and the postponers delay so long that they feel they have never reached a moment of conscious self-directed choice. The decision is made *for* them not *by* them.

The following case reports illustrate this process of becoming locked into donation by virtue of a pattern of postponement and stepwise decision-making. Though undecided whether to donate, the first donor cited below originally agreed to have a blood test; he then came in for the three-day work-up while still postponing the ultimate decision; and even

* As indicated earlier, in those cases in which a donor expresses a high degree of ambivalence to the physicians, he is usually told of the possibility of a medical excuse—that is, the recipient and family will be told there is a medical reason precluding donation on the part of the relative. However, not all ambivalent donors confide in the physicians, and others seem to find the medical excuse unsatisfactory because of the great need and hopes of the dying patient and the family.

two days prior to the transplant he, like one other person in the case series, felt the final decision still had not been made.

CASE Donor (brother donating to a brother)

At three-day work-up

INTERVIEWER. What did you say to his [the recipient's] wife when she first mentioned this to you? What did you think?

DONOR. I didn't know what to think. I still don't [laughs nervously]. I finally told her I'd go along [for the blood tests] if someone else did too. So then my sister Suzanne and I came [for the blood tests] [two years ago]. We talked some on the way home that day [the day of the blood test]. . . .We just kind of wondered if maybe he [the recipient] wouldn't be able to go on the machine [instead of a transplant].

(Donor indicates that his tissue matched the patient's a little better than did Suzanne's, but the issue was not raised again until the patient was hospitalized three weeks ago and then called him to come in for the three-day physical work-up.)

INTERVIEWER. You said he called you himself last week. What did you say then?

DONOR. He asked if I'd come in Monday morning [for the work-up].

INTERVIEWER. And what did you say?

DONOR. I said sure. I'd be there.

INTERVIEWER. What did you think about it?

DONOR. Well I wasn't so sure—but. . . .

INTERVIEWER. What would you say your feelings are about it?

DONOR. Well. . .how it will affect my life afterward. . .if I can still work like before. And I wonder what I'll have to go through.

INTERVIEWER. Have you talked to any medical people about it or haven't you done that?

DONOR. No. . .well they explained it all to us a couple years ago when we were here [for the blood test]. . .they told us quite a bit. But you know it was kind of a far-off thing then. They said they could maybe get some unrelated person by then. . .so. . . .

At two days before the transplant after admission, in answer to the questionnaire

INTERVIEWER. What did you say to [the recipient's wife] when she told you [about the need for a donor two years ago]?

DONOR. It wasn't definite he needed it then. . .I mostly just listened. I didn't give her an answer that night. I wanted to think it over. . .I think I'm still thinking it over.

Two pages later in the questionnaire

INTERVIEWER. When did you make your final decision to donate a kidney?

DONOR. I left it up to the doctors. I'm still thinking about it. I never did make a final decision. [indicates he still has major questions about the effect of the donation on future eating and drinking behavior].

The next case again illustrates this pattern of a donor arriving for blood tests along with other family members before having decided to donate, only to find out later that he is the best tissue match. The presence of other family-volunteers at first facilitates postponement; but by the time of the three-day physical work-up, the undecided donor is under more direct pressure because of building expectations of others.

CASE Donor (brother donating to a sister)

At time of blood test

DONOR. Well, the way I feel is I'll donate but I have some questions I have to have answered before I'll go through with it. . .I haven't had a chance to ask. [When my sister mentioned donation] I told her I couldn't really commit myself without talking to my wife. So I didn't sleep much that night. If I refused and something happened to her I'll never be able to live with myself. On the other hand if I give and something happened. . . .

Brother and children were tested. Brother was found to be a perfect tissue match.

At time of physical work-up

DONOR. She [the patient] called me up and she said, "You are the best possible type. . .identical. . .you are way better than [my children]. . . .Well, what could I say? My mind says for me to do it and my body says no, it don't want to. I don't know what to do. I told her I'd come in for the tests but I wasn't making any further decisions until I got to think more about it. . . .

INTERVIEWER. Did you sign up for the tests [the arteriogram, etc.]?

DONOR. Yes. I figured as long as I'm here. But that doesn't mean I'm [committing] myself anymore to the donor. . . .Well, I'm not making any decision until I go home and think more about it. I just came in to have my blood tested last Wednesday. . .I'm just not making any decisions yet. I think I'll tell [the son] that he has to come in for the tests first. He'll have to have the tests too. . . .Then we'll decide.

This was never done. The donor agreed to come in when the doctor called to say the transplant was scheduled.

Although only six cases clearly fit this pattern, 12 other donors (11%) who are coded as more consistent with another model* also demonstrated elements of the postponement pattern. Evasion of decision-making was evident, as were feelings of being locked into donation after early testing before a final decision was completely made. In fact one of these donors was responsible for the terminology we have been using here.

CASE Donor (son donating to his father)

At time of three-day work-up

DONOR. People who say you aren't committed to doing this when you take the blood tests or come in for these tests. . .to say you aren't committed at that point is poppy-cock! Once you come this far if they say you will be a good donor. . .you can't say no. You're locked in. I can maybe conceive of someone taking the blood tests and then saying, "No, I'm out." But once you are as far as I am, I'll bet you can't show me a single case where someone has taken the tests and been pronounced a good donor who has at that time said they decided not to do it. When I am, you accept it. You have to give.

Blood-Tested Relatives

Twenty-one percent of relatives demonstrated some element of postponement at the time of the blood test. Some, although not all, of these postponers indicate explicitly that they are following a stepwise approach; they are waiting to see whether they are the right blood type before really confronting the problem of whether they are willing to donate. In other words, if they turn out to be the wrong blood type or a

* All of these are coded as fitting the model of conscious deliberation.

less good match than someone else, they will never have to make the decision. In addition, some of them also indicate they are awaiting further information before deciding, a characteristic more appropriate to the deliberative model. Whether they will actually seek the information or will remain postponers is unclear at this point in time.

In the words of one of the stepwise decision-makers:

CASE Sister donating to a brother

Interview before results of blood test known

INTERVIEWER. Can you tell me. . .between the time when it first occurred to you that you might donate a kidney. . .and the time you decided to come for the blood test. . .how much did you think it over?

SISTER. How much did I think it over. . . ? Well. . .I think the way I looked at it. . .well, really not much. I didn't think it over much. In fact, the way I looked at it was that it was going to be a much bigger decision if I found out that I actually was a possible donor. We haven't found that out yet. If I found out the fact that I actually could donate, then I would have to think about it, I'd have to wait first and see if it's definite.

Postponement Among Nondonors

Postponement was not a pattern of decision-making we predicted among nondonors at the start of the study, but it appears quite frequently. In fact, it is much more prevalent among nondonors than donors. According to Table 8-4, 57 of the nondonors (24%) postponed deciding whether to volunteer until events seemed to make their nondonation inevitable. These nondonors considered donation and recognized that a choice might have to be made. But before they felt they had to make a decision, someone else volunteered or a cadaver was found, or they discovered they were the wrong blood type or a less good match than someone else. Of course, in reality the fact that another relative has volunteered to donate does not preclude volunteering oneself and determining who is the better match.

These persons did not appear to perceive their delay as a tactic to avoid donation. In fact many appeared willing to donate if necessary, although several of them were more ambivalent about donation. In all cases the nondonors did not perceive that they ever made a decision not to donate—events made such a decision unnecessary.

This group certainly parallels those donors who postponed ultimate decision while taking smaller steps leading to donation. In both cases decision was delayed, the actor let events transpire until he found himself either donating or not donating (see Figure 8-1). For this type of non-donor the process is a *drift*-process rather than a deliberative decision-process. This type of decision could be seen as compatible with the moral decision-making model.* The failure of the actor to volunteer seems to be partly *because he does not attribute responsibility to himself* (see Figure 8-1)—someone else in the family can donate, or a cadaver is a possibility. However, *other family members* do attribute responsibility to this relative and frequently wait to see if he will volunteer before taking action, whether that action is placing the patient's name on the list for a cadaver kidney or going ahead with another donor.

The following case reports illustrate this pattern of nondonor post-ponement. In the first case a cadaver transplant occurred before the nondonor felt he had made his decision. The period of postponement was five months from the time donation was first broached to this nondonor to the time of the transplant. During this period the patient concluded that none of his children were going to volunteer and allowed his name to be placed on the list for a cadaver kidney.

CASE Nondonor (son of a male patient)

After a cadaver transplant had occurred

NONDONOR. No decision was made that a person wouldn't do it. We were willing to donate but wanted more information. It was maybe yes or no. We never ruled out no and never said yes. . . .As far as I knew a kidney from one of the kids was never ruled out. I was never told he was going to get a donor other ways [i.e., from a cadaver].

In the second case, another family member volunteered and went through the testing procedures before the nondonor felt it was time to make a decision.

CASE Nondonor (brother of a male patient)

NONDONOR. A year and a half ago. . .a sister told me that my brother would need a donor. . . .We were thinking about the possibility of

* We have been emphasizing the instantaneous quality associated with donors' moral decision-making, because the model was used originally to apply to just this situation. However, as noted above, Schwartz (1975) sees the model as appropriate to all help-giving decisions whether they are made instantaneously or not.

donating a kidney. [I was away]. My brother wrote a letter suggesting that my mother would donate a kidney; her age was against her doing it, but she was willing. Later I understood that [one sister's] doctor said she shouldn't consider donating a kidney. . .so I think the [rest of the siblings] realized it would have to be one of us. We didn't talk about it. . . .We didn't think it was at that point. We didn't know how long it would go until it was necessary.

INTERVIEWER. Was there a point at which you made a decision about whether you would donate?

NONDONOR. Before I knew that, the point had been reached. The decision had been made and [another sister] had already offered and taken the tests.

The actual donor in this case indicated she had been waiting to see if the nondonor brother above would volunteer; when she did not hear, she herself went through the tests.

In other cases, information-seeking as well as decision-making was postponed.

CASE Nondonor (brother of patient; patient's son donated)

NONDONOR. I think my main concern was my family. . .whether I'd be able to function fully after and provide for them. I never got to the point of talking with any doctor about it. I'm sure he could have answered my questions. [The son] volunteered before anyone really had a chance to think about it. My wife and I talked about it. . .we didn't know what the donor had to go through but it never got to the point where we really had to find out.

In this case the son, though willing to donate, had originally waited for the patient's siblings to volunteer before proceeding with his own testing.

Postponement of decision and drift thus seems to be a frequent decision-pattern among nondonors. Latané and Darley (1970) show a similar postponement pattern in their altruism experiments among their experimental subjects who did not respond to an urgent call for help from a supposedly convulsive co-subject in another room. When the experimenter finally entered the room after ample time has passed, he concluded: "It is not our impression that they decided not to respond. Rather they were still in a state of indecision and conflict whether to respond or not" (p. 24). The very difficult decision may be postponed until it is too late to volunteer.

Postponement among Recipients

Once postponement was identified as a pattern of decision-making among potential donors, we noted that it seemed to apply to at least one other difficult decision being made. The wider applicability of the stepwise decision-making process is suggested by the manner in which several *recipients* decided whether to accept a kidney from the teen-aged or adult child. Once again we see the tendency to make smaller stepwise choices while postponing a final decision.

In general, as indicated earlier, parents found it particularly difficult to allow a child to take any risk to his life to save theirs (see Chapters 7 and 9). The role reversal was very stressful. Frequently only with insistence on the part of the child and encouragement by the physicians was the patient able even to consider the possibility. And then in at least three cases the parent was able to agree only to allow the child to be tested, while reserving final decision until later. Once the child was found to be the correct type, procedures were set in motion for further testing by the staff and finally the child donated.

DISCUSSION OF DECISION-MAKING MODELS

The Postponement Model

Of all the patterns, the *postponement of decision* model appears to be a particularly interesting one for future research, although it did not occur here nearly as frequently as the pattern of instantaneous choice. Leik (1971, p. 35) has posited that the most typical manner in which families handle existing problems may be to avoid dealing with them, rather than tackling their solution rationally. Our data certainly indicate that a substantial segment of blood-tested relatives and nondonors solve their problem by avoidance and postponement. A pattern of avoiding decision may be more functional than a direct refusal of aid for the continuing cohesion of the family unit (see Simmons and Klein, 1972, and Chapter 9).

Because of the great emphasis that has been placed on the deliberative model in the decision-making literature, the postponement patterns have probably not received their due attention. There *are* some conceptual forerunners for this model. Rapoport and Burkheimer (1971) and others (Ebert, 1971; Ference,1972; Noe and Ehrenfeld, 1973; Puscheck and

Greene, 1972) have written about sequential or deferred decision-making, and Luce and Raiffa (1957) have diagrammed a decision-tree with ever-separating branches to represent this type of thought process (see Simon, 1957; Taylor, 1965). Yet these conceptualizations by and large do not deal with evasion of decision-making, but with a more deliberative process. These writers depict each sequential step as an opportunity to gather more information in order to decide whether one wishes to proceed in a given direction. The information may be in the form of increased knowledge about probabilities and risks, or it may represent increased experience with the task at hand so that one can judge better if it is personally rewarding or costly. After each step a conscious decision is made to proceed or not toward the larger goal. We, however, are speaking not of increasing information with each step, but of a pattern of avoiding choice as long as possible. Each step is taken with the purpose of seeing whether one will or will not be compelled to make a decision, because the outcome of the stepwise action (in this case a medical test) may allow one totally to avoid the problem. Yet once halfway up the staircase, it suddenly becomes difficult to turn around and come back down, and therefore one feels compelled to proceed without ever having consciously decided to do so. Relative freedom of choice appears present at every stage in the Rapoport formulation whereas here the individual suddenly feels that he has no free choice.

Another conceptual forerunner of the postponement pattern is the incremental model that is utilized in Chapter 11 to discuss the development of federal funding for catastrophic illness. Analysts of government policy-making and legal decision-processes have stressed the notion of incrementalism, again in opposition to a more comprehensive optimizing method of policy choice (Etzioni, 1968; Janis and Mann, in press; Snortland and Stanga, 1973). Changes in policy are made in a series of small steps, each one of which is seen as an improvement but is only slightly different from existing practices. The final result of a long chain of such small steps may be very different from the situation any party would have wanted in the beginning.*

We noted earlier that some decisions such as family organ-donation are characterized by being embedded in a strategy or bargaining context in which the interests of relevant parties are in conflict. In the government or in organizations incremental decisions are particularly likely to be made in such bargaining contexts: Where there are conflicting parties, securing agreement to institute small rather than large changes is easier (see

* See Etzioni (1968) for a discussion of a mixed-scanning model that involves a combination of the optimizing and incremental process in the policy area.

Allison, 1971; Sisson, 1972). Similarly, if one's own spouse and one's dying brother have different attitudes about donation, one can more easily agree to the step of a blood test than to the sacrifice of a kidney. Janis and Mann (in press) view incremental decisions as satisficing ones, because the decision rules involve satisfying minimal conditions rather than attempting to maximize favorable consequences.

Despite this conceptual framework, comparatively little emphasis has been placed on the extent of incrementalism, sequential decision-making, or postponement in major life decisions. Yet, in 1960 Becker noted:

> Some commitments are not necessarily made consciously and deliberately. Some commitments. . .arise cresively; the person becomes aware that he is committed only at some point of change and seems to have made the commitment without realizing it. . .what might be termed the "commitment by default"—arises through a series of acts, no one of which is crucial but when taken together, constitutes for the actor a series of side bets [investments] of such magnitude that he finds himself unwilling to lose them (p. 38).

Several studies do indicate that other major life decisions outside of the family context may also be dealt with frequently through a pattern in which individuals delay making an important choice and instead take several smaller steps in one direction until they perceive themselves locked into that course of action. For example, Ginzberg and associates (1951) suggest that the process of occupational choice is often in reality a series of such small stepwise decisions. The process is seen as largely irreversible—once launched on a particular course of action, such as job training, the individual finds changing his goals increasingly difficult. He is restricted more and more by his previous decisions and expenditure of effort, time, and money (Crites, 1969; see also Miller and Form, 1951). Similarly, Matza (1964) posits that movement into a career of delinquency is better described by a theory of drift rather than a theory in which an actor commits himself and rationally plans such a career: "The delinquent sequence is itself normally a process of gradual development, beginning with minor offenses and proceeding slowly to more serious crimes. Consequently, the increments of sanction are sufficiently slight. . .so that each appears not much worse than the one preceeding it" (p. 188).

This stepwise process of decision-making can be applied even to the decision to marry. In his classic work Waller (1938) notes "the process of mating is one of the clearest examples of the summatory social process. . . .As the process unfolds each person becomes increasingly committed in his own eyes and those of others to the completed act" (p. 259).

A Comprehensive Flow Chart

Three patterns of decision-making have been delineated—an instantaneous choice made without conscious deliberation, a pattern of deliberation and conscious choice, and a mode of postponement of decision-making in which the decision-maker does not perceive himself as consciously selecting an alternative.

Before concluding this section, we will attempt to present a comprehensive flow chart that includes all three patterns as options and emphasizes the major distinctions at issue—the immediacy of the decision, the extent of deliberation, the degree of postponement, the conscious selection of an alternative. The extent of optimizing compared to satisficing is also noted (see Janis and Mann, in press; Kieren, et al., 1975, for other examples of decision-making flow charts).

Such a model must give an explicit place to the *costs* of helping the other party. One of the major reasons that so many potential donors postpone making a decision is that the physical costs both of donating and failing to donate are so great. If one were not risking one's life and health, if the commitment did not involve a great deal of pain and discomfort, or if obtaining a kidney were not so vital for the recipient, some of these postponers could more easily make a rapid or deliberative decision. The stakes on both sides are too high. It is an approach-avoidance conflict for many potential donors, and in such situations one could expect a final decision to be difficult and painful. Given the high costs of both donating and not donating, postponement and avoidance of decision should not be surprising.

As soon as the actor becomes aware of the decision that has to be made and *prior to any conscious weighing of costs and gains* or any information-seeking, he has a general perception of the overall level of costs and benefits involved. This perception may be inaccurate or imprecise, but nevertheless it is probably important. For example, *prior* to embarking on any deliberation, the actor has no difficulty distinguishing between the overall seriousness of the decision to buy a tie and the general importance of the decision to donate a kidney. This perception of the general level of costs and benefits may have an effect on the decision-making model used—on whether the actor chooses to spend time and effort on deliberating on whether instead he follows a pattern of postponement or of immediate choice.

In such an intense approach-avoidance conflict as the donation situation, where the costs of failure on both sides are so great, our impression is that individuals frequently wish to absolve themselves of the responsibility of the decision. Deliberation and a conscious decision emphasize the freedom of one's choice and one's responsibility for the choice. To hold oneself responsible for a potentially disastrous outcome is painful, however. In such situations persons are motivated to regard the decision as inevitable—as the only possible alternative, given the enormous moral obligation, or the social pressure, or the fact that another family member volunteered first, or the perception that this issue is not one's moral responsibility. Thus, while the outsider sees the potential donor as making a choice, the potential donor himself is likely to describe it as "no decision at all." When the stakes are very high on both sides, instead of expecting more deliberation as some hypothesize (Kogan and Wallach, 1967), we would predict less.

Thus a comprehensive decision-making model would have to take into account the individual's perception of costs as emphasized by the deliberative model as well as those additional variables stressed by Schwartz (1970b) in the moral decision-making model. All of these factors help to shape the speed of the process, the extent to which the actor considers the choice at all, the degree of deliberation, and the level of postponement.

Figure 8-2 is such a comprehensive model or flow chart. Diagrammed there and explained in the legend are the cognitive processes leading to immediate choices, postponement patterns, satisficing deliberative decisions, and optimizing decisions. The ability of the decision-maker to move between the postponement and deliberative modes is indicated. This flow chart is designed to be applicable to a variety of decisions to take action or refrain from action. However, the kidney donation situation is utilized as an example.

THE FAMILY PROCESS

The donor selection process generally involves two discrete types of decisions. The first is the one we have just examined—that is, each potential donor somehow either volunteers or fails to volunteer. A second process occurs at the family level.

Where there is more than one volunteer of the right blood type, the family must select one out of the pool to be the donor. In this part of the chapter we briefly describe the nature of this family-level decision-making. There is also a discussion of the degree of efficiency and conflict in this aspect of decision-making as well as an analysis of the type of family characteristics that are correlated with a smooth process of donor selection.

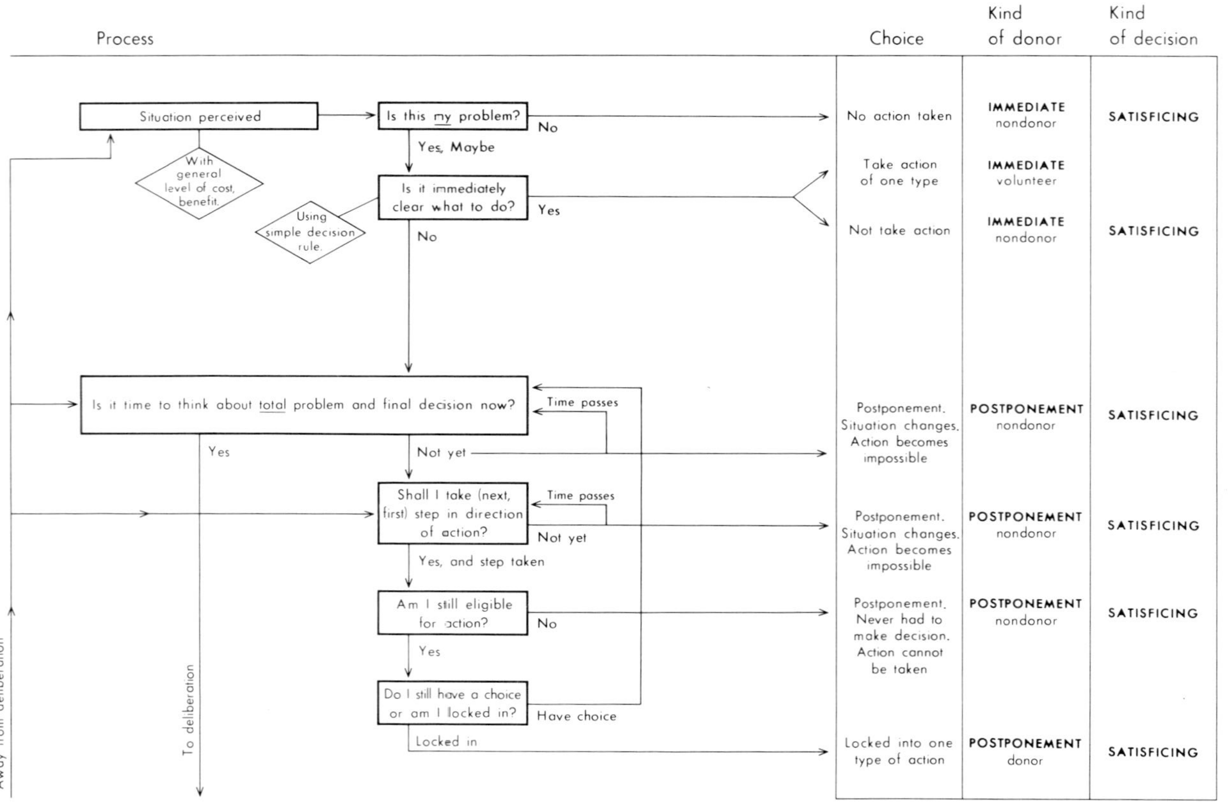

Process
Choice
Kind of donor
Kind of decision
Situation perceived
With general level of cost, benefit.
Is this my problem?
No
Yes, Maybe
Is it immediately clear what to do?
Using simple decision rule.
Yes
No
Is it time to think about total problem and final decision now?
Time passes
Yes
Not yet
Shall I take (next, first) step in direction of action?
Time passes
Not yet
Yes, and step taken
Am I still eligible for action?
No
Yes
Do I still have a choice or am I locked in?
Have choice
Locked in
Away from deliberation
To deliberation
No action taken
IMMEDIATE nondonor
SATISFICING
Take action of one type
IMMEDIATE volunteer
Not take action
IMMEDIATE nondonor
SATISFICING
Postponement. Situation changes. Action becomes impossible
POSTPONEMENT nondonor
SATISFICING
Postponement. Situation changes. Action becomes impossible
POSTPONEMENT nondonor
SATISFICING
Postponement. Never had to make decision. Action cannot be taken
POSTPONEMENT nondonor
SATISFICING
Locked into one type of action
POSTPONEMENT donor
SATISFICING

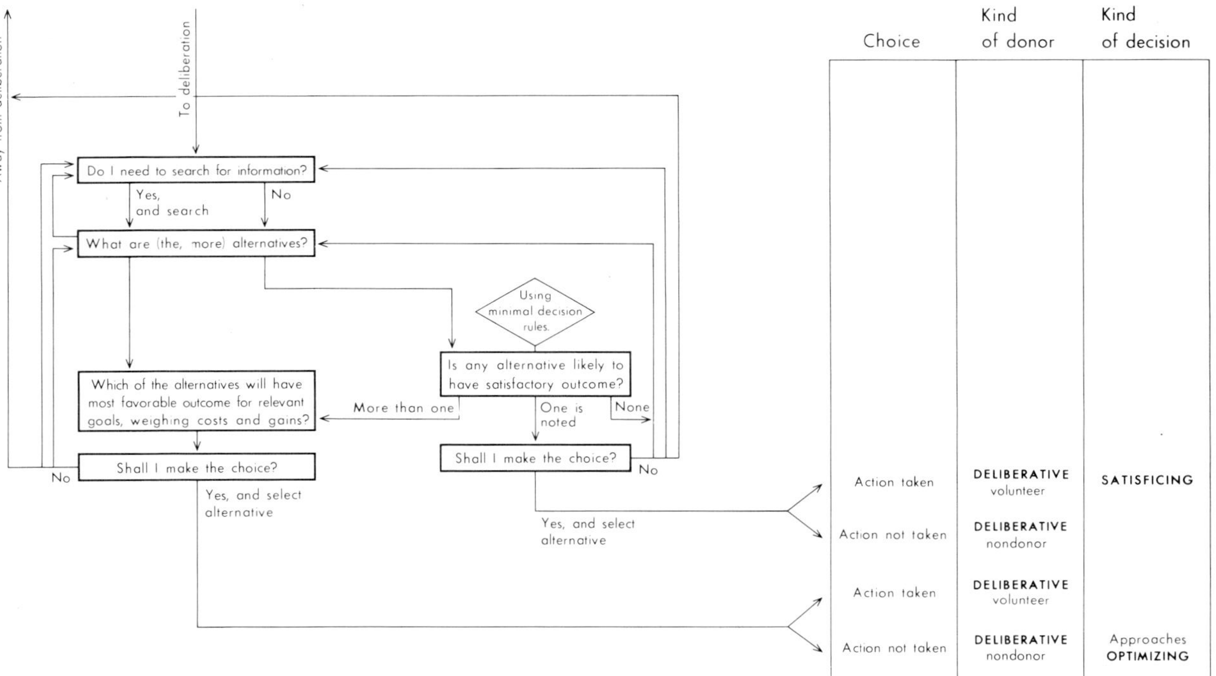

Figure 8-2 *Decision to take action or not: decision-making flow chart.*

Figure 8-2 Legend

Initial Steps and Instantaneous Decision. The individual first has to perceive and define the situation that could engender action on his part. If he perceives it, he also has some perception, perhaps inaccurate and imprecise, of the general level of cost and benefit involved. This general perception has an impact on all that follows. The decision-maker next must determine whether this is *his* problem or *his* responsibility. If he fails to ever ascribe responsibility to himself, he has in essence made an immediate, satisficing choice not to take action. Once he ascribes responsibility to himself, then according to simple decision-rules he decides whether the proper course is immediately clear (e.g., is it morally right or not?) If these decision-rules are clear enough, the individual may be able to make an instantaneous decision to take action or to refrain from acting. Again, this is a "satisficing decision" which may not feel like a "decision" at all to the party involved.

Movement to Postponement or Deliberation. If what to do is not immediately clear, the individual, according to this model, decides whether it is now time to think about the total problem and final decision. If he is motivated to evade the decision or if the time appears inappropriate to think about the total problem, he enters into a series of cognitive steps that may result in his fitting the postponement pattern. If instead, he believes it is time to think about the total problem, he moves to a series of steps fitting the deliberative pattern of decision-making.

Postponement. In the former case leading to postponement, the passage of time may cause the individual to reopen the question of whether he wishes to deliberate and he may at any time move toward the deliberative mode. However, he may drift and allow so much time to pass that the situation changes and makes a decision to *take* action impossible. Without making a conscious choice, the individual becomes committed to "nonaction." Or instead of drifting, he may consider taking a first preliminary step in the direction of action. This choice to take a first preliminary step is a decision in itself and all the steps mapped in this diagram for the larger decision could be applied. If he takes the preliminary step, he may then find himself ineligible for further action as in the case of a potential donor who makes the first step, has his blood tested and then learns he is the wrong blood type. In that case he will never have to make the larger choice at all.

If instead he is still eligible after the first step, he may perceive that this preliminary step has "locked him" into taking the final action without his ever making a conscious choice to do so. He may feel he no longer has any choice. If, however, he does not feel "locked in" he may then decide to proceed with the next step toward action. Or he may at this point reopen the question of whether it is time to think about the total problem; and he may move away from postponement toward the deliberative mode.

The Deliberative Mode. Once the actor moves into the deliberative mode, he may seek more or less information and generate one or more alternatives to evaluate. If he considers only whether one alternative is satisfactory according to minimal decision-rules and then makes a definite choice, he is a deliberator who has made a "satisficing type" decision. If instead he compares the relative costs and benefits of two or more alternatives before making his choice, then his decision approaches an optimizing one. The more thorough the search for information, the more extensive the attempt to generate alternatives and to compare them, the closer the decision approximates the optimizing model. In the process of deliberation, the decision-making may become difficult, the alternatives unsatisfactory, and the individual unwilling to choose. The individual may then reevaluate whether it is time to think about the total problem, and he may move back into a postponement pattern rather than make a final choice. Or, as this model also indicates, he may instead go back to his initial cognitive steps, redefine and reperceive the parameters of the situation to avoid

SELECTION OF ONE DONOR

Once several family members have been blood-typed, the procedure of winnowing down the choice to one person better fits a deliberative decision-making model or an optimizing model than does the individual's own "decision" to volunteer.

First of all, we should note that the majority of families never reached this stage of decision-making. Fifty-nine percent of the families had either no potential donor or only one person who was the correct blood type and still medically eligible after the blood testing. Thus this analysis is based on the 84 families where a donor pool did exist.

Second, the role of the "gatekeepers," the medical staff, may have been very large here. (see Fox and Swazey, 1974). If one donor was clearly a better match than the rest, that person received a direct call from the medical staff at this university and was asked if he wished to schedule the three-day physical exam. If he was an A-match, a perfect match, as 24% of the donors were, the enthusiasm expressed by the staff member was great, because over 90% of patients who receive kidneys from such a source have successful courses. In half of all the families at issue (42 out of 84) matching was a key factor used in selecting the actual donor out of the pool—that is, the relative gain to the recipient was a major factor in the decision-process. The family may have openly agreed on this criterion, or it may have been less a family decision than a matter of direct contact between the staff and the best possible donor.

Evaluating Costs

In addition to weighing the gains for the recipient, in the majority of families (49 out of 84) there was some attempt to decide for which member donation was least *costly*—for which family member donation involved less of a sacrifice or less difficulty. Although the underlying logic of weighing costs was the same in these families, the exact criteria and the conclusions reached often were diametrically opposed. One type of relative might be preferred in one family because the costs seemed relatively low, and the same type would be rejected in another family because the costs were perceived as too high.

---

the necessity for taking action. He may deny that the situation is one that calls for action, or that it is *his* particular responsibility to consider the problem.

This model does not outline steps that occur after the choice has been made by one of these cognitive processes. However, a choice once made can be reopened at any time before the final action is taken, and the individual can reenter the flow chart. Later evaluation of the decision can affect future choices.

The evaluations of age, sex, and stage in the life-cycle as criteria were particularly likely to vary among families. In some families (11 out of 84, or 13%) *women* of childbearing age were considered less desirable as donors, due to the fear that there would be a greater medical risk for them during future pregnancies if they had only one kidney; similarly in some families (16 out of 84, or 19%) *women* who had the responsibility of young children to care for at home were deemed less appropriate. In other families, however, females were preferred as donors, because the cost of the *men* taking time off from work was perceived as too great (17 out of 84, or 20%). The tendencies of some families to prefer males while some others prefer females seem to balance each other so that overall there is no sex difference between the actual donors and the other volunteers.

In some families *younger single people* were regarded most positively as donors because they had no family responsibilities of their own (10 out of 84, or 12%) or because older donors were felt to run an increased operative risk (8 out of 84, or 10%). In other families young single persons were viewed most negatively as donors because "their whole life was ahead of them," while the more mature family members were said to have at least lived satisfactory lives up to this point (17 out of 84, or 20%). In case of operative complication or death, an entire life would be compromised for the young person, rather than simply the end-portion. The cost for the youth would therefore be greater.

Although opposite arguments were posed in different families, the net result of these calculations was that among the siblings and children of the recipient, the person chosen as donor was more likely to be single than were the other volunteers (48% vs. 36%). The argument of lesser family responsibility appears to have been the overriding one in most families. In Chapter 7 we noted that volunteers and donors were more likely to be single than were nondonors, and here we see that the person actually chosen to make the sacrifice out of all volunteers was the one with fewest counterobligations to a family of his own. At every stage of the decision-process, donation is perceived as a conflict between obligations to the recipient and to one's family of procreation.

In attempting to choose the relative for whom the donation was the least costly, middle-class relatives are more likely to be selected than those from the working class. Sixty-four percent of male donors held middle-class jobs, in contrast to only 45% of the male volunteers who were not chosen as donors ($p < .05$).* In Chapter 7 we noted that both

* To rule out the possibility that a few working-class families with large numbers of volunteers are responsible for this difference, we randomly selected one volunteer per family to compare to the one donor per family. The class difference between donors and volunteers persisted (64% vs. 41%).

donors and other volunteers rated higher in social-class standing than did nondonors. The financial costs of being out of work or traveling to the transplant center probably were more difficult for the poorer family to absorb. To be able to give this extraordinary gift of a kidney, great life-resources are needed.

Other Criteria

Other than attempting to evaluate the relative benefit for the recipient and the cost for various potential donors, the family also considered certain normative and emotional criteria in selecting one donor out of the pool. Relatives who were more eager to donate or whose own family did not oppose the donation were more likely to be chosen. In addition, role considerations became relevant. Parents emphasized their greater obligation to donate when siblings and parents were both in the donor pool (10 cases):

CASE Interview with Mother of Recipient

Both parents and two siblings were volunteers of the right blood type

MOTHER. We're dubious about either of our other two children giving a kidney. We're proud of them, but as parents it's important to us to be the ones to give.

Types of Family Decision: Consensus and Conflict

Turner (1970) has classified family decisions into three types: (1) decisions of consensus—that is, decisions that leave everyone involved equally happy without any winners or losers; (2) decisions of accommodation in which agreement is reached but some members believe they have given in to others—there are winners and losers; (3) *de facto* decisions in which no active assent or dissent occurs, but events seem to determine outcome. He describes this last type of decision-making as follows:

> Many discussions finish inconclusively and are then decided by events. . . .Such decisions sometimes follow ineffectual discussions and sometimes occur in the absence of any group consideration of the question at all. What all such events have in common is that agreement is by the absence of dissent rather than by active assent, and, more important commitment is by the course of events rather than by acceptance (p. 100).

Clearly, the last type of family decision has strong parallels to what we have characterized as a postponement model. An action is taken without a conscious choice to follow that action. In this case an action is taken that has repercussions for at least two, if not more, family members without the family consciously attempting to make a direct choice. Turner notes that the *de facto* decision may occur because the area is too emotionally charged for open discussion. Frequently a single individual acts in this situation without either prior family blessing or active opposition. In 15% (13 out of 84) of the families the selection of the final donor out of the pool of eligible blood-tested relatives seemed to happen without explicit *family* discussion. As far as we could tell, there was no family discussion about the factors that would make one relative more appropriate than another. In some cases, but not all, these were situations in which the medical staff notified one donor that he was the best match and that donor arranged to proceed with the testing without first consulting other relatives.

In most cases, however, the process we have described of selecting one donor out of the donor pool is a conscious deliberate one rather than a *de facto* decision. In 49 out of 84 of the cases (58%) two independent coders agreed that family members *explicitly* compared the relative advantages and disadvantages of various donors.*

The question then arises whether the more conscious deliberative decision-making experienced by the majority of families is consensual, leaving everyone feeling relatively satisfied, or whether it is a process of accommodation in which some family members believe they have been overruled in the bargaining situation. According to the in-depth coding by two independent coders, the vast majority of decisions at this point are ones of consensus. Out of all these 49 cases in which there was explicit family discussion about the "winnowing-down" decision, in only five were some family members clearly unhappy with the outcome or was there any significant conflict of which we were aware. Thus 90% of these 49 families and 94% of all 84 appear to arrive at the choice with ease in the family; only five could be classified as instances of accommodation based on our information. In several cases (16) where consensus, was easy, each potential donor insisted he should be the one chosen; however, this type of disagreement tended to be easily resolved, frequently by leaving the final choice to the medical staff.

In sum, once the problem has reached the stage of selecting one donor out of a pool of willing volunteers, decision-making is usually not difficult. In addition, it tends to follow a pattern of deliberation more closely than does the prior individual decision-making.

* In the remainder of families (22 out of 84, or 26%) the pattern was not clear enough to be reliably coded either at the extreme of the *de facto* decision where there was no family discussion about the decision or at the other extreme of explicit family comparison of the various donors.

Effect of Type of Family upon Smoothness of Decision-Making

Although the selection of one donor out of a group of willing volunteers is not usually difficult for the family, many problems *in the earlier stages* of the donor search may engender family stress (see Table 8-5, left-hand column). Many of these problems are discussed in detail in Chapter 9. First, the recipient or those closest to him must communicate the need for a donor to the potential donors in the family. Families vary greatly in the extent to which this communication process is efficient and open. Second, once the information is communicated, the coordination of the various family members into the decision-process may also be more or less efficient. In fact, as we have indicated in discussing the *de facto* decision, there may be little coordination within the family at all. Third, one of the reasons the early stages of the donor search may be stressful is because of the unwillingness of some relatives to volunteer—families vary in the extent to which they include nondonors. The pattern of accommodation, described by Turner, in which some members are dissatisfied with the family decision frequently takes the form of the unhappy acceptance by the recipient and his closest supporters of the nondonors' unwillingness to volunteer.

Because families vary in the extent to which the entire donor decision-making process is smooth and free of stress, whether the level of stress is related to the type of family structure is of interest to investigate. We have not distinguished up to now among family types, although the families differ enormously in structure. In some cases there is one small nuclear family at issue; in other cases there is a large system of several interconnected nuclear families, for example. That is, in some cases the donor pool includes only relatives with whom the recipient lives; while in others members are involved who once shared a household but who now have set up their own homes; and in still other cases extended family members who never shared a household are involved, such as aunts, grandparents, or cousins. In some families the potential donors are all from one generation; in other families, they represent two or more generations. In certain instances all potential donors live nearby; in other families members are geographically dispersed. The recipient may be an adult or a child. Prior conflict may or may not mar the family history.

The question then is whether differences in family structure are related to the level of efficiency and consensus in decision-making. Table 8-5 indicates that in the following types of families decision-making is more efficient, communication less blocked, and the entire procedure less stressful: smaller families with fewer potential donors, families in which one or both parents are part of the donor pool or in which the recipient is a

TABLE 8-5 FAMILY TYPE AND CHARACTERISTICS OF FAMILY DECISION PROCESS—PEARSON'S CORRELATIONS [a]

	Family Type (N = 205)					
Characteristics of the decision-process [b]	Family size, number of potential donors	Number of generations involved	Geographical dispersion	Parent(s) among potential donors (for adult recipients)	Recipient is adult not child	Family reports prior conflict
Efficiency of communication	−.20*			.18†	−.18†	−.26*
Openness of communication	−.10		−.22†	.14‡	−.36*	−.24*
Presence of "noncommunication" (type of blocked communication)	.43*	.23*	.26*	−.22*	.20*	.20†
Efficient coordination of donor decision-process	−.23*		−.24*	.29*	−.27*	−.33*
Presence of "*de facto*" decision. No unified family decision-making	.27*		.34*	−.44*	.17†	.27*

Pressure to donate						
On donor				−.15†		
On nondonor	−.19†					
On someone in family	−.14			−.12		.15
All potential donors volunteer	−.14†	.12†		.28*	−.20*	
Potential donors unite against recipient	.16†					
Presence of family conflict	.16*	.10‡[d]	.20*		.12†	.28*
Presence of significant family stress[c]	.11‡		.13†	−.14†	.15†	.35*
Outcome happy for all	−.19*	−.13†	−.09[e]			−.19*

[a] Only correlations of ±.09 or larger.
[b] These judgments are based on coding of the in-depth family interviews. Only cases coded reliably by independent coders are included here.
[c] See Chapter 9 for a fuller discussion.
[d] This correlation disappears when family size is controlled.
[e] This correlation disappears when one controls for family size and whether the recipient is an adult or child.
$* = p \leqslant .01$. $\dagger = p \leqslant .05$. $\ddagger = p \leqslant .10$.

child, families in which no members are geographically dispersed, and families that do not report a history of major conflict prior to the transplant issue. In such families particularly, *all* potential related donors are likely to volunteer to donate. Furthermore, the outcome is more likely to be a happy one for everyone concerned when there are fewer potential donors in the family and when they are all from one generation.*

The only advantage that the larger family has over the small is that it is less apt to mobilize extreme pressure upon individuals to donate. The small family appears in most cases to be able to achieve a rapid, efficient, and satisfactory consensus; yet where consensus is not forthcoming, the pressure on the individual to donate can be more powerful. However, Table 8-5 indicates that such pressure is slightly less likely to occur if the parents are part of the potential donor pool—that is, if they are young enough to donate (under 65) and have no evident major diseases.

Having a parent among the potential donors appears to be a major advantage for a recipient and the family. This finding holds true both for the recipients taken as a whole and more surprising for the adult recipients considered alone (see Table 8-5). The great willingness of parents to donate and thus solve the entire problem is only a part of the reason for the great efficiency and volunteering in these families—that is, even in families where the parent does not become the actual donor, most of these correlations persist between the presence of a parent and the efficiency of the donor search.† The results suggest a greater cohesion among adult blood relatives when the mutual parent is still alive and of an active age.

The parents' (particularly the mothers') key role in this system of interconnected nuclear families is reflected in several ways. In half of the families there are one or two family spokesmen who attempt to round up donors for the sick patient. For married adult recipients, the parents,

* In Table 8-5 all correlations of .09 or greater, with one exception, are in the direction delineated above. (The one exception involves the small correlation between the number of generations involved in the donor search and the tendency for all potential donors to volunteer.) In addition, unless indicated otherwise, all relationships reported between geographical dispersion and the characteristics of the decision process persist when one holds constant family size and whether the recipient is an adult or child. When there was a relationship between the number of involved generations and a dependent variable, the findings also persist controlling for family size.

† Communication remains more efficient, open, and less blocked; decision-making more efficient and less likely to be characterized as *de facto*; and all eligible relatives are more likely to volunteer if a parent is part of the donor pool. There is no longer a significant relationship between the presence of a parent and the level of major family stress or the lack of pressure to donate. One correlation in the opposite direction emerges such that in families with parents present, the outcome is classified as less likely to be a happy one for *all* members ($r = -.16$).

especially the mother, and the spouses are particularly likely to assume this responsibility. In large families where the task of coordination was by definition more difficult, dominant individuals were likely to emerge who attempted to make family-level decisions themselves, and in half of such cases these individuals were the parents. The parents' attempt to protect the patient also extends to hospital visiting practices. When the adult patient entered the hospital, many had a fairly constant family visitor or visitors. Although usually the visitor was the spouse, in 18 cases the mother played such a role.

In sum, these data have suggested two polar types of families. At one pole stands the small undispersed family in which a parent offers this gift to a dying child and other family members follow parental example and rally around the child. At the other pole is the large geographically dispersed family of the adult recipient in which the patient's parents are no longer alive or are too old to be eligible as donors. This family acts less like a unified whole and more like a collection of separate individuals.

SUMMARY

A more important life-decision than whether one will or will not volunteer to donate a kidney to save the life of a dying relative is difficult to imagine. We have used this situation as a research site to investigate individual and family decision-making processes.

The in-depth analysis of the individual's perception of his own decision-making indicates that to most actors the term *decision* appears to be a misnomer. Insofar as decision-making implies a period of deliberation and a conscious choice of one alternative, most individuals do not feel as if they have made a decision. Although the gift of a kidney is a major sacrifice, the majority of donors (61%) appear to have known instantaneously that they would give the gift, and they report no conscious period of deliberation. Family members frequently verify the fact that these donors volunteered to donate immediately upon hearing of the need without time for deliberation. Approximately one-fifth of the nondonors also appear to fit this model of an immediate decision-maker who does not deliberate about alternatives.

A few donors (six) and about one-quarter of the nondonors follow another nondeliberative pattern—a pattern of postponement and evasion of decision-making. The donors postpone making the larger decision, while taking small steps toward action, until they feel locked into donation without having ever made a conscious choice to donate. Nondonors drift and postpone any final choice. Meanwhile the situation eventually changes and precludes the possibility of their donation. The hallmark of the postponement pattern is that the individual comes to feel committed to action or nonaction without ever consciously selecting that alternative.

In addition to the patterns of immediate decision-making and stepwise postponement, some donors (25%) and nondonors (31%) do fit a more classical deliberative pattern. They spend some time weighing pros and cons and they eventually arrive at a definite choice. However, their information-seeking tends to be quite scanty, given the major decision involved, and their deliberation often focuses on their conflicting moral obligations to the patient and their own families.

In general, the decision-making of the majority of potential donors appears to be of the "satisficing" type—an alternative is chosen that is good enough according to minimal decision-rules. Only the minority begin to approach an optimizing model where the advantages and disadvantages of more than one alternative are thoroughly explored and compared so that the optimal choice can be made.

Once a pool of relatives have volunteered to donate, a second decision-making process at the family level occurs. The pool of willing relatives has to be narrowed to one donor. This process is a more deliberative one, with most families discussing the advantages and disadvantages of each volunteer. The advantage for the patient of the closest match and the relative costs to each donor are compared and entered into the equation.

Once the problem has reached this point, the winnowing-down decision is usually made easily, with high consensus among family volunteers. Only in a few cases (five) could the decision be characterized as one of accommodation in which one family member emerges as a loser, the others as winners. Theoretically one might expect much bargaining and strategy at the family level, because the choice of one member as the donor relieves all other relatives from the need to sacrifice. Yet the strong emotional context of the family seems to work to produce consensus instead. In fact the temporary arguments that occur within families tend to take the form of each of several willing volunteers arguing that he should be the one to donate. Decisions of accommodation are more likely to involve an earlier stage in the process when family members become angry at nondonors, and volunteers' spouses become upset with the fact their husband or wife is going to offer a kidney. Such cases are discussed in the following chapter.

In a few cases (15%) the family decision-making process appears to be a *de facto* one—that is, there appears to be almost no family coordination or discussion, although one donor emerges from the pool. The final choice of one donor seems to occur because of the way situations structure themselves or due to individuals acting on their own or in consultation with the medical staff. Again, like the individual's pattern of postponement, this process is experienced by the participants as a non-decision. Although several different relatives have a key interest in the outcome, there is little coordination among them.

The nature of the families involved in the donor search varies greatly from one patient to another. At one extreme is the small nuclear family of the child. At the other extreme is the large system of several interconnected nuclear families all having blood ties to an adult recipient. Such differences among families appear to have a substantial relationship to the nature of the family decision-process. Small geographically concentrated families in which the parent is part of the potential donor pool or the recipient is a child appear to have major advantages. The decision-making in these families is more likely to be efficient and conflict-free and to produce a high number of volunteers.

The key role of the recipient's parents even after he is an adult has been noted. As indicated above, where such parents are present, the donor search is less stressful and more members volunteer to help in this way. The above findings suggest that the bonds among blood relatives of an adult remain more cohesive if the mutual parent is still alive and of active age. The parent, particularly the mother, is also likely to play the role of constant hospital visitor and of family spokesman for the recipient, informing family members of the need for a donor. The role of the parent is thus considerable in protecting the adult child in trouble, in organizing family sacrifice, and in promoting family cohesion after the children are grown.

Throughout this volume the question of the ethics of using living related donors has been an important policy issue. The study of the decision-making of such donors certainly indicates that for the majority of donors the decision is a rapid, easy, and strongly motivated one. While a critic may question the lack of deliberation for such a major life decision, most donors themselves feel comfortable, probably more comfortable, without extensive deliberation.

9

FAMILY STRESS IN THE SEARCH FOR A DONOR

ROBERTA G. SIMMONS
KATHLEEN SCHILLING
LINDA KAMSTRA

The picture of the donor search that has emerged throughout our analyses is a positive one for most families. A high proportion of potential donors actually volunteer to donate; the decision-making process is an easy one for most donors; and the long-term social-psychological consequences for the majority of recipients and donors are favorable. Yet the data from those families we followed intensively indicate that in a minority of cases the donor search generates major stress: In 23% (46 out of 197) of the families where there was a donor search, two independent coders agreed on the existence of major stress. At the other extreme the two coders agreed that in 34% of the cases there was virtually no stress. In the remaining 42% of the families, either the coders felt that there was some insignificant stress or discomfort associated with the donor search (28%);

or they could not completely agree on the level or existence of stress (14%).

Our object in this chapter is to analyze the nature of the major stress that did occur in families, although in some cases milder problems are also discussed.

The close examination of this stress should facilitate an evaluation of the overall policy to use living related donors. It should also contribute to a greater sociological understanding of family behavior in a crisis situation. There are three kinds of stress during the search for a donor: (1) the distress experienced internally by individual family members, (2) the conflict within the potential donor's own nuclear family, and (3) the conflict or tension within the part of the family that includes the recipient and the potential donor (the mutual family). Each of these kinds of stress will be explored in turn.

INDIVIDUALS' INTERNAL STRESS

The Donors

In Chapter 6, the internal distress experienced by a few of the actual *donors* was reported in some depth. Out of the 46 cases of major stress, seven involved highly ambivalent donors.* As discussed in Chapter 6, in two cases where the kidney transplant was successful, marked ambivalent feelings about the donation still persisted at a year posttransplant.

Although routine interviews were not held at a year after the transplant with donors whose kidneys had been *rejected* (see Chapter 6), our impression from our occasional interviews with such donors is that their internal distress and grief was more extreme (see Chapter 6, p. 169). One unexpected reaction was guilt that their kidneys had not been adequate. In one case the guilt appeared major; in another, transitory.

CASE Donor of rejected kidney is patient's father

Interview with patient's husband after the doctors announce that rejection is certain and a second transplant necessary

> HUSBAND. Betty's dad is an alcoholic. Or when he gets down he drinks a lot. Betty's sister thinks we shouldn't let him know about the transplant. See her dad gave the first time, and he thinks it's his fault Betty is rejecting.

* Often major stress in a family had more than one source. Thus some of the examples cited in different sections of this chapter refer to the same families, although there was an attempt to use examples from many different families.

From patient's brother (the second donor)

INTERVIEWER. How do your parents feel about your donating? Your father?

BROTHER. He was quite upset that she lost the kidney. [Probe] Dad, he feels that it is his fault. . . .

INTERVIEWER. What did he say?

BROTHER. He was blaming himself. . . .

INTERVIEWER. What kinds of things would he say about it?

BROTHER. He'd just say it was his fault, that's all. I told him it wasn't.

* * *

CASE Donor of rejected kidney is patient's sister

Interview with donor's mother

INTERVIEWER. How did Peter's sister feel about the removal [of the rejected kidney]. . .from the standpoint of being the donor?

MOTHER. I think. . .at first she didn't say much. . .like the rest of us, she was more worried about his health, if he would come through. The doctors talked to her way before they realized it was definitely not going to work and convinced her it wasn't her fault. . .it was not the fault of her kidney. And we talked to her too. So she took it very well.

Interview with donor

INTERVIEWER. Well, how are you taking all this?

SISTER. I was pretty upset when I first heard about it, but then I talked to Dr. C., and he told me it wasn't my fault. The kidney was perfect when they took it out of me, and it worked perfectly for a month.

The Nondonors

Severe internal distress is as rare among nondonors as among donors. In only four cases were we aware of extreme guilt on the part of a nondonor, although for 48 of the 222 nondonors for whom we had information (21%) there was indication of milder guilt feelings.

The case of most extreme guilt involved a married daughter (Brenda) who had agreed to donate to her mother but who became extremely anxious and angry the night before the transplant after she was admitted to the hospital and some minor errors were made by the surgical resident. She alternated between indicating at some points that she was too fearful to donate and at other times that she wanted to continue with the donation. The donor's doctor decided she could not donate in her psychological state and gave her a false medical excuse so that the recipient would be unaware of her unwillingness. Her guilt at having backed out was considerable, as documented by relatives who were aware of the true circumstances.

CASE Interview with Brenda's brother-in-law

BROTHER-IN-LAW. It was terrible for Brenda too. You know she's done a couple of things that are completely out of character for her. A few days after her mother went home, her dad took her. . .[the mother] out shopping. . .Brenda heard they were there and it's only a little ways from her house so she rushed right over there and followed them around like a little puppy dog. That's not like her at all. . .and another thing she did which is out of character for her. She went out and bought some [presents] and gave them to [several of us]—that's not like her. It said, "I'm sorry, I love you, I need you, etc."

Interview with Brenda's husband

INTERVIEWER. How do you think all this will affect Brenda?

HUSBAND. I think it's gonna take a long time. She seems to be better, but she has nightmares. The other night she had one that her mother was cut up in four pieces. It's always been so morbid for her.

INTERVIEWER. Do you think Brenda might be willing to talk to us about her feelings about all of this?

HUSBAND. I don't know. She's always been exceptionally cool. I've never seen her so upset. Her hands were cold, her blood pressure was up. . . . She couldn't sleep for days and days. Now she has nightmares. She never talks about it any more though. She had another nightmare. . .the people in this town kept accusing her of kidnapping this friend of hers. The friend in the dream was this friend of hers that had spent the night with us once when she [the friend] had a fight with her father. The fact that this friend had a

> fight with her father seems significant to me. [The father in this case had expressed some anger initially when Brenda said she wished to withdraw from the donation.]

Less severe guilt was indicated by many other nondonors, who either told us directly they felt guilty or demonstrated guilt indirectly. The indirect manifestations were interesting. One nondonor raced to the hospital after hearing that his sister had received a transplant with a cadaver kidney and now volunteered to have his blood tested in case the cadaver kidney were rejected and a second kidney were needed. Another nondonor volunteered to help build a house for the recipient.

Thus whether the potential donor decides to volunteer or not, ambivalent feelings about the issue can cause internal distress.

Ineligible Relatives

Ambivalence about donation may also upset relatives who do not themselves expect to donate. A family member who is ineligible or is less eligible than others may suffer at the prospect of one of his close relatives donating to save the life of another. In fact relatives report being caught in a role conflict between their loyalties to the donor and recipient. Parents of donors are particularly likely to feel torn, because in some cases their tacit or actual permission is assumed by the donor.

CASE *Interview with mother (one son is donating to other)*

INTERVIEWER. How do you feel about having Clyde donate to Harry?

MOTHER. It's a horrible dilemma. You don't want to sacrifice Clyde, but you want Harry to be able to live. It has to be Clyde's decision. I just wish it were. . .over with.

* * *

CASE *Interview with elderly mother (one sibling is donating to her brother)*

INTERVIEWER. When did you find out that your daughter would donate her kidney?

MOTHER. Last winter I'd figured out about it. She said to me, "Brian is sick and I'm going to give him my kidney." I thought she was funning me, but it soaked in finally.

INTERVIEWER. How did you react to that?

MOTHER. Oh, how else? I was scared. I felt bad, but I knew I couldn't talk her out of it. And I don't know if I would want to because I want Brian to live too.

INTERVIEWER. What did you say?

MOTHER. Nothing. I was just kind of in the middle, a sandwich. I didn't want my youngest hurt, but I wanted Brian to live too.

INTERVIEWER. Kind of a hard place for a mother.

MOTHER. Oh yes. Before I came here when I was home I felt terrible. I cried all the time so I decided to come here. And now I have gotten my strength. I know if I cry I'll upset my son, so I don't.

INTERVIEWER. Did you try to discourage or encourage your daughter?

MOTHER. No, I didn't. How could I? She wouldn't listen and anyway I'm not sure I'd want to. I'm really in the middle.

The Recipient

The recipient may suffer from the same ambivalence. In six of the 46 families in which the donor search was extremely stressful, the source of the tension was the recipient's guilt at accepting a kidney and/or the difficulty he had in asking for one. As indicated earlier, parents find it particularly difficult to accept a kidney from a child:

CASE Mother who repeatedly said she wanted a cadaver kidney, but whose daughter volunteered

Interview with recipient

RECIPIENT. [I guess my youngest daughter will be donating.]

INTERVIEWER. Oh, have you talked to her about it?

RECIPIENT. Well, yes, just when I first heard she was here and [she] said right away that she would give. [Started to cry.] But I didn't want her to. She has four children. Goodness, here I go again. The doctor said he was going to take up a collection and buy me a sponge.

INTERVIEWER. Just take your time, we'll be all right.

RECIPIENT. [Crying]

INTERVIEWER. What is it that bothers you?

RECIPIENT. Well, it's what happens to the family. After all, my daughter has four children of her own and I hate her to take this chance for me.

In some cases the situation became more upsetting for the recipient, because there was a sibling who could have donated instead of his own child, and that sibling did not offer.

CASE Daughter donating to father

Interview with Father

INTERVIEWER. When you first found out about the transplant, who did you at first think would donate?

RECIPIENT. My daughter was the first to offer, but I knew the blood relationship was closer in my sisters. I had hoped one of them would be the donor. And they're older and if something happened they'd have less time to lose.

INTERVIEWER. Do you now feel you should be getting a kidney from someone other than [donor]?

RECIPIENT. I don't have any specific person in mind, but I'd rather have someone else. I consider the possibility of not having one, rather than asking her to make that sacrifice.

INTERVIEWER. Why do you think it's harder for you to ask your daughter to donate than your sister?

RECIPIENT. Because she's younger. I just hate to ask her to do a thing like this. To go through this.

Some recipients, however, also felt great guilt at taking a kidney from their siblings. A particularly stressful case involved a situation in which the recipient had rejected the first kidney from her brother, and then her sister offered her a kidney for a second transplant.

CASE Interview with sister volunteering to donate

INTERVIEWER. How do you think [the recipient] feels about accepting [another] kidney from someone in the family?

SISTER. I don't know. We haven't asked her, she's been so depressed. I

> know she said before her first transplant if this one didn't work she wouldn't take one from anyone else. We told her, "You don't have anything to say about that." She was feeling guilty. She had these dreams where everyone in the family died. I don't know if she thinks she killed them. But she was always talking about her execution. . . .

Recipient distress prior to the transplant was not solely a matter of guilt. In seven of the families exhibiting major stress, the cause was the fear felt by the recipient or his spokesman that no donor would be forthcoming, and that the recipient would therefore die. Hurt at the family rejection was difficult for the dying patient who watched other recipients receive kidneys from related donors.

CASE Patient, none of whose relatives have volunteered

Interview with recipient's wife

INTERVIEWER. Well, how does [the recipient] feel about the family now? Has he said anything?

WIFE. He gets upset by it. At first it really upset him, but then he just didn't talk about it anymore. He did talk about it on the way here Tuesday. He got pretty upset. . . .We both knew Don [another patient] and his wife from Station 22, and you know his sister donated. And then there's a new patient on Station 22. . .Pearson. My husband knows his family. . .well he knows his mother, and his mother is donating. . . .It really bothers my husband that they're willing to donate, but not *his* family. It almost seems like to him that everyone else's family is willing to donate. . . .If they'd only talk to the doctors here. But they just won't do it.

In a hospital such as this one where related donation is encouraged, the patient who does not secure family volunteers becomes particularly aware of how the level of his family's love compares to that of most patients. In everyday life such clear comparisons are not possible.

CONFLICT WITHIN POTENTIAL DONOR'S FAMILY OF PROCREATION

As noted in earlier chapters, the potential donor frequently reports that the major factor against donating is his obligation to his own nuclear family, to his own spouse and children. In fact the spouse of the nondonor is particularly likely to be opposed to the donation (see Chapter 7) and to believe that the nondonor's obligation to his own family of procreation precludes donation.

Thus for many potential donors, the stage is set for a conflict of loyalties. As discussed earlier, the potential donor is liable to find himself in a role conflict between his obligations to the recipient and his family of origin on the one hand, and to the family he has created on the other. The issue here is whether conflict between the potential donors and their spouses and children over donation assumed major proportions. In seven cases the conflict between a potential donor and his or her spouse was classified as a major family stress: Four of these cases involved the actual donor, three involved volunteers, and none concerned nondonors. The opposition of the nondonor's spouse, though common, did not seem to lead to marital conflict, because spouse opposition simply reinforced the nondonor's personal feelings of reluctance.

The most severe case of conflict between a donor and her spouse ultimately resulted in divorce.

CASE Sister wishes to donate to her sister; her husband is opposed

Donor interview prior to the transplant at the time of blood test

DONOR. Well, I feel like I really want to do it. I did right from the start. But my husband was really against it. He really doesn't want me to do it *at all*. It was really quite a [bad time], but he finally said it was my decision. I was so mixed up in my mind I almost went in to see a psychiatrist. One day I just couldn't get anything clear in my mind and I thought I was going crazy. It really is a big decision to make.

INTERVIEWER. Yes it is. Your husband didn't want you to donate?

DONOR. No, not at all. . .but he finally said it was my decision, so. . . .

INTERVIEWER. When you felt that you were upset, or however exactly it was you felt. . .what feelings made you want to go, or think that a psychiatrist might help you?

DONOR. He was just *so* negative about it. I didn't know what to do. Like I thought, I don't want my sister to die. . .and if I didn't donate and something would happen to her. . .I'd feel just awful. I might even [crack up] or something. . . .

INTERVIEWER. Do you feel the subject of you donating or not is resolved with your husband, or isn't it really?

DONOR. No.

INTERVIEWER. He still doesn't want it, but he said it was your decision.

DONOR. Yes.

INTERVIEWER. What exactly is your decision?

DONOR. I want to do it, and I will if I can.

INTERVIEWER. Do you feel you have or will have any feelings on your conscience about making a decision your husband openly disapproves of, or is this something that will not bother you?

DONOR. No. . .well, what do you mean? No. . .I mean, he's so unreasonable. He just can't understand the way I feel. I think I'm right. . .I'd rather he went along with me, but. . .he never will.

INTERVIEWER. Do you think this difference of opinion has had or will have a serious influence on your marriage, or won't it?

DONOR. I don't know. I don't think so now. Not after it's over anyway and [he sees it's alright].

Later interview prior to the transplant at time of donor work-up after husband agreed to let her donate

INTERVIEWER. Do you think it would have been difficult for you to go through with donating knowing he was against it, or wouldn't it have bothered you too much?

DONOR. I don't think I would have.

INTERVIEWER. You don't think you would have [agreed to] donate. What would you have done, or what were you doing taking the tests when he was still against it?

DONOR. I was hoping that he would give in if I acted like I would do it whether he wanted me to or not. But, well. . . we were talking of a separation because of this. It just wouldn't have been worth it. I mean, even for my sister. I never could have done it. It wasn't worth it. . . .

INTERVIEWER. What I'd like to understand is if your talk of separation at this time was a result of only the disagreement over the donation, or if it was that in combination with other previous stress between you and your husband?

DONOR. I really don't know. I know it was *mainly* this. That was the real disagreement. The only important one. All marriages have rocky roads, and ours is no different. . .but it was because of that I wanted to donate and he didn't want me to.

Donor's husband prior to the transplant

INTERVIEWER. You mentioned that this whole thing almost caused a divorce? How did this come about?

HUSBAND. She thought I was bullheaded. . . .

INTERVIEWER. I see. . .Was your marriage a stable one before this or was this just another strain on top of others?

HUSBAND. It was not the perfect marriage. But it was the first outburst in a long time. . . .

INTERVIEWER. Did you say that you told her that you thought this might lead to a divorce?

HUSBAND. No, I didn't. She filed on me. She was being pulled on both sides. Each side was pulling her really hard. Her family on one side and me on the other. She was swaying one way and the other. And then she filed and she moved out Monday to Wednesday—three days. She said she didn't want to have to go through this. On Wednesday she was going to turn to me, but I could see it was. . .there was a deep down strain and that we could never have a marriage after that. So I [came here to see the doctor]. After my talk with the doctor today, I just feel relief. He really eased my mind.

Three months posttransplant

INTERVIEWER. How does [your husband] feel about it [donating] now?

DONOR. [Long pause.] I don't have a husband.

INTERVIEWER. What happened?

DONOR. When I came home he threatened to kill me and punched one of my teeth out and gave me a black eye. So I told him to get out.

INTERVIEWER. Why did he do that?

DONOR. I don't know.

INTERVIEWER. Well, did this happen because of your donating, or was it because of something else?

DONOR. Because I donated.

INTERVIEWER. How do you feel about him doing that over your donating?

DONOR. I really don't feel that bad that I told him to go. Now I know that if anything ever went wrong in the future, he'd do the same thing probably.

INTERVIEWER. Do you ever have any regrets about donating because of the trouble it caused you with your husband, or not?

DONOR. No. I'm still glad I did it. If I didn't, for the rest of my life I would have regretted it.

This fury of the husband when his wife violated his wishes may have been in part due to traditional sex-role expectations. The fact that the wife attempted to make this decision on her own challenged her husband's masculinity.

The following similar case of major conflict involved a female volunteer and her spouse. In this case the volunteer was not used for medical reasons. The husband clearly demonstrated pathology when speaking of the possibility of his wife donating to her brother. In fact he requested to speak to a psychiatrist about the issue and did so some time after this conversation with the sociologist.

CASE Interview with volunteer's husband

HUSBAND. I called my wife and told her no. She came before I did, and I told her I didn't think she should go through with it.

INTERVIEWER. What did she say?

HUSBAND. She didn't say much. . .I remember everything. Physical control I did not have, but mental I did. So I told her, you know. . .I didn't want her to do it, and the following day I got in touch again and I gave her pretty much the same answer.

INTERVIEWER. What did your wife say?

HUSBAND. She said she had to. She had to go through with it. Then I had some real hard thoughts. . . .I was ready to look into a divorce.

INTERVIEWER. Uh-huh.

HUSBAND. I thought of suicide myself.

INTERVIEWER. What did you think?

HUSBAND. I thought of my own commitment, my marriage vows "for better or worse.". . .So I thought, OK. . .I made a commitment. I have to live with it. So my thoughts changed. They turned to. . .like I reached the bottom. I dropped. I felt like there was nothing to look forward to. I felt like doing violence against her and against her brother.I resent the fact he's so avidly for it. I honestly can't conceive how any brother could ask it of his sister. . . .I am fearful for the operation itself, and the scar. To me, I've wondered how that will affect me in the future. Under normal circumstances, an appendectomy. . .there's no choice. That's not objectionable. For me, with the scar. . .it's just going to be a reminder of everything every time I look and feel. A reminder of something done without my approval, and possibly, I'm not sure, against my will. It may affect our sex life. This is all a mental strain. . .my mental strain. I can understand too her feelings. I know she'd like to do this. I'd like to respect her too. But. . .it's hard to see really the right answer, it's perplexing. I don't know, you know. . . .

In this extreme case, the husband would regard the scar as a constant reminder of a choice made by his wife against his will, as a challenge to his masculinity and a threat to their sex life.

Two of these last cases are *extreme* examples of a very common role conflict. In several cases the wife accepted the right of the husband to forbid donation and there was little conflict between them.

All opposition to the donation did not involve traditional sex-role expectations or male spouses: Several wives also opposed their husbands' desire to donate.

In most situations, however, the opposition of the wife or husband did not lead to major conflict. In the case of the nondonor such opposition usually seemed to reinforce their own predilections not to volunteer. In the case of the donors several spouses (nine) expressed the norm that the decision must be that of the individual involved and they themselves should not interfere. In some other cases the donors indicated they were able to convince their reluctant spouses by asking them what they would do if the situation were reversed and their family were in need of a donor. By the time of the donation almost all spouses (at least 82%) were supportive of the donor and remained so posttransplant.

The spouse is not the only family member who may oppose the donation. The donor's children also may raise significant objections. In only one case was the opposition of other family members severe enough to lead to major stress. This was a case in which a grandmother was donating to her son's child and up until the last minute she was pressured both by her daughter and by her brother-in-law not to donate.

CASE *Interview with donor's daughter*

INTERVIEWER. In your family was there any time in which bad feelings arose between any family members because of the transplant or because of the need for a donor, or because someone in the family did not offer to donate?

DAUGHTER. When I went down there [the night before the transplant] I tried to have it stopped. I tried to talk her out of it. I called her on the phone a couple of times.

INTERVIEWER. How has that caused bad feelings?

DAUGHTER. They think I was butting in where I wasn't supposed to.

INTERVIEWER. Who indicated that to you?

DAUGHTER. My dad [and my brother]. . . .My dad called me up about two weeks ago and told me my mother was in the hospital with bleeding ulcers and I was the cause of it.

Interview with donor posttransplant

DONOR. [My brother-in-law] didn't think I should go ahead with it. He thought I might harm myself.

INTERVIEWER. Did he tell you this personally or did you just hear it?

DONOR. He called here the day before the transplant. He really upset us. He talked to my husband and my son and myself.

INTERVIEWER. What did he say?

DONOR. He thought it was going to cost a lot of money. It was really upsetting to all of us.

INTERVIEWER. I'm sorry. What else did he say?

DONOR. Oh, that medicine can really mess up your life.

INTERVIEWER. What did you say?

DONOR. I told him I'd never live with myself if I didn't. . . .I think he thought I'd harm my health, be a cripple for life or something. It was very upsetting.

INTERVIEWER. Was there anyone [else] who suggested any problems about giving a kidney or who tried to discourage you from donating?

DONOR. [My daughter.]

INTERVIEWER. What did she say?

DONOR. She just said "I'm not in favor of it, Mom."

INTERVIEWER. Did she say why she felt that way?

DONOR. I didn't give her a chance. If I had I think I would have broken down and cried.

CONFLICT AND STRESS IN THE MUTUAL FAMILY

Internal distress and conflict between potential donors and their spouses are less evident sources of major stress than are conflict and tensions within the mutual family—that is, the family that includes the recipient and the potential donors. There appear to be three issues that generate stress within the mutual family: (1) the emotional relationship between those less willing to donate and the members who wish them to donate; (2) the communication problems that arise because of the need to request a donor; and (3) problems of gratitude between the actual donor, the recipient, and their respective families.

CONFLICT INVOLVING THE LESS WILLING FAMILY MEMBERS

Anger Toward the Nondonor

Anger and ill-feelings toward the nondonor are not rare during or after the donor search. Failure to volunteer a kidney carries a real cost in terms of closeness to other family members. Forty-three percent of the cases of major stress (20 out of 46) involve anger toward the nondonor. Expressed in another way, in 10% of the 205 families (20 out of 205) ill-feeling toward a nondonor reached a major level. Even when major problems did not emerge, there were some hard feelings against nondonors in a substantial minority of the cases. The qualitative coders find that one-third of the nondonors were the object of some anger, irritation, mild or severe hostility, expressed by at least one family member during our investigation.

These ill-feelings remain as a permanent cost of nondonation: Even at a year posttransplant 17% of donors and 9% of recipients agreed with a multiple-choice statement saying that they "can't help feeling a little angry at those others in the family who might have donated." Furthermore, after the transplant the donor and recipient became much closer to each other while the nondonor remained considerably less close. Pretransplant 56% of the donors viewed themselves as "very close" to the recipient; and this proportion rose to 75% after the transplant. Yet a month after the transplant only 39% of the nondonors claimed to be this close to the recipient. Table 9-1 shows an increase at a year posttransplant in the discrepancy between the recipient's feelings toward donors and volunteers on the one hand and the nondonors on the other: At a year after the transplant the recipients felt "very close" to 79% of the donors and to 67% of the other volunteers, but only to 36% of the nondonors. As Table 9-1 shows, recipients reported being less close to nondonors than to donors prior to the transplant, but the discrepancy is considerably greater at a year after the operation.

TABLE 9-1 RECIPIENT'S FEELINGS OF CLOSENESS TO VARIOUS RELATIVES

	Percentage of relatives to whom recipient feels "very close"				
	1	2	3	4	
	Of actual donors or prior donors	Of volunteers or verbal offers	Of excused or ineligible relatives	Of non-donors	Discrepancy between donors and nondonors (Col. 1 minus Col. 4)
Pretransplant	65% (96)	65% (192)	59% (153)	42% (182)	23%
1-year posttransplant	79% (75)	67% (151)	54% (127)	36% (185)	43%

Where the anger against the nondonor reached major proportions, cases were similar to the following:

CASE A female recipient, none of whose siblings or parents volunteered to donate

The patient's husband became involved in arguments several times with them over their refusal to come in and talk with the doctors. Following these exchanges, the entire family stopped calling and visiting. In an interview with the patient's husband, after the patient was finally put on the list for a cadaver kidney; the following was said:

INTERVIEWER. Did you talk to [the patient's brother] or his wife about it?

HUSBAND. No. I haven't talked to anyone about her. I just don't mention it. It's too frustrating.

INTERVIEWER. . . .What about [the patient's] parents. Have they expressed any more thoughts about her illness or need?

HUSBAND. No. I don't talk to them about it. They don't mention it and I certainly don't bring it up.

INTERVIEWER. . . .Have they said anything about her being on the cadaver list?

HUSBAND. Not really, but I think they've accepted that. . .at least they're going along with it without saying much. I've only seen them three or four times since she came home though, which is kind of a good thing, because even if I try not to think about it when they're not around, as soon as I see them I get frustrated. But I *will not* say any more about it. There's no point in beating a dead horse, and it won't help our relationship any for the future [when and if] this is all over.

. . .Her mother really runs the whole family, and the whole family is the same. Whatever she tells them they just swallow, and they won't even talk to the doctors about it. That's what really burns me. I wouldn't care if only they'd come and talk to the doctors about it. Just listen to what they had to say. But they won't, so. . . .When this first all started her father talked like he might want to help and maybe was even thinking about donating. At least he asked some questions like how long the donor is in the hospital after the operation. . .but then after a while we didn't hear any more from him about it. Of course her mom was the one who talked him out of it. She expects everyone to think just like her.

INTERVIEWER. Did you ever talk to her dad about it after he mentioned it?

HUSBAND. No. He never would talk about it again. Her mom is the head of the house and that's it. I think they're scared. It's so frustrating for me. They won't listen to anything I say and it always just winds up in a big battle, and her mom is always right!

Typically, whether the anger was major or not, the nondonor or the nondonor's spouse was described as selfish.

CASE Sister donated, father was a nondonor

Interview with donor

INTERVIEWER. You had mentioned to me before that you didn't think your father would consider donating. What has he said about his feelings about donating?

DONOR. Nothing, but my opinion would be that he wouldn't.

INTERVIEWER. Why do you think that?

DONOR. He's just selfish. I don't blame him but he wouldn't even consider it I don't think. Like my younger sister went through agony and was relieved when she couldn't. At least she considered it!

* * *

CASE One son donated to his mother, a daughter was a nondonor because her husband was in opposition

Interview with donor's wife

INTERVIEWER. Why do you think [nondonor's] husband had a lot to do with it? What were his concerns or worries about his wife donating?

DONOR'S WIFE. I don't think he was worried. He's just selfish. He's just the type that don't do anything for anybody. He felt it was his wife, and she ain't gonna give anybody anything.

Thus, in the eyes of those willing to give the gift of a kidney, the unwilling family members are guilty of violating an important family norm. If a relative is unwilling to help his kin or at least to consider helping, he is often viewed as a less worthy person, as inherently selfish.

In addition to characterizing the nondonors as selfish, the angry family member frequently was hurt and surprised by what he defined as a lack of caring. The patient or his spouse felt abandoned at a time of great need. The blow was particularly difficult to tolerate when it appeared to deviate from the norm of reciprocity, as in the following case where the recipient had previously come to the aid of one of the nondonors:

CASE *The patient's mother had been burned in a fire a few years ago; and the patient (Lilly) was totally responsible for her care during the recovery period. Now when she needs her parents' help she can't understand why they aren't willing. Furthermore, the parents will not allow eligible siblings to donate.*

PATIENT. I don't have one, a donor, you know. My 18-year-old sister was typed. She matched, but my folks wouldn't let her. They are against it. She is a minor and can't do it. . . .

INTERVIEWER. Is there any reason why your folks are against it?

PATIENT. Possibly cost. Whenever anybody goes in to the hospital it costs money. Yet Dad can get a new car.

In other cases the anger was less at the nondonor's failure to donate than at his inability to be clear and direct about his refusal (see discussion of communication problems below) or at his complete neglect of the patient (see discussion of isolation below).

In two cases the family member angry at the nondonor was a potential donor himself who was placed in a more vulnerable position because the person whose "role" it was to donate did not offer. In one case the donor, a child of the recipient with several children of her own, was angry at the recipient's brother who had no small children but did not offer. In another case a nondonor brother was angry that the recipient's son whose "place" it was to volunteer had not relieved the other family members of this responsibility.

CASE *Nondonor brother*

NONDONOR. Some of us were kind of disturbed with some people in the family.

INTERVIEWER. You were disturbed? For what reason?

NONDONOR. Because some weren't even tested. Some of us thought my younger brother should have done it because he's not married. I thought [the patient's] son should be the one. Her own son should have done it. . . .We all felt her son should have done it.

Although the angry family member was often quite bitter when he talked to us, he usually had not voiced this anger directly to the nondonor. In 14 out of 20 of the families where anger toward nondonors reached major levels, the angry family member had not communicated his feelings openly to the party concerned. The possibility of restoring family cohesion was thus left open (see below).

Nondonor Anger Toward Family

The nondonor may have reciprocated his relative's hostility with or without the larger family becoming aware of this. According to the qualitative coders, in one-fifth of the families containing nondonors—that is, in 21 families—nondonors voiced hostility or irritation toward some family member. In seven of these families this anger constituted a major stress. We may have learned of this hostility directly in our interviewing or indirectly through another family member. Of course we could be underestimating the degree of temporary and hidden anger felt by the nondonors. Although our conversations with the donor and other family members were extensive and intensive, the nondonor may have talked with us for only an hour. If he chose to conceal his feelings to us and if he did not express them to other family members, we would not be aware of them.

About half of the nondonors who were irritated were reacting to what they felt was too much pressure to donate. While other family members may have regarded the nondonors as failing to fulfill family help-giving obligations, the nondonors sometimes perceived the recipient as unreasonable in his expectations for help. Some nondonors explicitly rejected the idea that they had any obligation to donate. In four cases the nondonors felt that donation was too much to expect of them and that they should not have been asked at all. In most cases, however, the nondonors objected not so much to being asked but to being pressured.

CASE Nondonor sister to recipient

SISTER. I'm like an identical twin [according to the matching]. As soon as the family found out about that it was dumped in my lap, and I was the donor! But at the same time, I felt that I have two little kids at home to consider.

Later in interview

INTERVIEWER. You mentioned earlier that when the family found out you were an identical match they sort of "dumped it in your lap." Do you mean that you felt pressured to donate, or what?

SISTER. I was being very pressured, and it was going into my lap.

INTERVIEWER. Who, in particular, pressured you?

SISTER. Nobody in particular. Everybody just kept calling me and saying [we gotta get Lois into surgery soon], as if I hardly had any time.

Anger of Less Willing Volunteers

Anger at pressure to donate was felt primarily by the nondonors, but this also was the major source of stress for donors in two families and volunteers in one family. The following case was a situation of a parent attempting to pressure one daughter (Harriet) to donate to one of her other daughters (Lynn) because Harriet was an A-match (a perfect match) unlike any other member of the family.*

CASE Interview with potential donor's husband

HUSBAND. It really got hectic then. . . .We went again then to see the doctor, this time with Susan [the patient's other sister] too. The first time we conversed with the doctor he had said that Susan was alright too. Harriet was an A, Susan was a B. The only thing we could see was Lynn's chance and when it boiled down to it, Susan could do it. The three of us discussed it quite at length in conversation with the doctor and we arrived at the decision that Susan would be the one. That was all that really amounted to. . .then. . .we told the decision to Harriet's mom. The family was all at the hospital that night. Harriet's mother wanted to know if she was going to donate. Harriet and Susan told her that Susan was going to. Well. . .she got all upset. She didn't like the decision. She said she didn't think we were taking Lynn's best interest in mind.

Personally, I think she was unfair. . .because we did think of Lynn. It really upset Harriet, and I think right then she kind of resigned herself to it. She knew she was the best match. . .and, if Susan went through with it, and then Lynn rejected, she'd think it was all her fault. I don't think it was right of [her mother] to jump on her like she did. She was really upset. Oh. . .in the middle of all this her mother went down and got another doctor and brought him down. . . .It kind of put the doctor on the spot. I mean, it was a pretty heated situation. There were a lot of bad feelings. And everyone was tired. . .it was all very uneasy. This poor guy was brought into the middle of it, and he was supposed to explain. I think Harriet's mom

* A-match donors are usually more not less positive toward the donation (see Chapter 6).

> felt we hadn't understood what it meant to be the best one. The doctor didn't say too much, nothing we hadn't heard before. But after all that fuss Harriet finally said she'd do it. . .to save any more argument.

After Harriet made the decision to donate and was prepared to go through with it, her mother, probably feeling guilty, decided to refuse to let her donate and insisted on doing it herself.

HUSBAND. Actually there were two decisions. One that Susan would be it, and one that Harriet would be it. And then both of those were shoved back in our face. I felt pushed around!

INTERVIEWER. Do you feel there are bad feelings now in the family?

HUSBAND. Well, when [her mother] said all that to us that night. . .and it made me feel like she didn't think we knew how to make decisions. . .you can't forget things like that. I can say I don't have any bad feelings now, but I will always remember that night. I don't care what happens, I just won't forget it. Harriet has agreed with me.

When one sibling is the recipient and the others are potential donors, the role of the parent is often central. The mother is frequently a spokesman for the recipient and organizes the family donor decision-making. In some cases, as noted earlier in the chapter, the parents can prevent all siblings from volunteering. In others the parents themselves feel torn between the needs of the two siblings. In this case, a less frequent one, the parent pressures the siblings to volunteer. The children may resent the pressure on many grounds, one of which is the parent's continuing to make decisions for them despite their entry into adulthood. (Out of the 11 families in which pressure to donate constituted a major stress, the parent of the recipient and the potential donor was the offender in four cases. In five instances the recipient himself was guilty of pressuring his siblings.)

Nondonors View Donor Search As Stressful

Thus, although pressure to donate has been a source of anger for some volunteers and donors, it is more likely to have constituted a major stress for nondonors. In fact the nondonors view the donor search in general as more stressful than do other family members. On the questionnaire they are three times as likely as donors to agree that donation stimulated bad feelings within the family (23% vs. 7%). Furthermore when asked, "For many families it is easy to decide. . .who will donate. . . .For your family was it very difficult, somewhat difficult, a little difficult, or not at all difficult," 51% of the nondonors answered that it was "somewhat" or "very difficult," in contrast to only 18% of the recipients and 11% of the donors.

In addition, the nondonors were more likely to see the family communication process as blocked. Both donors and nondonors were asked the multiple-choice question:

> When your family was thinking or talking about the donor question, do you think (the patient) was told
>
> ——most things you were thinking or talking about
> ——only some of the things
> ——hardly anything the family was thinking about the donor question.

Fifty-eight percent of the donors felt the patient was well aware of most of others' thought processes, in comparison to only 40% of the nondonors. (This difference persists when the type of blood relationship to the recipient is controlled, and all the above differences remain if we restrict the number of nondonors to one per family as in the sample of random nondonors.)

Isolation of Recipient by Nondonors

Therefore, a large proportion of the major stress in these families involves anger expressed toward nondonors and to a lesser extent the nondonor's perceptions that pressure has been applied on him to donate. In some cases the conflict between nondonors and family is worsened because the nondonors begin to feel uncomfortable in the presence of the recipient and therefore avoid contact. At a time when the recipient is very ill, hospitalized, and in need of all types of family help, the nondonor avoids the patient, escalating whatever negative effects nondonation has already had on the relationship.

CASE Posttransplant interview with wife of a recipient

INTERVIEWER. Do you think your sister-in-law [the nondonor] feels guilty about not donating?

WIFE. I was talking about that with my brother. He said maybe she was feeling guilty and that's why she didn't visit when Dick was in the hospital in March and April. And even when we were home they didn't come to see Dick.

The qualitative coders were able to document 40 nondonors who reacted in this way (or 18% of those nondonors for whom we have clear information). Twenty-eight of these came from 11 families for whom the donor search constituted a major stress.

Even after the transplant the nondonors are less likely than volunteers to contact the recipient or the donor when they are in the hospital recovering from the operation. We listed all potential donors in the family and asked both the donor and recipient to indicate whether each person had visited them, telephoned, written, or made no contact during the recovery period. The nondonors were less likely to have visited and more likely to have made no contact at all with either party. Twenty percent of all nondonors had failed to contact the recipient in the first three weeks posttransplant, compared to 14% of family members who were excused from donating and only 3% of volunteers. These differences persist when prior emotional closeness to the recipient is controlled. Thus the donor search itself appears to lead the nondonor to avoid contact with the patient at a time of particular need.

Not only the recipient, but also the donor can be hurt by this isolation.

CASE Brother donates to brother; six siblings are nondonors

Interview with wife of a potential donor who had been excused

INTERVIEWER. Has [the donor] heard from his brothers or sisters recently?

SISTER-IN-LAW. [Tom, Jean, and Rita are the only ones who have had contact with him. Tom called Rita and she told him to get flowers and everything for the donor.] But he hasn't had a card or a telephone call from any of the others. I think they feel guilty.

INTERVIEWER. How does the donor feel about not having heard from his other brothers and sisters?

SISTER-IN-LAW. I think it hurts him that none of them have called him or anything.

Negative Feelings Toward Ambivalent Donors

Family anger at the nondonors and the nondonors' reaction of anger and withdrawal from the patient have been identified here as major sources of stress. Is anger at *donors* who demonstrate ambivalence also a source of major difficulty? As noted in Chapter 6, when the recipient perceived the donor as ambivalent, antagonism was likely to result at least temporarily.

The following case was the only one of this type classified as a major family stress.

CASE A sister had been worked up and accepted as a donor, but when the date for the transplant was set she refused to go ahead then because there was not enough time notice. Several months later she did donate, but in the interim the recipient and her husband became angry and upset.

Interview with recipient's husband before transplant

HUSBAND. It's just real hard cause we don't know where we stand now, and the hospital doesn't know and nobody knows. It's just kind of disgusting. . . .

INTERVIEWER. How does [the patient] feel about [her sister]?

HUSBAND. I think she's kind of disgusted with her. If she'd just say no. . .we could go ahead and either get [the brother] or get a cadaver. If we hadn't been waiting we probably could have had one by now. It's been about four months. . .What my wife and I are both thinking now is that if she does give we'll never hear the end of it.

INTERVIEWER. What do you mean?

HUSBAND. Well, just that anything little that might go wrong with her after this she would blame [on the donation]. She'd never let us forget.

The reluctant gift is less appreciated, even when major stress is not involved. Donors who had scored higher on the ambivalence scale prior to the transplant receive less gratitude from the recipient a year later ($r = -.15, p = .09$). They also are less likely to experience an improvement in their relationship with the recipient at a year posttransplant. Although 63% of the unambivalent donors report their relationship as closer than before (in answer to a multiple-choice question), only 43% of the ambivalent donors indicate such a change.

Conflict among Potential Donors

In this section, we have been reviewing the major family conflict that involves relatives who are less willing to donate. Not only is there mutual anger between unwilling relatives and the rest of the family, but in four cases of major stress, several ambivalent relatives appear to be in conflict with one another as to who will be the donor. Each hopes the other will be the one who actually will donate. The following case concerns one of the seven ambivalent donors cited earlier.

CASE The brother of recipient becomes the donor in a family where the recipient's son was also blood-tested. The brother was the best match; the son was also possible.

At the time of the donor work-up

BROTHER. I told my brother I thought his son should do it. He said, "You don't have to." That's what they all say—his son, his daughter. . ."You don't have to do it." But you do. If a man's drowning you don't have to save him but you probably would. . . .I don't like this position, and here I am. I don't like it at all. I feel his son should come in for these tests too, and after he has the tests then we can talk about it and make a more rational decision. Maybe he wouldn't even pass the tests, and then [I would do it and that would be it.] But I don't think anything should be decided until we're both tested. . . !

After some further conversation

INTERVIEWER. Does the son know how you feel?

BROTHER. Yes. He says, "You don't have to do it." [That really burns me.] When my brother called me and told me I was supposed to come in, I didn't know what was going on and I didn't want to say too much to him, so I called the son right away. I said, "Why did they call me in? Why aren't you going?" He said, "But you're the best [match]." I said, "Yes, but you could do it too. Why don't we both go in and have the tests and then we can talk it over and decide." He said, "I don't think they'll do that. It costs money you know." Yes, I suppose it does, but I still feel he should come in too with me. He said, "You don't have to go." They know when they said that what position it puts me in. They know I have to then. What can you say. . .?

After further conversation

BROTHER. [The son is] chicken. . .! He's really chicken, and I don't think it's fair!! He gets out because he's scared, and his father excuses him because they didn't call him in!!

Major stress involving competition between potential donors was not always an issue of unwilling family members. In one case the severe conflict was between two donors, both of whom wish to donate. The competition was generated by earlier family difficulties.

CASE Recipient (Louise) has two sisters and a mother who were tested. A sister is the donor

Interview with the donor sister

INTERVIEWER. How does your mother feel about your donating?

SISTER. She's kind of [jealous] I think.

INTERVIEWER. Why do you think that?

SISTER. I think she sees it as a competitive thing [for Louise's love].

INTERVIEWER. Has she said something, or done something to make you think this?

SISTER. It's just that she seems hostile about me being the donor instead of her.

Later in pretransplant questionnaire

INTERVIEWER. Was there anyone who was upset because he or she couldn't donate?

SISTER. My mother.

INTERVIEWER. Why was that?

SISTER. I don't know. One theory is that she wants to compensate for some of her own guilt. [Probe] Guilt as a mother. [Probe] I don't know what she'd ever done to feel guilty about, and I think she feels some guilt because of our relationship. I was in psychotherapy as a result of our relationship. Although she's always encouraged achievement and success, she's envious of anyone who achieves it. She was very jealous, particularly of my sister Helen because she's [somewhat successful], and she sees me [getting what I want out of life]. I think she sees this as a form of achievement.

INTERVIEWER. Donating?

SISTER. Yes.

COMMUNICATION PROBLEMS

Problems in the mutual family not only involve conflict with less willing donors and conflict between potential donors, but also difficulties in communication. Blocked communication in the mutual family is one special type of stress generated by the donor search, particularly by the need to request a donor. In 25 of the families where there was major stress it was a problem, though not necessarily the most intense one. These communication difficulties are analyzed in some detail both to clarify this common problem and to understand family communication processes in general better.

The communication process begins when the physician informs the patient or his spokesman of the need for a related donor. This spokesman tends to be the patient's spouse or mother. Somehow the patient or those closest to him must then communicate the need for a kidney to those relatives eligible to donate. Potential donors must be "asked" to donate, and subsequently a "response" is expected. Yet if the relative feels ambivalent or negative, this response becomes problematic.

Although communication patterns in decision-making have been extensively studied in the small-group laboratory situation, (Bavalas, 1950) and in large-scale organizations (Guetzkow, 1965), there have been few studies of the communication patterns as "normal" families make major decisions (Epstein and Westley, 1959; Hill, 1965; Morgan, 1968; Ruesch, 1957). The transplant situation provides a unique opportunity to observe family communication during such a major potentially stressful situation.

From our qualitative interviews we gathered a picture of considerably blocked communication channels both during the "request" stage and the "response" stage (see Simmons and Klein, 1972).

The Request Stage

After they identify the possible candidates for donation, the first problem for the recipient and perhaps his spouse is to inform the relatives that a donor is needed. If only considerations of efficiency were involved, the most rational procedure would probably be to contact each possible donor, explain the situation, ask whether he wished to donate, and request a reply one way or the other by a given date. In this way, if no family donors were available, the patient would know quickly and be able to have his name placed rapidly on the list for a cadaver-donor.

In many families a process like this does occur. Yet a strong norm inhibits this process at the outset. The norm expressed by a high percentage of the patients is that one should not *ask* for a kidney, one should wait for a volunteer. Recognizing the risk involved to the donor and the sacrifices he must make, the patient does not think he should be responsible for pressuring the donor into a decision. Thus patients and their spouses frequently feel under considerable constraint in communicating their need for a donor. To enhance the patient's chances for survival, they must somehow inform the relative that he could donate, yet they cannot be direct; they must hint.*

In some cases, despite the patient's attempt to conform to this norm, the pressure on the relative appears to be quite direct.

CASE A 30-year-old patient

PATIENT. I just told them I needed a donor. I wouldn't ask. If you ask you put someone on the spot.

INTERVIEWER. Could we go through this again, from the time you first mentioned donorship to your brother?

PATIENT. I called him and told him that mother had volunteered to donate but "if they won't accept mother, you'd be the only one."

In other cases, however, the request is a less direct one but just as obvious.

CASE A 35-year-old woman whose brother was the donor

INTERVIEWER. How was the question of a donor discussed?

DONOR. Well, my sister said to us right away she'd never ask any of us to donate. She said it was too big a decision to ask anyone to make. . .to ask of anyone.

Later the donor's wife was interviewed.

DONOR'S WIFE. I was down here and Jane was fussing about it and said she would never ask anyone. So I told her she wouldn't have to ask, that Steven had already volunteered.

Other patients attempt to communicate the request through joking.

* See Chapter 6 for a discussion of the directness of the request for a donor as it relates to family pressure, and Chapter 7 for an analysis of the differences between donors and nondonors in this regard.

CASE A 20-year-old boy talking about a sister, who never did volunteer to donate

PATIENT. I think Brenda would do it. . .When we're kidding around and I ask her if she wants to give me her kidney, she says no. But if I ask her serious, she'd do it. . .I know she'd do it.

Interview two months later with the sister

SISTER. Martin has never seriously talked to me about it. When my mom was going to donate he would say to her kiddingly "I don't want your kidney, I want *her* kidney [meaning sister's]."

In still other cases the request is made so indirectly that it is not clear whether the message has been received or not. In several instances the relative later claimed he did not realize he could donate or did not realize the need was imminent, while the patient has assumed that the lack of a response is a refusal or he is left unsure whether to ask for a cadaver donor or not.

CASE A 50-year-old man whose donor was his sister

Interview with wife

WIFE. They [the doctors] told me it was my job to ask every member but. . .I just didn't want to do it. I thought it was a very awkward situation to put a person in and as I was preparing myself to ask as a last resort—how I would do it and when would be the best time—in the midst of all this she offered.

INTERVIEWER. During your conversations, did Edith make any comments about the donation?

WIFE. I think I did most of the talking and she did most of the listening. . . .It wasn't like we were discussing it, I was just giving her information and hoped she would understand that we wanted her to offer, that I wanted a response, but I wasn't getting it.

INTERVIEWER. You were hoping that she would offer so you wouldn't have to ask?

WIFE. I was hoping I wouldn't have to ask but I didn't think it would work because it had been several days and I was trying to find a way to ask.

In this case the sister claimed that the reason she had not offered earlier was that she had not realized she was a potential donor; she had thought only brothers could donate to brothers. In other words, the indirectness of the request either prevented its being perceived clearly or allowed the sister to avoid making a decision.

CASE Patient communicated little information but seemed to assume, when no immediate response was forthcoming, that all siblings had refused

PATIENT. They all know I'm here. They all know I'm going to have a transplant. If they were going to donate, wouldn't they have called by now?

INTERVIEWER. How do you know that your brothers and sisters know that a donor is needed?

PATIENT. Oh, they know. My mom reads about it in magazines and in the newspaper. They know more than I do probably.

INTERVIEWER. [later] So your brothers and sisters haven't yet refused. . . .

PATIENT. I could call tomorrow and get a No.

Yet a few days later, after his wife had spoken to some of the family more directly, a sister volunteered and another sibling indicated she might consider donation.

Whether the indirect request is obvious enough to be accurately perceived, its very indirectness allows the relative not to respond: "If you ask, you put someone on the spot. They have to say something. But if you just leave it open, just make a statement, they can say nothing."

Tables 9-2 and 9-3 show that the "request" for a donor is most frequently made in a form that does not require an answer, as noted in Chapters 6 and 7. For those cases in which the initial approach to a possible donor is clear enough to code, only about 10 to 12% of the potential donors appear to be approached in a way that forces a direct answer. The largest proportion is informed only about the need for a transplant—that is, the donor-need is *assumed* to be obvious rather than explicitly mentioned. Another large proportion seems to be told about the need for a related donor, but no question of their willingness is directly posed (Table 9-2). Over time, as indicated earlier, the majority of potential donors appear to receive only such indirect requests. However, when an immediate offer is not forthcoming, another sizeable proportion of relatives are subject to a more direct approach (Table 9-3). Although the

TABLE 9-2 FIRST APPROACH TO A POTENTIAL DONOR—QUALITATIVE CODING[a]

	Donors (N = 94)		Nondonors (N = 127)		Blood-tested volunteers (N = 29)
Asked directly—an answer required					
Told to donate	2%		1%		—
Asked if would donate	4%	12%	11%	13%	10%
Statement, hard to avoid[b]	6%		1%		—
Asked more indirectly—answer not required					
Told "someone" in the family will have to donate	6%		1%		3%
Statement made about need for a donor	19%		32%		24%
Statement made about definite, or tentative need for a transplant; donor need only implied	42%		24%		45%
Ask for less than donation (ask to have blood test, to think it over)	12%		11%		—
Avoidable hint or joke[c]	10%		17%		17%
Donor need stated plus "You can't donate"	—		1%		—
	100%		100%		100%

[a] For donors and nondonors, this classification was added once the coding began and was not coded on the first cases done. Those potential donors who thought of the donor-need themselves and were not "asked" initially, are not included in this table.

[b] For example: "If you'd donate, you'd save me." "John needs a transplant; you're the only one with the right blood type." "The doctors would like to consider you as a possible donor."

[c] For example: "John needs a donor, I am willing to do it." "John needs a donor, mother can't do it." "I'm waiting for a cadaver since (no one can, Sam can't) donate." "I wouldn't take your kidney."

TABLE 9-3 REQUESTS TO POTENTIAL DONORS OVER TIME–QUALITATIVE CODING

	Donor (*N* = 72)		Nondonor (*N* = 289)		Blood-tested Volunteer (*N* = 49)	
Always asked directly—an answer required	14%		14%		10%	
First directly then more indirectly	0%		1%		5%	
First indirectly then more directly	35%		15%		28%	
Always asked indirectly—no answer required	51%		69%		58%	
Total clear, reliable cases	100% (57)		100% (163)		100% (40)	
Percentage of unreliability out of total	14%		16%		12%	
		21%		43%		18%
Percentage unclear out of total	7%		27%		6%	

unreliability for donors and volunteers is within reasonable limits and although many different family members were carefully interviewed about this point, as noted before, we must regard these data with some tentativeness. Slight changes in wording could turn what was reported as an indirect statement into what actually was an unavoidable question.

The Response Stage

The distinction being made here is between the request that forces a response and the request that allows the potential donor to say nothing. In fact, *lack of response* is a very common pattern of behavior in these families. Frequently the potential donor handles this difficult situation by saying nothing—he neither refuses, accepts, nor indicates he will consider the situation. He does not make excuses; he simply does not respond. This failure to respond may persist indefinitely, or in some cases for a period of time until a donor volunteers. In 30% of the cases in which there were eligible relatives, some potential family donors clearly showed this pattern of nonresponse, a pattern we term noncommunication; in 12% more of the families the evidence was less clear but pointed in this direction. Fourteen percent of the nondonors never responded at all to the request, at any time in the donor search.

In all of these cases of noncommunication the story is similar.

CASE *A 19-year-old girl; her 20-year-old brother was the donor*

DONOR. She just asked if I would give her one of my kidneys. I didn't know what to say, so I didn't say anything. [Then later]. . .she asked me again and I didn't say anything. But when I found out how sick she was I said okay.

CASE *A 30-year-old recipient talks about one married sister*

PATIENT. My sister in Pennsylvania has been pretty vague. Whenever I've written to ask her she doesn't answer about it. It's like I hadn't asked the question.

This noncommunication can persist for several months.

CASE *A 56-year-old father whose married children were potential donors*

Interview with the recipient

PATIENT. I saw Paul first because he was here. I told him that I was going to have a transplant and that the doctors said to line up donors.

INTERVIEWER. What did Paul say?

PATIENT. He didn't say anything at all.

Later interview with Paul's wife

INTERVIEWER. Did he [the patient] ask Paul if he would donate?

DAUGHTER-IN-LAW. No, he would never do that. He would never pressure anyone. He just said that if any of the children wanted to, they could go in to be tested.

INTERVIEWER. What did Paul say?

DAUGHTER-IN-LAW. Nothing.

INTERVIEWER. Has Paul ever said anything to you about it?

DAUGHTER-IN-LAW. Yes, I brought it up with him. . . .I asked if he would donate. He said he couldn't donate and didn't want to talk about it. I didn't bring it up after that.

Interview with Paul after the transplant

PAUL. One brother didn't have the right blood type. . . .My father mentioned [to me] about who else could donate.

INTERVIEWER. What was it that you said about it?

PAUL. I didn't say anything at the time. It was kind of brought up and then dropped and we talked about other things. We never really discussed it.

The lack of response by the relatives can be very uncomfortable for the patient and his spouse.

CASE A 45-year-old female patient

Interview with her husband

INTERVIEWER. Have you thought any more about what you will do about the donor question?

HUSBAND. She keeps hinting and hinting [to her brothers and sisters] but nobody says anything.

INTERVIEWER. How does she hint? To her brother Thomas, for instance?

HUSBAND. Like she [says she] wouldn't want his kidney anyway, because he's so mean or something.

INTERVIEWER. And what would Thomas say then?

HUSBAND. Nothing.

INTERVIEWER. Well, after your wife says something like this hint to one of her family members, what do they say next? Do they ignore it, or change the subject or mention some reason why they aren't so well themselves, or walk away, or what?

HUSBAND. They just kind of leave it hanging up in the air. They just laugh, kind of—you know. They don't say anything. She doesn't ask them, so they don't have to say. She just jokes and they laugh.

INTERVIEWER. Have any of them said they wouldn't?

HUSBAND. No, but none of them said they would, either. They're kind of on the fence.

INTERVIEWER. Have any of them said they'd think about it?

HUSBAND. No, they don't say anything.

Potential donors who wish to postpone the difficult decision-making and avoid the entire problem find noncommunication comfortable.*

CASE Brother of a potential transplant recipient who later became the donor

Interview at time of blood test

He had heard of the possibility of a transplant a year before, put it out of his mind, and is now telling of when it became definite.

BROTHER. This was probably just last month. They had been at our house. In fact, they came over to our house one night and we had company there. So they came back the next day because they wanted to talk about it. There were always people there, so they couldn't talk confidentially. Then they came back that noon. That's when she really said she'd have to have it.

INTERVIEWER. What did you say when your sister said to you that she'd have to have a kidney?

BROTHER. I don't know if I said anything. It's really something. You don't know what to say.

INTERVIEWER. Right, I can understand.

BROTHER. It kind of knocks the wind from your sails. You know it has to be done. But you don't want to admit you know this.

INTERVIEWER. Did you actually not say anything or did you change the subject, or what?

BROTHER. I think we sat down to eat dinner.

INTERVIEWER. What did you think when you heard what the patient said?

BROTHER. I think I knew it was coming. I knew that's what she'd need. You suspect it all along. You're aware of the time coming, and

* In fact 67% of those nondonors who followed a postponement decision-making pattern demonstrated noncommunication, in contrast to 39% of those who made an immediate decision not to donate and 33% who were classified as following a pattern of deliberation (see Chapter 8).

you're afraid the time is coming closer. . .and one day you see their car, and you know the time has come.

INTERVIEWER. Was it awkward for you that day, not saying anything, or wasn't it really?

BROTHER. Not really. I went back to work. I just kind of put it out of my mind somewhat.

Of course there are also a great many families in which the immediate response is quite direct. This is usually the case when the relative who is contacted volunteers immediately upon hearing of the need, as did the majority of donors (see Chapter 8). Relatives who demonstrate the pattern of noncommunication are frequently those who never volunteer to donate.

In summary intensive study of the family communication patterns in the search for a kidney donor has revealed that in a sizeable minority of cases communication is considerably blocked. Many transplant patients do not believe they should ask directly for a donor, and many potential donors who have not yet volunteered do not appear to communicate any feelings about donation to the patient. In fact, the coders classified communication as generally "very blocked" between recipients and 6% of the donors, 50% of the nondonors, and 15% of the blood-tested volunteers.

What are the consequences of this noncommunication? We cannot assume that closed communication channels are totally maladaptive in this situation.

Our impression is that during the long period prior to the transplant the stress level of the patient in many cases is increased by the noncommunication. In 65% (25 out of 46) of the families classified as cases showing major stress, there is clear noncommunication during the donor search, in contrast to only 10% of the families with no stress. The uncertainty may be particularly difficult for the recipient, especially before he feels free to apply for a cadaver donor. As the wife of one patient said, "Well, he'd like to know one way or another, but he won't say anything. I say to him, 'I wish they'd shit or get off the pot;' put it in plain language. He agrees with me, but he won't say it himself."

The period of time before the patient receives his transplant may be lengthened by this uncertainty. In addition, to maintain this noncommunication, some relatives find themselves unable to maintain any contact with the patient.

However, if the relative feels he cannot make the sacrifice of donation, the fact that he does not refuse outright serves some important functions. It allows him to save face and to avoid directly insulting or hurting the patient. When asked, "Why do you think you did not discuss this?" one patient's brother said, "Well, I suppose you're a little scared to face him and tell him you're turning him down"; another patient's daughter said, "I just didn't know how to tell her I didn't feel I could donate. . . .It's kind of hard to say that to a person who's lying there and that's their only hope; so I just never brought it up."

The indirect request of the patient, by allowing the potential donors to avoid replying, also protects both the patient and the relative from a direct insult and severe embarrassment. In many extended families the ties can be very fragile and might not be able to sustain such a direct blow. Or the relationship may appear too important to endanger by an open refusal. In the words of one sister who did not communicate her doubts: "I try to put myself in her place. How would I feel if someone came and told me, 'I'm not going to help you.' I think I would resent him the rest of my life."

Noncommunication also allows the *undecided* relative to avoid either committing himself or refusing prematurely.

CASE Interview with son of recipient

INTERVIEWER. How did you find out they would consider family? Can you tell me who told you that and what they said?

SON. I was sitting in her room with my Dad and my older brother. . . anyway, we were sitting there and I was looking at the paper. I heard them talking about it. It really threw me for a loop. Just out of the blue. I didn't know they were even considering it.

INTERVIEWER. Was your mother telling it?

SON. No, my dad.

INTERVIEWER. What was he saying?

SON. Well, because we figured no family could do it, my two sisters-in-law had said they would do it. I just heard him say that they would be ruled out, but there was a chance the family could. He said the family would be better. It just came out that we were eligible anyway. I don't know how I felt then. Mixed up!

INTERVIEWER. What did you think?

SON. It kind of shook me.

INTERVIEWER. Did your brother say anything?

SON. No he didn't. He didn't say anything, not really. He's my one brother who has diabetes and I was the only one there besides Mom and my brother.

INTERVIEWER. What did you say at that time?

SON. I didn't say anything.

INTERVIEWER. Did you just keep reading the paper, or what? Did you say anything?

SON. No, I didn't because before I said I'd do it I wanted to be sure. So I didn't say anything.

INTERVIEWER. Was it awkward not saying anything?

SON. Yes, a little. My mother was laying there in bed. I just kept reading.

INTERVIEWER. Did you feel they expected you to say something, or wasn't it like that?

SON. Yes, I think my mother kind of hoped I would. I don't know if she expected it or not, but I think she probably hoped I would.

The long-term consequences of this pretransplant noncommunication are discussed below.

One might expect the pattern of noncommunication identified here to be generalizable to a wider variety of situations in which one extended family member asks help of another. This block in communication may be maladaptive from the point of view of the efficiency and rapidity with which the problem that generated the call for help can be solved. Yet the noncommunication may have positive functions for family cohesion and individual comfort.

PROBLEMS OF GRATITUDE

Family tension because of less willing donors and blockages in family communication thus constitute areas of major stress in the mutual family, that is, in the family segment that includes the recipient and potential donors.

The expression of gratitude between donor and recipient is the final major source of stress in the mutual family to be discussed. In Chapters 3 and 6 we noted that the issue of gratitude did not constitute a problem for the vast majority of donors, because they received abundant praise and thanks. Nor did *most* recipients feel overburdened by enormous debt, although some cases of guilt were noted. In three instances, however, the donor's anger at receiving too little gratitude was defined as a major stress. Where the donor received little gratitude, anger at being manipulated and used seemed to develop. In addition to the cases reported in Chapter 6, the following case is illustrative:

CASE Recipient who rejected her brother's kidney

Interview with a sister after rejection

SISTER. She didn't even seem to appreciate what Irv did. . . .She wasn't even very nice. She acted like his kids were brats. . . .I think too the doctors advised against her driving. She just said to heck with that, and she was driving all over. She didn't care. You feel, why be cut open if she isn't going to take care of herself. . . .

INTERVIEWER. How do you think Irv feels now about having donated?

SISTER. I think he kind of regrets it.

INTERVIEWER. Do you? Why do you think that?

SISTER. He said to me once he kind of regretted it. Because she didn't appreciate it, and he said, "Now it's just in the garbage." Then the deal with his kid when she called [the kid] a brat. His kid was pushed off on other people while [Irv and his wife] were here [in the hospital]. I'd think she would consider that affect on [the child]. But it doesn't seem like she appreciated Irv at all.

Two patterns appear in the few cases where gratitude issues lead to anger. First, as in the above case, the donors felt as if they are "suckers." when no appreciation is forthcoming. Second, as illustrated in Chapter 6 (see p. 174) and earlier in this chapter, if the donor either demands too much gratitude or acts ambivalent about the gift, the recipient becomes angry, belittles the gift and the donor, perhaps labelling him as selfish. In one case the mother who had been conscious of her daughter's ambivalence at donating to her, reacted with anger when the daughter complained postoperatively. "[I said to her]'I didn't tell you about my labor pains.' And that shut her up." The recipient, angry at the daughter's earlier demands for gifts and expressions of gratitude, attempted to cancel the debt by reminding her that as a mother she had once suffered bodily pain to give her life. The daughter, instead of being perceived as donor of an extraordinary gift, is defined as reciprocating the mother's prior sacrifices. The parallel of childbirth and kidney donation is emphasized once again.

Many donors appear anxious to avoid conflicts over gratitude. Some state emphatically that they do not want the recipient to feel overburdened by guilt and indebtedness.

CASE *Brother who donated to brother*

I don't make him feel he should pay me back because he doesn't owe me anything. . . .I don't want him to feel grateful. I don't want him to feel anything. He doesn't owe me a thing.

In particular, parents of young children are happy to see their children accept their giving as a natural act, without undue expression of gratitude.

CASE *Mother who donates to a 12-year-old daughter*

Five days after the transplant in the donor's hospital room

INTERVIEWER. Has Carol talked directly with you since the transplant about how she feels about your donating or not?

MOTHER. No.

INTERVIEWER. What do you think she feels about your donating?

MOTHER. Well, I'm sure she's very grateful because she knew it was life or death. I haven't pushed for her to see me before I'm better because I don't want my condition to have any effect on how she feels. If she is grateful fine, but that's not the reason I did it. The only reason I did it was to give Carol life and I don't ever want it pointed out that her mother did this great thing.

CASE *Mother who donated to her eight-year-old daughter*

MOTHER. I think to her it's just one of the things a mother does. It's no big deal to her. We watch "Girl in my Life" on TV. I said, "Why don't you get me into that program?" She said, "What did you do?" [Laughs]

INTERVIEWER. Did she express any gratitude to you about donating or wouldn't that be like her?

MOTHER. I guess so. We're kind of close. I don't think she has to. I think kids just take things as they come.

Some donors become upset with indication that the recipient feels indebted; they see the closeness of their relationship jeopardized by it.

DONOR FATHER. If I were going to be hypersensitive, I would suspect he almost resents that he got in a position where he's beholding to me.

In summary, indebtedness is a potential problem for donor and recipient. Usually, however, a great deal of gratitude is voiced, which seems to add to the donor's general exhilaration at donating. One donor who told us she was "delighted" every time she thought about the donation also reports happily:

> My brother [the recipient]and his wife bought me a sofa and chair just to show their appreciation for what I did. They know I couldn't afford it. They have said that no amount of money could ever be enough for what I did.

But where such gratitude is not expressed easily, donors are less positive over the long run (see Chapter 6). At one extreme when the recipient is thought to take the gift for granted, the donors feel manipulated. At the other extreme where the feeling of debt on the part of the recipient is too great, the donors are saddened by the barrier to closeness that has arisen. Finally, if the gift is given with reluctance or with clear "strings attached," the recipient feels less gratitude and in the extreme is angered. The dynamics underlying these patterns are discussed further in the concluding chapter.

LONG-RANGE OUTCOME OF STRESS

We have documented in detail the distress that does occur in some cases during the donor search—the *internal* ambivalence of potential volunteers, the internal guilt of the recipient, the *conflict between* potential *donors and their spouses*, the conflict and stress within the *mutual family* as feelings of anger are directed toward and reciprocated by less willing family members, as the need to request a donor results in blocked communication, and as problems of gratitude emerge between donor and recipient.

The stress generated in 46 cases is indeed dramatic. Yet, as noted earlier for most families the donor-search generates no clear or significant distress, and for many donors and recipients the donation proves to be a highly rewarding emotional experience. In addition, the stress that does occur must be examined relative to the other events occurring at the same time. The stress arising from the donor search may be temporary, coinciding with and perhaps exaggerated by, the crisis of fatal illness in a family member. The tension of the illness may in itself leave key family members emotionally vulnerable and unable in the midst of crisis to solve the donor problem with equanimity. Central family members may have difficulty coping with any major decision at this time of grief and anxiety.

Perhaps the most important question is what happens after the period of crisis has passed, after the patient is successfully transplanted and the donor issue resolved in one way or another. What are the long-range consequences of the donor search? Do the wounds opened pretransplant leave significant scars for the family?

We have noted that a lesser closeness to nondonors and a residual anger toward them does remain in a sizeable minority of families (17%) at a year after the transplant. Also, in some cases gratitude toward donors who give reluctantly is less than that directed toward more willing donors. Yet if we attempt to examine the families in which there was major stress during the donor search and in which the transplant was successful, we find few where the stress level still appears significant one year later. Out of the 46 families where there was significant stress originally, 34 of the recipients are relevant for this analysis—that is, they were actually transplanted and maintained their new kidneys for at least a year.

In only two of these 34 cases were we aware of major distress at a year posttransplant. One case involved the ambivalent donor reported earlier who was glad to have helped the recipient but still experienced major anxiety about his own physical well-being and great anger toward other ungrateful relatives. In the second case the recipient remained very bitter toward one nondonor and had severed contact with her, and the donor also reported residual anger and lack of contact with this nondonor.

In addition to these two cases, there were two others in which some active negative feelings were still evident, although they no longer appeared to reach major proportions—One involved resentment of nondonors, and one concerned a donor's irritation at the lack of gratitude expressed by the recipient.

Finally, in two cases discussed earlier in which the husbands opposed their wives' donation, no major active distress was evident at a year, but the donation had a lasting effect on the donors' marriages. The first is the case in which the donor and her husband were divorced after the donation, and the second involves a situation in which the woman began to redefine her role as a result of having made a decision to donate against her husband's will:

> My husband hated the whole idea. He's gotten better about that. But if the transplant was part of awakening my self-consciousness, it also made my marriage definitely more difficult. . . .He was always telling me he wanted me to be more independent, but he doesn't.

Thus out of the 34 families at issue, two still show some major distress, two some moderate levels of hostility, and two show permanent marital scars. However, we may have overlooked some persistent problems. Our information at a year posttransplant is usually based only on interviews with recipient and donor. Although these interviews explore family stress, problems of which these parties are unaware would be missed, particularly internal feelings of nondonors.

REINTEGRATING THE FAMILY

In most families there was a definite tendency to forgive prior transgressions after the transplant and to attempt to reintegrate the family. In some cases this attempt was quite conscious, as can be seen by a comparison of pre- and posttransplant interviews.

CASE The recipient's wife had been angry because her husband's sister had criticized her for mentioning the possibility of donation

Pretransplant interview

WIFE. I talked to my sister-in-law and immediately got a lecture about opening my mouth too much. . . .As soon as I got there I got a lecture from his sister that I was too openmouthed and that I shouldn't lay all the cards down on the table at once. . .[The sister said] "You just shut up."

INTERVIEWER. Has there been any conversation with the family since then?

WIFE. No. Not only that, but they haven't even offered to donate blood. My family has offered to donate blood already. . . .

INTERVIEWER. Were you surprised [the sister] wasn't donating?

WIFE. I was surprised that I got bawled out.

Two months posttransplant

INTERVIEWER. [reviewing the same story] Did you tell your husband what your sister-in-law said?

WIFE. He was right there. . . .But I don't believe in holding grudges. Forgive and forget. . . .There's no use fighting about it now. Your feelings just get hurt and everyone gets unhappy.

The wife then explains that the sister has offered much practical aid to the patient since the transplant.

CASE At a year posttransplant, another recipient tells of a conflict with his wife three months after the transplant as to treatment of a nondonor sibling

INTERVIEWER. Was there anyone in your family who might have been able to donate a kidney to you but for some reason didn't offer?

RECIPIENT. Yes. . .Joan. After she came for the tests, she said she'd be back in ten days to finish the tests and we never heard from her again. . . .

INTERVIEWER. How do others in the family feel now toward those who might have donated but didn't? Since the transplant does the rest of the family seem to be closer, less close, or is there no change?

RECIPIENT. Less close. My wife. She didn't want to even see Joan when she came to visit [after the transplant] or send her a Christmas card. But I explained to her that it was water under the bridge. . . . She's OK now.

There is an elation that follows a successful transplant, an elation that frequently permeates the entire family. In this type of mood the feelings that arise during the tense pretransplant period dissipate and can be forgiven and forgotten, especially because in many cases these feelings were never communicated directly to the party concerned.

The nondonor can attempt to reintegrate his position by offering aid. In a small number of cases (11 cases) the nondonor gave gifts or money to the donor or paid some of his expenses. Forty-seven percent of the nondonors to whom we spoke said they had helped the recipient by taking care of his children, driving him to and from the hospital, giving him money or a place to live, or cleaning house. In these cases, through gifts of less importance than a kidney, the nondonor attempts to reestablish his old position. The gift of a kidney is repaid with an intensified emotional closeness, although many recipients believe no adequate exchange can be made. The nondonor cannot expect like-gratitude back for his gifts; he can expect only to counteract some of the loss he has sustained by making clear to the recipient that he was unwilling to suffer a major sacrifice on his behalf.

DENIAL OF PRIOR CONFLICT AND NONDONATION

This tendency to close up ranks in the elation of posttransplant success coincides with the psychological motivation of the recipient to avoid the painful recognition that some family members may not have cared enough to donate. At a year after the transplant some recipients definitely appear to be trying to "cover up" the fact that certain members of their family failed to volunteer. Whether they are distorting reality for themselves or for outsiders like us is unclear. In reality, 59% of families contained at least one nondonor, and prior to the transplant 56% of patients who were to have successful transplants reported the existence of nondonors in their families. Yet at a year posttransplant, in answer to the same multiple-choice question, only 31% of these same recipients indicated that someone in their family "could have been tested but was not."

Further evidence of this process of denial is obtained from the coding of the qualitative material from those families in which there was either nondonation or conflict over donation. At three weeks after the transplant 10% of recipients from such families showed clear evidence of trying to cover up the nondonation or conflict, and this proportion rose to 18% at a year posttransplant.

The following cases illustrate this process of denial. Patients upset pretransplant about the indecision and nondonation of some relatives appear able posttransplant to repress these prior problems and tell us that all eligible relatives volunteered.

CASE Two of the recipient's siblings were nondonors

Pretransplant the recipient talks about her siblings and expresses sorrow about the nondonation of one of them

Pretransplant

INTERVIEWER. I believe you said the first time I talked to you. . .you felt that James had talked Lucy and Helen into it [volunteering to donate]. . . .Is that right?

RECIPIENT. Yes. I still think James probably talked Lucy into it.

INTERVIEWER. How did you feel about it. . .thinking that James had probably talked Lucy into it?

RECIPIENT. I think that's probably the reason why Helen is here [alone]. . . [one of the reasons]. Lucy probably backed out. [Interviewer detected a tear here.]

INTERVIEWER. I think you also said that at one time Lucy said to you she thought it would be all right if you remained on the machine, instead of having a transplant?

RECIPIENT. Yes.

INTERVIEWER. How did you feel when she said this?

RECIPIENT. Well, I felt quite sad. . .to think she would want me to continue on the machine.

Three weeks posttransplant

INTERVIEWER. When your family was thinking or talking about the transplant and the question of finding a donor, did they talk to you about it directly and clearly, or did they only hint at it indirectly?

RECIPIENT. They really all just said, "We'll donate!"

INTERVIEWER. Who said that?

RECIPIENT. All my brothers and sisters and children.

Thus, in many cases the recipient and family attempted to deny the fact that some members of their family had not volunteered.

In cases where the nondonation *was* recognized posttransplant, stress was still avoided, because the recipient accepted the nondonors' reasons as compelling. For 11% of the nondonors, according to the qualitative coding, the recipient indicated that the decision not to donate was understandable and excusable. In this regard several recipients stated that they were uncertain whether they themselves would have donated had the tables been reversed.

THE ROLE OF NONCOMMUNICATION

Noncommunication appears to facilitate the ability of the recipient later to distort reality and to deny the prior unwillingness of relatives to donate to him. In many families the "request" was made indirectly in the form of a hint, and the potential donor acted as if he had not heard the request and made no definite reply. This pattern of noncommunication may have aided the process of reintegrating the family and denying nondonation. The nondonors' ability to give help to the posttransplant patient and to resume interaction may have been easier when the requests for a donor, the refusals, and the temporary indecisions had not been directly voiced, and when the patient's anger at his relatives had not been communicated. The indirectness of the earlier communication may have helped both the recipient and the nondonor to minimize the latter's prior unwillingness.

There is evidence that families that utilized noncommunication prior to the transplant were more likely to deny nondonation after the transplant. Thirty-eight percent of the recipients from families in which there was obvious noncommunication pretransplant showed evidence of "covering up" nondonation at a year posttransplant, in comparison to only 7% of recipients from other families. (Only families in which there were non-donors or conflict over donation were included in these calculations.)

ROLE OF THE CRISIS IN ENHANCING FAMILY COHESION

Crisis, in this case the crisis of fatal illness and the need for a major family sacrifice, can expose and further weaken the most vulnerable linkages within the family. Distress, hurt, anger, and conflict all may intensify at this period. Yet the family seems quite able to reintegrate and smooth over the problems once the initiating crisis is over. Scars remain but are hidden and denied.

For a few family members, however, the crisis period does not act to aggravate old wounds but to heal them, at least temporarily. Old petty differences may be overlooked in the face of the potential death of a mutual loved one. Shared concern can bring new closeness. For some relatives, the attempt to use the crisis to heal relationships is a conscious one.

CASE Donor's wife hopes transplant will bring her closer to husband [Jonathan] and her in-laws

Pretransplant interview with donor's wife [concerning her in-laws]

DONOR'S WIFE. We just don't communicate well. They don't approve of me and my life. They don't like me. . . .They have never approved of me and my marriage.

INTERVIEWER. How has Jonathan been with you here this time?

DONOR'S WIFE. I think we've been closer, believe it or not. I feel we're closer somehow. I'm just hoping it will stay permanently. I feel like I'm here mostly just to support him and not for any of the rest of the family or to worry anybody. I think maybe Jonathan is growing up a little with all of this. He's really quite a little boy. But I feel like he's a little more sensitive somehow. Our marriage isn't what you'd call the most perfect. It's pretty shaky in fact. I just hope we can stay as close as we are now for a while anyway.

Posttransplant interview

INTERVIEWER. How are things with you and your mother-in-law?

DONOR'S WIFE. Well, surprisingly I think we're getting on quite well! I think it's better than ever before. But you know, I don't think the family's ever been this close before. It sure has brought everyone together. Everyone just has to keep reminding each other to [keep together and not quarrel or snap at each other.] You know, it's easy to snap, and sometimes not really mean it. . .but I think everyone's really very good, really. Especially Jonathan.

INTERVIEWER. He's been especially good?

DONOR'S WIFE. Well, yes. [He's just been] so much warmer or something. He's been really good to me up here.

INTERVIEWER. [I'm happy to hear that.]

DONOR'S WIFE. Yes. I just hope it lasts. He's really a different person. I think he's less self-centered and. . .just warmer.

In some cases the increased closeness vanishes after the transplant, along with the crisis of illness:

CASE The recipient is a preschool child [Sally] whose parents have had a difficult marriage

Pretransplant interview

FATHER. It [the marriage] would have been worse without Sally. She takes up so much of her time. [My wife] doesn't go out for sports or clubs like some women. . . .So if she didn't have Sally to keep her busy, she'd have more time to complain about me [and find fault with the marriage.] And with the transplant and everything the doctors are always forcing us to be together, talking to us together, [asking questions of us together].

Interview one year posttransplant

INTERVIEWER. We had a long talk last year and you told me that you were having some problems in your marriage. How is that?

FATHER. The same.

INTERVIEWER. Has the transplant affected or changed this?

FATHER. No.

INTERVIEWER. You told me last year that for a while the transplant seemed to bring you and your wife closer together.

FATHER. That was just at the time, for a short while.

INTERVIEWER. But the transplant has had no long-term effect on the marriage?

FATHER. No.

Even in families where there are no major problems, the transplant and donation crisis may intensify family closeness by reasserting important life-values (see Chapter 6).

CASE Sister is volunteer

SISTER. . . .Another thing is I can't believe how much closer this has brought our family. We were always close, but we're definitely closer now.

INTERVIEWER. How has it brought you closer?

SISTER. Everybody always just would come and go in the family. We'd never sit and talk. Everything was all fun and games. Now we sit and we get our feelings out, and we tell each other now we care. Just the last month and a half all of us have been together so much. This Thanksgiving was the first time in my whole life all my family sat down to a meal together. I mean, like on holidays, some would be there at noon and then leave and some others would come later. But the family was all together. It's really great.

> And it's funny. . .little things. . .you do for each other that you know mean a lot to the other person, and they aren't anything. . .but we never did them before.

In fact, we asked both nondonors and donors the following question: Do you think your family has been brought closer together by the transplant experience or not? Although donors perceived a greater increase in family cohesion than did nondonors, the majority of both groups characterized the family as closer after the transplant. Fifty-nine percent of the nondonors, 62% of the random nondonors,* and 71% of the donors answered that the family had grown closer.

SUMMARY

Although the donor issue is not a problem in the majority of cases, stress during the donor search was major in approximately one-quarter of the families. Primary causes of stress were the hurt and anger felt toward nondonors and the nondonors' angry feeling that they had been pressured to donate. By and large, however, neither type of anger was expressed directly to the person who was its target.

Other issues generating major stress, albeit in only a few cases apiece, involved donor ambivalence, nondonor guilt, recipient guilt at accepting a kidney, recipient fear that a kidney would not be forthcoming, mutual relatives' distress at seeing two loved ones (donor and recipient) at risk, communication difficulties in asking for a kidney and understanding the response, and problems of gratitude between recipient and donor. In addition, there were two examples of severe conflict between volunteers and their own spouses, who were opposed to donation.

The communication problems involved in requesting a kidney are of particular interest to the study of social interaction. A pattern was identified that probably occurs in many situations where one party asks a favor of another, and the latter wishes to deny the favor without jeopardizing the relationship or embarrassing the favor-seeker. The request is made so indirectly that it can be ignored. When the second party ignores the request and does not respond, the person making the request is not sure that the question was heard at all. Although this pattern may have favorable long-term consequences for the particular relationship, uncertainty and stress may be intensified at the time the favor is needed. In the

* See Chapter 7. Because there is only one donor per family, a sample of random nondonors was selected limiting the number of nondonors also to one per family.

case of the donor search the recipient does not know if he will obtain a related donor at a time when speed of decision is essential.

Thus, the crises of fatal illness and the need for a family member to make a major sacrifice produced major stress in some cases. Yet this stress of the donor search appeared temporary in all but a few cases of successful transplants. Once the crisis had been successfully resolved, a process of denying and minimizing past conflict and nondonation, or at least trying to forgive these prior insults, began. Although there was a long-term cost in terms of a lesser closeness to nondonors or ambivalent donors, these feelings were not openly discussed and there appeared to be an attempt to reintegrate the family.

It has been hypothesized that the earlier barriers to full communication—the failure of many nondonors to make their refusals clear, the fact that anger was not expressed directly between recipients and nondonors may have facilitated the later denial of past problems and reintegration of family.

For members of some families, the transplant crisis did not intensify conflict, but was an opportunity to overcome earlier family tension and to institute closer relationships. Whether anticipated or not, the successfully handled crisis was perceived by the majority of donors and nondonors to have the effect of making the family a closer one. Where the transplant was a success, increased family cohesion appeared to be an unintended consequence.

It is difficult to weigh the gains for the majority of recipients and donors against the severe, temporary tension focused mainly on nondonors in a minority of families. This issue is discussed to a greater extent in the concluding chapter. However, it should be noted that the absence of a donor search might not have reduced the overall level of stress in these families. If living related donors had not been used, many recipients who have survived would not have done so. The stress associated with an increased level of kidney rejection and death might have equalled or surpassed the stress of the donor search.

10

THE CADAVER DONOR AND THE GIFT OF LIFE

JULIE FULTON
ROBERT FULTON
and ROBERTA SIMMONS

Stress and ethical dilemmas are elements that are present in almost all aspects of organ transplantation. In the drama of transplant surgery the stresses and ethical problems encountered by the family of the cadaver-patient are often overlooked. To illuminate this aspect of transplantation we undertook a small exploratory study of families whose relatives had served as cadaver organ donors at the University of Minnesota Hospitals.

In this preliminary research we were interested in exploring the impact of the cadaver donation experience on the family as a unit as well as its impact on the individual family members. In particular we focused on the family members' perception of the decision-making process, their emotional reactions to the death and the donation, and their assessment of the problems the donation may have caused for them as well as the benefits it may have provided.

The size of the sample as well as its diversity means that we can claim only an impressionistic quality for the findings. Nevertheless, this study is the only one of its kind, and the issues suggested by the findings are important even in preliminary form.

METHOD

THE SAMPLE

We defined as our basic population all families whose relatives had served as cadaver donors at the University of Minnesota Hospitals during the period for January 1971 to May 1972 and who, at the time of the interview (a year and a half later) still lived within a 20-mile radius of the Twin Cities of Minneapolis and St. Paul. Seventeen families met these criteria, 12 of whom were subsequently interviewed in an unstructured open-ended interview. Three families refused to be interviewed, and two families agreed to be interviewed but failed to appear at the scheduled times. Among the families interviewed there was one extended family unit in which there had been two separate accidents resulting in two separate donations.

We also have included, for purposes of this analysis, earlier interviews conducted with two families whose relatives had served as cadaver donors prior to January 1971.

We attempted to interview all members of the donor's immediate family who were in the Twin Cities area as well as other relatives who played a significant role in the decision to donate. The sampling restriction as to residence and the stressful nature of the interview's subject matter meant that several potential respondents were lost. A total of 35 relatives from 14 families were interviewed: Spouses, parents, siblings, grandparents, and in-laws were among those who participated. The respondents ranged in age from eight to over 65.

Only families who agreed to the cadaver donation were interviewed. Family processes may have been different in families where the donation was refused.

THE CADAVER-PATIENTS

Table 10-1 shows the age, sex, and cause of death of the cadaver donors. They are predominantly male, young, and single. The sudden unex-

TABLE 10-1 CAUSE OF DEATH OF 15 CADAVER-PATIENTS[a]

Sex	*Age*	*Cause of death*
Self-inflicted injury		
Male	21	Suicide (gunshot wound to head)
Male	26	Suicide (gunshot wound to head)
Congenital weaknesses		
Male	24	Aneurysm
Male	30	Aneurysm
Male	8	Aneurysm
Female	$3\frac{1}{2}$	Pneumonia following open heart surgery
Accidental injury		
Male	19	Two-car collision
Male	16	Car-truck accident
Male	15	Car-train accident
Male	20	Motorcycle accident
Male	20	Motorcycle-car accident
Male	6	On bicycle, hit by motorcycle
Male	17	Fell off car trunk when car started to move in parking lot
Female	15	Pedestrian, hit by car
Female	10	Suffocated in snowdrift while playing

[a] Only three patients (all male) were married, and each of them was the father of young children.

pected character of their deaths is evident. In no instance were these the only children in their family; the average number of children was 4.6, slightly larger than the national average.

DISCUSSION

THE USUAL DONATION PROCEDURE*

The "usual" donation procedure is somewhat difficult to describe because during the time in which these interviews were conducted,

* For more detail about the technology and procedure of cadaver donation, see Chapter 2.

several changes in the donation process took place. These changes were instituted either as a result of technological improvements in the storage of organs or as a result of the information obtained from our respondents in the early interviews. For example, some of the first interviews revealed that relatives were anxious to know the time of death of the cadaver-patient and time of the transplant operation, and they wished some knowledge about the person to whom the organs were given. As a result of our informing the transplant service of these concerns, a program of telephoned and written communication was established with the family of the cadaver-patient. Later interviews with other families, therefore, did not reflect the same areas of concern.

In addition, the invention of a kidney preservation machine, which allows plasma to be circulated through the removed and stored kidney for two to three days, means that the brain-dead patient himself no longer has to perform a storage function while the transplant recipient is prepared for surgery. Most of the families interviewed in this study were interviewed before the advent of this machine, and in these cases the cadaver-patient had to be transferred from the admitting hospital to the University Hospital where he/she was reevaluated by a new team of neurologists and, if brain death were confirmed, was declared by them to be officially dead. Various machinery subsequently artificially maintained his/her circulation, respiration, and kidney function for hours or days until one or two suitable transplant recipients could be located, transported to the University hospital, and then readied for the transplant by a 7 to 10 hour hemodialysis. The resultant waiting period for the family members (who usually did not accompany the cadaver-patient to the University Hospital) was often extremely long and difficult.

Currently (and as was the case for some members of our sample) no such transfers are necessary. Brain death is declared at the original hospital by the local physicians and shortly thereafter a University surgeon arrives to remove the kidneys and place them in the preservation machine. The waiting period, after death is declared and before the family can claim the body, has thus been significantly shortened. In this respect, therefore, the first and last families in our sample had somewhat different experiences.

In other respects, however, their experiences were similar. In almost all cases of cadaver-patient organ donation, the cadaver-patient is a young person in otherwise good health who is the victim of a severe and ultimately fatal accidental injury usually directly involving the head. In almost all cases the patients suffer sudden and irreversible brain damage at the time of the accident and are comotose or actually brain-dead by the time they arrive at the hospital. In most of the cases studied here the patient was taken to a local hospital, examined by a local physician, and placed on machines to maintain respiration and circulation of blood. The patient was kept on these machines for several hours or in some cases several days even though all neurological evidence indicated that the brain had ceased to function. The family frequently maintained a 24-hour vigil at the hospital during this uncertain time, returning home only for short periods or for brief rests. As soon as the attending physician was certain that recovery could not occur, he informed the family that the patient was essentially dead (i.e., brain-dead), although the official "declaration" and signing of the death certificate had not yet occurred.

Generally this was also the time that the physician first suggested the idea of donation to the family, although he may have mentioned it earlier as the hopeless prognosis became increasingly apparent. After having made the suggestion of donation, the physician usually left the family alone to discuss the possibility among themselves. If the family agreed to donate, another physician from the University Hospitals arrived to explain the procedure more fully and to obtain the appropriate legal forms permitting the donation.

Subsequently the declaration of death and the completion of the death certificate occurred before the organs were removed and while the machines were still maintaining circulation, respiration, and most important, kidney function. Thus in reality the "moment of death" was not physiologically different from the time that preceded or followed it: A declaration of brain death, in other words, occurs at an arbitrary moment in time and serves merely to label a situation that has occurred one or more days before and to define as permissible the cessation of the respiratory and circulation machines as well as the possible removal of organs for transplant purposes.

Once the organs were removed from the cadaver-patient, the family was notified and, subsequent to an autopsy, they or the funeral director were able to claim the body. A transplant did not relieve the family of any expenses they might otherwise incur, although once the patient was declared officially dead and permission to use the organs had been granted, the transplant service assumed all expenses for the cadaver that were incurred within the hospital. Expenses up to that point, however, were assumed by the family and the later disposition of the body was also their responsibility.

THE PERIOD PRIOR TO THE DECISION

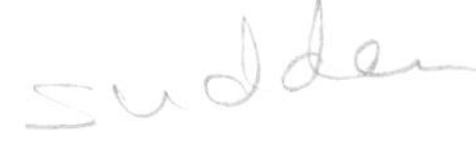

The Suggestion of Donation

Most of the family members interviewed were unprepared to accept the death of such young persons. The suddenness of the event as well as a refusal to relinquish hope were significant factors in the initial response of family members to the idea of donation.

In 12 of the cases* the initial suggestion to donate organs was made by the physician in the local hospital to which the patient had been taken. In the other three cases the donation was brought about (1) by the suggestion of a hospital staff member who was a friend of the wife of the deceased; (2) by the parents themselves in a case in which the mother's brother had been a cadaver-donor the year before, and (3) by the cadaver-patient himself who had written a suicide note directing that his entire body be given to the University.

This suicide note raises an important question: Among those particularly eager to donate their organs or bodies, is there a higher than normal proportion of suicidal persons? In the larger Minnesota series of 210 cadaver-donors there have been 20 suicides† but only in the above case was the staff aware of a suicidal note requesting body donation. There was an additional case in which a patient with a nonfatal self-inflicted gun wound arrived at the emergency room with a note pinned to him stating, "Give my kidneys to (a local celebrity who was being evaluated for transplantation)."

Flanagan and Murphy (1973) systematically studied the causes of death over a three-and-a-half-year period among all persons who had previously arranged to donate their bodies upon death to the medical school and whose bodies in fact had been received by the department of anatomy. They found that the proportion of suicides was indeed higher than expected in a general population of like age. Body or organ donation in these cases may have functioned as a last "noble" act to give meaning to an otherwise disappointing life and to raise a deflated self-image (see Blachly, 1969). However, Flanagan and Murphy's data indicated that no suicide occurred within two years of the original agreement to donate and that suicide was the cause of death for only a small minority of all body

* Since the 14 families yielded 15 cadaver-donors, there were 15 separate events and decisions to be made. Throughout this part of the analysis the total number of cases, therefore, is considered to be 15.

† This involved the series from 1971–1975. Eight of these suicides are only presumed, because the deaths were caused by drug overdose or carbon-monoxide poisoning rather than a self-inflicted wound.

donors. Thus suicidal donation occurs, but only rarely in the total population of body donors and even more rarely in the population of organ donors.

In most cases the idea of donation was not originally activated because of the patient's prior desires but because of the physician's suggestion. Given the family's state of shock and disbelief following the accident, it is not surprising that *they* were not the ones to suggest the donation. An additional reason for the physician suggesting organ donation may be that it helps him to inform the family that the patient will never recover. The suggestion, in other words, becomes tantamount to a declaration of death.

Initial Response to the Suggestion of Donation

Therefore, the reactions of the relatives to the physician's suggestion of donation may reflect more than just their feeling about the donation *per se*; their initial response may also reflect their readiness or willingness to accept the inevitability of the death. In at least half of the families interviewed, one or more of the relevant family members experienced initial reservations about the donation but then changed their mind in the time they had to think about it. Of the 35 respondents considered individually, four indicated they were definitely against the idea of donation initially, five needed time to think about it because they had some serious reservations, three said they were ambivalent, and 23 felt basically positive toward the idea.

Thus although the majority were immediately disposed to donation, approximately one-third needed more time before they were prepared to permit the donation. Eventually each of these persons—or at least each of the *relevant* decision-makers—came to accept the idea of donation. The determination of who among the possible decision-makers *were* relevant decision-makers is of interest.

Which Family Members Were Included in the Decision

The *living* donor's decision to give his *own* organ to a relative can be made without the concurrence of anyone else. But interpersonal strictures mitigate against a person unilaterally deciding to donate the organs of a dead relative if there are other survivors who may be affected by this decision. The exception to this rule seems to be the case in which the cadaver-patient is married, for then the surviving spouse may be viewed as legitimately making the decision alone. In only one of the 12 cases in which the patient was not married did a surviving relative make a unilateral decision to donate organs. This was a case in which the parents of the dying child had been divorced and the custodial parent made the decision without consulting the other parent, who, she implied, had ignored the family and therefore had not earned the right to be consulted. The decision to donate someone else's organs, therefore, is usually a group decision. What becomes critical in the decision process is the determination of whose wishes prevail. Who among all possible survivors are felt to be the legitimate decision-makers with regard to the question of donation?

In fact, there are strong normative feelings about the right to decide such an issue. Usually marital ties are the strongest and blood and age factors also play significant roles. If the patient is married, the spouse, in both a normative and a legal sense, is seen to be the major decision-maker. This holds true despite the fact that the marriage may be of short duration and despite the fact that the parents may also be present.

In each of the three cases in which the cadaver-patient was married, the wife became the primary decision-maker, although this fact presented difficulties to the parents in two of the three instances. In one of these two cases, the wife made the decision to donate the organs and swore the physicians to secrecy because she was afraid of the response of her husband's father. In the other case the family members felt distressed that the decision seemed to be left up to the wife because she had been estranged from the patient. Although the wife was willing to make the donation and the physicians felt that legally her permission was sufficient, both she and the physicians were responsive to the feelings of discontent among the husband's family members. Together the physicians and the wife decided that unless all the family members agreed, the donation would not take place. With some difficulty, the husband's parents and siblings decided to "allow" the donation.

In the third case of a married cadaver-patient, the legitimacy of the wife's authority to make the donation decision was accepted by her husband's mother who was with her at the time. However, the patient's mother was "thrilled" by this choice, because she had previously signed an organ-donor card herself. She intimated that if the wife had not approved of the donation, she would have remained silent. In fact, when the wife agreed to donate the kidneys and the pancreas but refused to donate her husband's eyes, the mother was somewhat surprised but said nothing because of her belief that this was properly the wife's decision.

If the patient was not married, the strength of the blood ties seemed to determine which relatives could be "legitimate" decision-makers. Parents figured prominently in the decision-making processes of the remaining 12 cases. In four cases parents alone made the decision for the donation. In two other cases the parents included the siblings in the discussion but indicated that they would be willing to donate even if the children were not willing. Their inclusion was an apparent attempt by the parents to be considerate of them as family members rather than to respond to any of their contradictory feelings. In one family, for instance, the mother reported:

> We [parents] *knew* right away, but didn't *decide* right away so as not to hurt my older daughter and my father. We let it sink into them. . . .Now the older girl thinks it was her decision. If she had said no or something, I think her father and I would have gone on anyway. My father didn't express any opinion, he said, "It's your son."

In these cases the disapproval of other family members would probably not have made a difference to the parents in the final decision.

In four other cases the parents specifically wanted to include siblings of the cadaver-patient in the decision-making process. These interviews suggest that the parents were truly concerned about the responses of their children and would not have decided to donate if family consensus on the donation could not be reached. Age of siblings was a factor in these and other cases, however. The parents were careful to include the older children in the decision but never considered the opinions or feelings of the younger children. The age cut-off seemed to be around 14 or 15 years; anyone younger than this was not seriously included in the donation decision.

Despite the weight that the parents may place on the feelings of older children, the siblings themselves may be uncomfortable in the decision-making role. In one such case the brother of a cadaver-patient said, "Why my parents said, 'Well, what do you think?' I didn't want to say. I felt it should be my mother and father's decision. I think this was also kind of the case with my sister."

Although there is normative uncertainty about the role of older children in the decision-making process, the role of grandparents seems clearly defined as irrelevant. The opinions offered by grandparents frequently reflected traditional beliefs and strong objections to the proposed transplantation. Larger surveys have also indicated that older persons are less positive toward organ transplantation and toward nontraditional methods of handling death (see Chapter 2, and Simmons et al., 1974). In seven of the cases one or more of the grandparents expressed a profound resistance to the idea of the donation. One respondent said, "My mother had absolute fits. She is extremely religious and she feels you are given one set of organs and if something goes wrong with them, that's it. Horrible to go putting somebody else's organs in another body. She'll never come around." Obviously, since each of these interviews was conducted because the family did agree to donate organs, the resistance of the grandparents was overcome or, more likely, ignored. In one case in which the grandparents expressed strong objections, an 18-year-old son stood up in the hospital waiting room and announced, "The decision is on the basis of what we [that is, father, mother, and older sister] want, and whether you [grandparents] want it or not doesn't matter." In several other cases the irrelevance of the feelings of grandparents was also clear. One father reported, "Well, my wife's mother did say something but we shut her off real quick on that. It was our decision and she would have had nothing to do with it." Sometimes family members were significantly upset by the disapproval of grandparents, but their nonsupport did not dissuade them from their final decision. In none of our cases was the opinion of the grandparents specifically sought. Whether grandparents played a larger role in cases where parents did not allow donation remains to be investigated.

Usually, then, among the family, only the closest blood relatives or the patient's spouse are included in the decision-making process. In two out of the three cases in which the dying child had a stepparent, the stepparent was left out of the decision-making. But the data indicate that in an intact family *both* of the parents of the unmarried cadaver-patient must ultimately agree if the donation is to take place. As one mother said, "If he says no and I say yes, I'm not going to push my yes. After all, if there's any disagreement, it has to be the no one, then." Another mother made it very clear that the possible objection of her husband was crucial in her thinking:

> If there were going to be one death in the family, this boy would probably be the most important one to his father. They identified with each other very closely. . .their walk, their speech, and the things that they did. If he would have objected at all I would never have said yes.

Type of Decision-Making Process

In the discussion of the decision-making of the living *related* donor we classified both family and individual processes. At the family level evidence was found for each of the three types of decisions identified by Turner (1970): the decisions (1) of consensus in which all family members come to support the final choice; (2) of accommodation in which some family members feel their opinions have been overridden; and (3) *de facto* decisions in which the event appears to occur without the family as a unit arriving at any definite choice. Based on this small sample of 15 cadaver-donor decisions, almost all families seem to achieve consensus at least among the immediate relatives. In 11 out of the 14 decisions in which there is enough information for us to make a judgment, consensus within the immediate family was evident, although there was some opposition from grandparents in five of these cases.

In the cases in which the patient was married and both the spouse and parents were potential decision-makers, the situation became more complex. One of these cases was responsible for the one clear instance of accommodation in which the parents felt they had acceded to the wishes of the wife despite their own predilections. Another involved a type of *de facto* decision in that the wife made the choice without consulting any other interested family members.

In one family the decision-making resembled the postponement and *de facto* decisions described for the living related donors. In this case the parents of the dying child were leaning toward the donation but anticipated their conversation with the *University* physician as one that would help them to arrive at a final choice. They took what seemed to them one step toward donation by requesting the interview. Yet because most families have arrived at a decision prior to their contact with the University, the University physician defined the situation differently. To the physician, his task was to further explain the procedure and secure the signatures of the willing parents. The net result was that the parents felt prematurely locked into the donation, although they were also motivated in that direction.

Out of the 14 situations that were clear enough to categorize, four induced significant family stress during the decision period above and beyond the grief all were experiencing. These situations have all been described: (1) the above family that felt locked into donation; (2) the family in which the parents were angry at the estranged wife; (3) one family in which the grandparents' opposition was strongly expressed and was upsetting to the parents; and (4) the family in which the wife concealed the donation from her husband's family. In the latter case the cadaver-donor's brother who suspected the truth expressed great anger to the wife.

At the *individual level*, family members who perceived themselves as having a decisive role in the choice* appeared divided between relatives who reported an instantaneous decision (nine relatives) and members who spent some time deliberating (13 relatives) about the decision.† In

* Many relatives, particularly younger siblings, reported that they were informed of the family's choice rather than asked for their view.

† Two of the authors independently classified these decisions. There were two additional cases in which the coding was unreliable. Overall, given the fact that this classification is

addition to these two groups were the two parents cited above who described a postponement and stepwise type of decision-making. The net result was that in six families the decision appeared to be immediate; in five families the local physician was given an affirmative answer within two hours; and in four families the decision took from 12 hours to two to three days.

Thus, as in the case of the living related donors, individuals seem to vary in their approach to major life choices; many make such decisions immediately and easily without conscious deliberation, while others attempt to deliberate at greater length.

Role of Friends, Medical Staff, and Clergy

The question of outsiders' influence in the decision-making process is relevant. Did those who deliberated about the decision turn to any type of expert for advice?

Although in some cases friends were present throughout the ordeal and their tacit approval was clear, in only three cases were we aware of a larger role on their part. In all three cases the friends were either medical personnel themselves or were closely affiliated with medical staff and thus felt free to argue in favor of donation. The major nonfamily member involved in each process, however, was the local physician himself, and his primary role seemed to be to initiate and explain the idea of donation. In two cases the physician also assumed the role of temporizer: He refused to accept immediate consent from the potential donor's family and directed them to think the issue over more carefully.

In three cases local physicians assumed a more active role in urging the donation in order to help families bring themselves to turn off the machines. One father reported that the physician said to him:

> When do you want the machines turned off? Your whole family is here now and you have been going through this for three days. We're just conducting a charade. We could do this for the next two weeks. The hospital bills are very high. If it's comforting for you to sit here and hold her hand when she's in a coma, O.K. She's breathing, but she's essentially dead. You might as well agree to the fact that she's dead. It's costing like $700 to $800 a day to go through this.

The clergy played a supportive but not influential role for these families. Their role in the decision process seemed to be more a matter

---

based entirely on reports a year or more after the donation, our certainty concerning it is much less than that for the living related donors.

of supporting a decision once made than of providing information or guidance in making the decision. In almost all of the cases either a hospital chaplain or their own clergyman was in contact with the family at the time of the decision-making process, but in only three families out of 15 were the clergy said to have had some role in the decision-making process. One of these families was concerned whether brain death was approved by the Catholic church; another wanted to make certain that their child's religious salvation would not be compromised. Several of the families were of the Catholic faith and stated in the interview that they were aware at the time of making their decision that the Catholic church approves of organ donation, so they did not seek out this information. Generally families who did seek out the opinions of the clergy were relieved to find that the clergy approved of what they were thinking and feeling,* but several did not feel that the clergy's opinion was particularly relevant in their eventual decision. Half of the families did not consult a clergyman about the decision.

Thus the decision to donate cadaver organs is a group decision made by key family members in a crisis situation. At the time of the decision these key members, both at home and in the hospital, are likely to be surrounded sporadically or continuously by other individuals who are normatively defined as having less right to make the choice but who provide emotional support—the hospital medical staff, clergymen, friends, younger children in the family, grandparents, in-laws, stepparents, and so on. Of these persons only the grandparents are likely to express an opposing view.

The factors that make the decision easy for these key family members, as well as the factors that make it difficult for others, must be explicated.

What Factors Made the Decision Easy?

Prior Knowledge of Transplantation. Only one family indicated that they knew nothing of transplantation prior to this incident. In fact transplantation had been a subject of family discussion previously in seven families; and in these discussions five of the cadaver-patients (all male and all over 17) had indicated their desire to donate organs in the event of their death. In view of the fact that four of the sample of cadaver-patients were 10 years of age or younger, it is interesting that five of the remaining 11 had expressed some prior interest in donation.

In these cases the decision of the family was made easier because once

* The position of most Christian churches is one of acceptance and support. The Orthodox branch of the Jewish faith, however, does not condone organ transplantation, although the Conservative and Reform branches are positive toward such a gift.

the issue of donation was raised, they remembered the cadaver-patient's own desires concerning the subject. A father reported:

> It's a funny thing. We had talked about organ transplants no more than two weeks before. He said he would like to do something great with his life. Our thought went back to that conversation. I guess I was feeling that that was about as great as you can do when you are going to die. If one accepted this as terminal within a matter of hours, it's just logic. If he is going to do anything great and if he's going to contribute, it's going to have to be our decision. I think that made it easier to feel as we did. That he had a desire to make a contribution of some kind and that he had expressed it.

Even though the patient's expressed interest in donation did not lead the family to suggest the gift themselves, the recollection of such wishes did facilitate their decision to allow the donation. In addition, several of the family members said that prior to the death of the cadaver-patient, they too had a desire to donate their own organs. In the majority of these families, in other words, transplantation was neither an unfamiliar nor an unacceptable idea. Sometimes, however, desires for donating are felt to be highly personal and are not discussed among the family members. In one case the husband and the wife each felt privately that they would like to donate their own organs and had felt so for some time before the death of their child. Only during the decision process with regard to the organs of the child was each made aware of the feelings of the other.

Altruistic and Empathic Motivation. Altruism and humanitarianism play a major role in the family members' decision to donate. A few of the respondents said that in the decision process they empathized with the recipient's family and thought about what it would be like if their own child were "lying there, waiting for an organ."

One wife was convinced by hearing of the need of some patients for the kidneys. "I figured if he had two good kidneys there are two people who need them to stay alive with their family. I said O.K. It took maybe an hour. I don't know what he would have said [the dead husband], but I figured if he could save two lives, I'm going to do it."

A mother said:

> It was horrible for me, just that short time from Friday to Saturday night. A neighbor who worked in the emergency room sort of convinced me that it was better not to try to keep him alive on machines and to donate. She said, "They don't experiment or anything." All I could think was, "If he's going to die, why not give someone his kidneys?" A doctor from the University came and told us that if you could see the difference in these peoples' lives after a transplant. . .well, it really made me feel good.

Usually families of cadaver-patients are not informed about the identity of the specific recipient at the time they are asked to make their decision. Some respondents reported that they had had to envision a potential recipient in making their decision. The fantasized recipient was generally a child of the same sex as the cadaver-patient. In reality, however, children in need of transplants usually receive organs from a living related donor, which means that the majority of patients who need cadaver organs are adults. Whether a realization of this fact would have affected the decision of these families cannot be determined with these data. Titmuss (1971) reports, however, that there *is* a reluctance on the part of the young to donate their blood to their older relatives. He found, in other words, a directionality to altruistic giving: The usual direction is from old to young rather than from young to old.*

The apparent need to regard the beneficiary of the donation as young and similar to the donor was reinforced even in indirect ways. In one case, for instance, in which a parent was told that one of her child's kidneys would go to a woman with a child, the comment was made that it gave her great satisfaction to know that some *young person* would possibly not lose their mother because of this donation.

Feelings about Immortality. Certain feelings about immortality also sometimes made the decision to donate an easier one. At least five of the survivors took comfort in the idea that part of the cadaver-patient would still be alive. In the words of one mother:

> I think we generally got approval from most people but kind of like "Isn't that nice of her to do this?" I didn't do it because I thought it was nice to do. I did it because I thought [crying], I guess, something to help him [son]. Perhaps he was alive as far as I was concerned. So his death wasn't totally a death.

A sense of extended life was echoed in the words of another father. "Well, it's a funny feeling. In a sense you think they're still around and yet they're not. [As long as his kidneys still function] he isn't dead down there."

Another family viewed the transplant as a continuation of "life" in another way. The mother explained:

> We had the privilege of having all the children in on the decision. There was very little discussion. The decision was "yes"; we really didn't have to go into it much at all. Then my nineteen-year-old son had this beautiful thought that it

* As noted in Chapter 7, among potential living related donors, parents whose children need a kidney are the most willing donors. However, the recipient's older siblings are not more likely to donate than are their younger siblings, and the recipient's children are more willing to donate than his siblings.

was two transplants. As her family who knew her joy and knew what her life was, it was up to us to do a psychological and a spiritual transplant. The doctors would do a physical transplant and we would live her joy and implant it in others.

The Second Medical Evaluation. Donating organs for transplantation may sometimes be motivated by a refusal to regard death as a *finality*. In addition, before the preservation machines were invented, willingness to consider donation may have been prompted by a refusal to accept death as a *reality*. The desire to have access to University facilities and personnel for a second medical evaluation in the hope of a cure played a significant part in the decision of some families. One father said:

> Of course, I think you always hold on to that last strand of hope that maybe the people at the University could find something. So actually, that *was* another reason for agreeing to donation: another review of the case. That was definitely a factor in it at that stage. This, too, I used in talking to my wife. A slim hope. You're sure you're not basing your decision on the findings of one place.

Relief from Deciding to "Turn Off" Machines. Once the death was accepted as a reality, the prospect of donating organs was felt by some family members to be a solution to their dilemma of when to turn off the "life-maintaining" respiratory and circulatory machines. In a way the decision *to* turn them off was made by them, and yet they were relieved at not having to decide *when*.

One father said:

> He [the physician] put the termination in very clear light, and the fact that he hated to be the person that would turn off these machines. I don't think he would hesitate to take the responsibility, but, I mean, he's a human being too, just like the rest of us. We didn't want to put him in that position. So [with the decision to donate] everything just pretty much fell into place.

The mother in this case describes the situation more emotionally. When they had to put her son back on the machine to sustain his breathing, the doctors told her that it was "sort of a waiting game." "You mean," she replied, "waiting to decide who's going to turn the switch off?" and the doctors admitted, "Well, sort of like that." Then, said the mother, the doctors began "tossing it [the decision of when to turn off the machines] back and forth like a football." Finally she asked, "Well, is the ball game really over?" and one doctor replied, "Well, yes, unless you want to sustain him on the machines, which isn't really much of a choice, for his sake." For some period of time, while this realization set in, the family paced the halls asking questions such as "Who's going to play God here?" When one of the doctors suddenly seemed to realize that organ donation would be an alternative and suggested this, the mother said, "We [she and her husband] both just jumped for joy. The pressure was off of us, you know. It was just like a shot in the arm. We both even smiled."

What Factors Make the Decision Difficult?

Problem of Brain Death. In each case, as in all cases of transplants using cadaver organs, the patient experienced sudden and irreversible brain damage at the time of the accident. Sometime later the family was told that, despite appearances of life, the patient was dead because his brain had ceased functioning. Without the artificial respirator, he would not be able to maintain a heartbeat or respiration. The concept of brain death, however, was sometimes very difficult for family members to comprehend in the presence of other signs of viability such as breathing and a pulse rate. One woman said, "[My husband's] mother couldn't get it through her head—she felt that as long as his heart was beating and he was breathing, he was alive."

A definition of death relying upon the absence of certain neurological signs not only is a departure from the traditional definition of death (i.e., no heartbeat or breathing) but also is a departure from the concept of a "moment" of death. Brain death suggests a death process, something extending both forward and backward from the moment of a verbal declaration. According to Muller (1967), "Although law speaks of death as a moment in time, in reality, it is a series of physical and chemical changes starting before the medical-legal time of death and continuing afterward." To decide at what point in this process they wish to discontinue the efforts to keep the other systems functioning has been the task of the family or physician. But many family members, tied as they are to an "instant" notion of death, are reluctant to make any such decisions until they are told that this "instant" has taken place and that their relative is "dead."

One mother reported that the physician said to her, " 'We wanted to approach you about a transplant. Would you consider it if her organs were still intact?' He did a beautiful job of presenting it but she hadn't been declared dead [as far as we knew]. It was kind of a shock." Paradoxically, therefore, the suggestion of donation becomes this "announcement," and the family is then led to realize that the decision to discontinue "life-saving" measures will soon be made. The family members seem to have had to deal with both "kinds" of death in their response to the initial suggestion of donation: They have to accept the emotional shock that the *instant* when life ceases and death begins has already passed; and they have to confront the fact that part of the *process* of death is still to occur.

Several respondents commented that it was difficult to talk about taking organs (or making funeral arrangements) when the patient still seemed alive. The 14-year-old sister of a cadaver-patient (who was not included in the donation decision) said,

> That night we discussed what we were going to do and someone said that they were going to donate some of his organs. And I was just shocked. You know he's dead but he's still alive. I was just shocked, I couldn't believe it!

Doctors may also be aware of the problems families have with the notion of brain death. One mother reported that after she gave permission for the body to be used and after it had been transported to the University, she felt the doctors kept her from seeing her son on the machines for fear that this would affect her decision to donate. She reported:

> I said to the doctor, "Should we come over?" because usually if someone is dying, you want to be with them. But the implication I got was, it's too late, there's no practical value; technically, he's dead. But I got the feeling that because he would still be on the machines it would be harder for me and that maybe they felt I would change my mind if I saw him breathing and looking like he was very much alive. I realized that he would still have to be hooked to the machines to be mechanically alive until the surgery and that's probably what they didn't want me to see. Maybe if I saw it I would say, "No, I don't want to give my permission yet."

Not being present at the "instant" of death is difficult for some family members. In our culture this moment has assumed a sacred and fundamental quality and its absence is disturbing. As one mother said:

> For the most part, people said, "Well, great." They thought it was a tremendous thing to do. But I think the majority of them say this not knowing that you give up their organs before their heart has stopped beating. My mother died seven months before he [son] did and I stood at her bedside and felt her pulse until it was completely gone. It's a different kind of thing when you walk into a room and see the kid is breathing. You know the difference.

Actually "parting" with the patient when he or she does not seem to be fully dead was thus a problem for many of the survivors. Usually this reluctance manifests itself in a delay in the decision process while the surviving family members come to terms with the alternatives. Although most survivors did not go to this extreme, one mother admitted, "You know, you have second thoughts too, [such as]I could bring him home on one of those machines. . .I could take care of him. It's funny the things that go through your mind 'cause you don't want to give him up."

An 18-year-old sister stated that she never had any regrets about the decision to donate. Rather, she said:

> I think it was harder trying to decide at what point we would say that he was dead when he wasn't. But I never felt that they should just have kept him on the machines for an indeterminate period, just to prolong his life so that he could exist. I knew that this wasn't the kind of life that he would want to live. And I felt that rather than being a vegetable all his life, or being in a coma, or whatever, I think that would have been harder on us if that would have been the way he would have lived.

The word *vegetable* is mentioned in several of the interviews. Although the family member may not have been able to comprehend the notion of *death* from the definition of brain death, the extent of the brain injury slowly penetrated their thinking to the point that they were able to talk about the continued existence of their relative (were the machines to be kept on) in terms that seemed to them to mean a subhuman condition.

Sometimes, however, the definition of the patient as a potential "vegetable" ("subhuman" but "alive") brings with it other religious and ethical problems for the survivors. One respondent, a mother, said:

> I had this terrible feeling when he was lying there. I would rather see him dead than incapacitated for the rest of his life because it would break his spirit. And this was sort of a death wish on my part and I really felt (and I've been real depressed about this at times) that I wished him dead, you know, and that maybe my wish was strong enough. I feel a real strong communication with the higher power in that you have to be careful sometimes with what you ask.

Another father confided:

> The one reluctance I had [to the donation] I think may have been kind of a religious question—wrestling with the concept of death, either as I am used to thinking of it or as one might legally define it, as a plain death. I guess basically in my mind I wondered, "O.K., if we, by our decision, are going to terminate his life, where is he in terms of salvation?" I don't have any guilt feelings, but I wonder if we were short on patience.

Several relatives could only partially accept the certainty of brain death and felt some guilt at making the decision that would absolutely ensure death. A mother elaborated:

> I guess I have no regrets other than the fact that I would have liked to have a better knowledge of what could have happened to him had he been left the way he was. Of course, they did tell us it would have been 24 hours and this type of thing, but I guess you always have the question that man isn't always right. You always hear about the miracles and this type of thing, where a doctor thinks that someone is just about dead and he lives. I guess you kind of have some of these things in the back of your mind.

Two other mothers put their feelings even more bluntly. One lamented "I think the hardest part is the fact that she didn't die. I had to tell them to 'pull the plugs,' I willed her to die." And another said, "There he was, right around the corner, still breathing on a machine and we were signing his life away in here."

Their decision to allow donation and the cessation of the machines is an irreversible one, while the condition of the heartbeating cadaver appears capable of being reversed despite physician's assurances to the contrary.* However, the decision not to donate or the failure to consider the decision would also be irreversible. Most of these cadaver-patients, in reality, would not function indefinitely on these machines. The condition would continue to deteriorate; their hearts would arrest; and the transplantable organs would become useless. In the words of one wife who was very conscious of the irreversibility of the decision:

> The donation was the only good thing that came out of his death. I've been very thankful that someone mentioned it to me, and had it been later, and I hadn't done this and had someone said to me, "Did you ever donate his kidneys?" Then I would have felt bad. I would have felt like I really goofed up the one chance I had, and if I goofed up, that's when you can't make up for it.

Predecision Waiting. Time is a factor that plays a significant but complicated role in the donation experience of the families. The fact that the accidents usually occur suddenly forces upon the survivors a demand for an immediate transition in thinking. Most respondents would have liked more time for this mental transition, but the time needed to observe the patient in the hospital before the neurologist informs the family that brain activity has definitely ceased can seem interminable for waiting family members. In an ongoing lifetime a few hours or days may seem insignificant, but in the lives of these responding family members the waiting was almost uniformly described as "endless."

One woman said that the time it took to wait was "like a lifetime. It was like an eternity. There were so many good things, it was handled well, it

* See Chapter 2 for discussions of controversies within the medical community concerning brain-death.

really was, but of the things that stood out in my mind, the hardest thing to endure was the length." Another woman said, "I can remember my mother saying over and over, 'You're moving too fast, don't make these decisions. Why are you deciding on this so fast?' Well, to me, it wasn't fast. It was like an eternity we had already been through."

Timing. The timing of the decision process seems to be extremely crucial. Not only must the decision to give the organs be made within a reasonable period of time (so as not to jeopardize the organs unduly), but also the family must be given sufficient time to overcome their initial feelings of shock and disbelief. Because the request for donation is frequently tantamount either to a declaration of death or to an announcement that the case is hopeless, family members sometimes respond only to the announcement rather than the request. The grief at the realization that the patient's condition is in fact hopeless is so overwhelming that the donation issue cannot be handled at that moment. In fact to be making future plans of any type appears in some cases to be inappropriate before the shock of the death or impending death has been assimilated.

Thus in some cases the initial negative reaction to donation was not necessarily a negative judgment of donation but rather a feeling that this was not the time to consider such issues. One father remembered telling the doctor:

> There's such a shock to think that there's no hope for her living, that I can't bear to make such a decision right now. . .After about a day, I'd say, when the whole idea kind of developed in my thinking, then I was a little more apt to consider it on a rational basis, that it might be a worthwhile thing to do.

There seems to be in the brain-death donation experience certain stages of acceptance and awareness that family members go through that somewhat parallel the grieving process (but in the donation process the timing is, of necessity, accelerated). Dealing with the family members as if they are in one stage of grief when they may in fact be in another, can lead to strained communication. The 18-year-old brother of a cadaver-patient summarized:

> [The doctor] was just saying "If she's going to die, then I think you should think about this.". . .But as far as my mother and father, it was way too early to say something like that. . . .There were certain stages you go through the whole time, and each thing needs a little bit of time. It seems kind of ridiculous, but maybe just an hour, maybe after each thing, an hour or half-hour. . . .When my sister came [from out of the country]. . .well, she was at a different stage than us [the rest of the family who had been together in the hospital since

> the accident]. You know, it was strange to try and talk to her, well and try to explain things. And then other people would come, well like at the funeral. . .home. . . .You know, we were grateful and could talk about it so easily [the death and the donation] and friends of ours. . .couldn't believe the way we were talking. We were just in a different stage.

Even when family members experience the accident and the hospital events at the same time, their stages of personal acceptance may differ greatly from one another. In one case when the parents were approached with the idea of organ donation, the father agreed to the transplant and the mother refused. The father told the physician no and the physician went away but said, "I'll be around anyway in case you change your mind." The father commented, "The only thing I can say is if he [the physician] had talked much longer after the first refusal, he never would have gotten it. It was the wrong time and the wrong place."

Limited Information. One of the reasons that some families felt they needed more time to decide is that despite knowledge that transplantation existed, they really knew very little about the *details* involved. Although local physicians were able to satisfy the queries of many individuals, five respondents who were very anxious to have their questions answered found that the medical staff did not seem to have time to give them the answers they sought. One father said, "I think the initial reaction was that we wished we knew more about it so that we could have a better basis for making a decision. The doctor didn't stay long or provide much information."

One mother suggested an educational approach for other donors. "I would think that a pamphlet or a brochure [for the family to read in the waiting room] would allow them not only to be clear in their own minds as to what certain procedures are but also help answer the thousands of questions they are asked by friends and relatives." Donors' families need information not only for their own decision but also to help them explain the process to interested others. Such a booklet has been recently issued by HEW.

Attitude toward Special Body-Parts: Body-Image. A decision to allow the donation of any organs at all for transplantation is the first decision that must be considered by the family, but in addition, they can decide which organs they will allow to be donated. A willingness to donate certain organs was arrived at without too much feeling of body disturbance or body mutilation, but the idea of removing certain other organs sometimes aroused great emotion. Most respondents did not have any feelings one way or another about the spleen, pancreas, liver, or kidneys. But hearts and eyes, particularly, were organs of the body that sometimes provoked very strong images and association; these organs possess special significance even after death for many people.

Two families specified that the heart could not be taken. Because heart transplants are not being done at the University of Minnesota, no family was asked specifically to give up the heart; yet these families felt so strongly that the heart should remain with the body that they wrote in this qualification on the permission form themselves.

Unless specifically excluded, however, the permission signed by the family did allow for the removal of the eyes. Family members were not always aware of this when they signed the waiver, and two families became quite upset when they learned from their funeral director that the eyes had been used. Even though the body, if it were viewed, would have the eyes closed, it was important to them that the eyes remain with the body.

THE SHORT-TERM PERIOD FOLLOWING THE DECISION

We have been focusing on the positive and negative aspects of cadaver donation prior to the family's decision to donate. The short-term period after the decision was made also presented many sources of stress for the donating family. Much of this stress was automatically alleviated with the introduction of the preservation machine which shortened the time period between the decision-point and the hour the body was made available for the funeral director. What used to be a matter of days has been reduced to a few hours. Nevertheless, a consideration of this stressful period in the early days of organ donation is enlightening.

Contact with the Physician Representing the Transplant Service

As soon as the local physician learned of the family's willingness to donate, he notified the University, and a representative of the transplant team was sent to speak with the family and secure their signed consent. One would predict that this type of contact would engender some stress, and for respondents from three families it did. Despite the family's desire to help save another life through donation, it could be hypothesized that at some emotional level, the transplant physician might represent a type of predator. These were the persons who were going to "use" and invade the body of their loved one and then stop the machines that now maintained appearances of life. To give one's signature to this physician would make the *process* of death inevitable. Furthermore, the physician was a stranger who had no personal attachment to them and who had not been on the team that had tried to save their relative's life. It is not surprising therefore that the anxiety and grief and anger at such a tragic death is sometimes displaced onto such a stranger, who seems to represent only those who are to benefit from the death.

From the point of view of the transplant physician, the contact is also stressful. To have to intrude on the grief of strangers to ask a favor is difficult. In addition, the time pressures of the transplant service also impinge on him. He is aware of the great machinery of effort about to be put into motion once the signed consent is obtained. To ensure that the recipients and staff are prepared before the scarce cadaver organs lose their usefulness will mean an around-the-clock effort for many members of the transplant team.

The transplant physician must have a special sensitivity to cope well with such a situation. As one woman said, "I felt after speaking to the doctor that he was a person who made me feel very comfortable about it. I'm sure not every person is really qualified." Understandably, not every physician is equally well-qualified to deal with all of these pressures—respondents from three families characterized the physician as "pushy," a "little bit cold," or "greedy." One father was particularly unhappy with the way the doctor handled the request for donation. He said

> He [the physician] was pretty direct and wanted to know if we were interested in going ahead with it; you know, kind of like a business problem. I guess they evaluate if they want him or not. I wish they'd made up their minds before they asked us. He was kind of basic. He kept saying he realized it was hard, but he didn't show it. He seemed anxious to do it—almost as though they wanted to go right at it, as though life would run out. At one point he made the comments that he wanted the kidneys because they were scarce. It was like buying an automobile.

The brother of a cadaver-patient also objected to what he felt was the commercialism of the physician's approach to obtaining his brother's body-parts: To him it seemed "almost like stripping a car."

One mother felt pressured by the physician's impersonal manner:

> I think he [the physician] was a little bit cold in a way. He met us out in the hall and asked, "Will you sign this?" I think possibly he could have sat down a little bit with us because when he asked us in the beginning about donation, it was the kidney and the spleen and that was all. And then he comes with this sheet of paper and all these other things are mentioned and at the time we were really

> pressured into it, you know, "Hurry up and sign this," without really having time to talk it over.

Duff and Hollingshead (1968) describe similar situations when the physicians have had to request autopsy permission from grieving families.

Waiting for the Transplant to be Completed

The time period after the signature was secured and before the body became available was especially difficult for cadaver-donor families, particularly before the institution of preservation machines. Normative and practical uncertainties made the situation stressful. Where should the family go? Should they visit the "body" in the University hospital? Was the donor in fact "dead?" What was happening to their relative during the waiting period? Had the transplant been completed? Several funeral directors also indicated their displeasure with the uncertainty. Their questions as to when the body would be available only increased family discomfort. Transplantation had interrupted the customary accepted practices of death and had prolonged a period where the distinction between life and death was ambiguous.

The proper behavior during the waiting period was unclear for several families and was not clarified by the staff. The mother of a married cadaver-patient described her experience in the hospital as follows:

> Well, we just seemed to be waiting for that person with those bloody forms for hours and hours. [After the person came and they were signed] we just sat there. Nobody said, "Why don't you go home" or anything. I think we sat there until three o'clock in the afternoon. Somebody kind of just shut us off and let us go. Finally I just said, "I don't know why we don't go home, do you?" and she [patient's wife] said, "I don't think they'll even miss us."

The transplant staff did not encourage family visitors when the cadaver-patient had been transferred to the University Hospital and death had been declared, but they also did not refuse visitation prior to the operation. In three cases relatives regretted not having a last look at the patient. One mother felt she would have liked to have been allowed to sit through the transplant operation with the cadaver-patient son rather than to leave him before he was "finally" gone. A grandmother was very upset that her grandson was alone at the University Hospital for testing and organ removal. She kept saying to the parents, "Well you don't just leave. I'm going over there and stay then. You don't just leave a child." Again, the difficulties people have with the definition of brain death and their need to know a specific time of death are clear.

The fact that originally families were not told when the operation was over was seen as a problem by some. They felt that they should have been called as soon as it was over to stop some of their worries and waiting. In their mind, apparently, the death was not truly final until after the operation was completed, despite the prior declaration of brain death. One mother suggested that the hospital should keep in periodic touch with the family by telephone if they were not asked to stay at the hospital.

> The hospital should respond every few hours or so. They can say, "We're awfully sorry we told you 12 hours or 24 hours but it looks like it's going to be more. We want you to know that we're doing everything we can to see that your son's body is returned."

As a result of information gained from early interviews in this study, phone calls to the family during this period were made part of the customary procedure.

Although there is no way to assign a moment to death in the case of brain death, one father was somewhat upset when the time of death on the death certificate disagreed with his understanding of the time death had been declared. The uncertainties and discrepancies inherent in this period were sources of stress for several individuals.

After the Transplant: The Body-Image. After the transplant was completed, two families experienced difficulties because of feelings about autopsies. The fact that an autopsy would be done following a transplant was clearly spelled out in the consent form signed by the family. However, in the particular state of grief and confusion in which the survivors found themselves, the likelihood was great that even if they read what they were signing, they would not clearly understand it at the time or fully remember it afterwards. These two families did not realize that an autopsy would further delay securing the body and when they became aware of this, they were upset. One father wondered, why if the death was certain, as he had been informed, should an autopsy be necessary?

Some funeral directors reacted negatively to the transplant donation and made their displeasure known to the family. Their major dissatisfaction was with the delay and uncertainty in being able to obtain the body, and the various problems this delay presented them in their funeral preparations.* As one father noted:

> Particularly. . .we were getting a lot of pressure from the mortuary. We couldn't get the body out of the hospital. They didn't get it until after 5:00 p.m.

* This problem has been partially alleviated by the use of the preservation machine.

> The funeral director told us he was concerned because the tissues were drying out and they couldn't get the face back to normal.

In a few cases when the family expressed displeasure at the cadaver's appearance, the funeral director deflected blame onto the transplant or the autopsy.

Almost all of the families interviewed (12 of the 15) put the body on view either at the funeral home or at the funeral ceremony or both. In five families there were specific complaints about the appearance of the cadaver. In one family this was blamed on the mortician, but in four families it was blamed on the experience in the hospital and on the procedures necessary for the transplant operation. One mother said, "Even if that look were normal, we would naturally associate it with the transplant." Some of the others felt that the head or face did not look right partly because the lips were swollen from having had tubes in them and the face was puffed. Many of these patients, however, had had direct injuries to the head which in and of themselves might have been disfiguring.

The Funeral. In some other ways the donation made the funeral a more positive experience than it might otherwise have been. In two cases the fact of the organ donation was mentioned by the clergy as part of the sermon at the funeral service. This official praise was comforting to the concerned family members, as was the praise of friends at that time. In the words of one of these mothers, who had discussed the sermon with the minister the night before the funeral:

> The minister read this into the sermon. . .I wanted him to get across in there loud and strong. . .that there has to be some meaning. . .that it [the death] wasn't just a wasted thing, and so [the minister] weaved this through his sermon. . . .[My son] was. . .an outstanding leader. . .and so there had to be some meaning for why He would take a boy who's never been in trouble. . .and so I think this transplant was a good substitute. . .just to hold everybody together.

Subsequent Hospital Errors. A new medical technology is most likely to become instituted first at a large, impersonal, bureaucratic medical center. Such a bureaucracy is resistant to change. When cadaver donation first became instituted, all bills related to the donation itself were to be paid out of the transplant research grant. Yet in the beginning the centralized billing office found it difficult to create procedures that would identify the cadaver-patients quickly enough to prevent bills from being sent directly to the donor families themselves. Although this is no longer a problem, two of the early families found the postdonation period stressful because they were erroneously billed for transfusions, transportation, and for hospital stays of the cadaver-patient during the period of transplantation. Even though these errors were later rectified, family members found this particularly upsetting for two reasons: First, because it indicated to them that their loved one had been through additional "trauma" and second, because they felt that it was gross neglect on the part of the hospital to bill them after they had given the hospital such an important gift. The recipient of a gift is expected to reciprocate with gratitude not "inconsideration," and the hospital was defined as one of the recipients of the gift of life.

THE LONG-TERM REACTION TO CADAVER DONATION

Throughout the period in which the decision to donate is made and the transplant operation is performed, the concerns of the family have been largely focused on the cadaver-patient. In the weeks and months that follow their focus begins to shift. The long-range issues associated with the donation center more clearly on the welfare of the survivors, particularly with their own grieving processes. Our question was whether the donation eased or intensified the grieving process. Were the long-term attitudes toward the donation primarily positive or negative?

Overall Evaluation

Although the donation was not equally salient to all family members a year or more after the death, most respondents appeared to hold a primarily positive attitude toward it at the time of the interview. Table 10-2 indicates that 23 out of the 28 adults were still favorable toward the donation. Whether this proportion would have been reduced had we been able to interview all the families in the targeted population is a question that cannot be answered here.

For all five of the ambivalent or negative respondents, the negative reactions were very much attributed to the transfer to or administrative problems at the University Hospital. Two of the respondents were from the families that had been erroneously billed by the University, and one of these persons had also been upset by the lack of communication from the hospital during the time they were waiting for the transplant to be completed. Two others were the parents who reported that they had felt "locked into" donation before completely making up their minds; and at this point they were concerned they had not been patient enough. A

TABLE 10-2 RATINGS OF ATTITUDES OF CADAVER-DONOR FAMILY MEMBERS 1 YEAR OR MORE AFTER THE DONATION[a]

	Adults		Children under 14	Total	
Clearly positive attitude	(17) 60%	82%	(7)	(24) 68%	85%
Primarily positive with a few slight reservations	(6)[b] 22%			(6) 17%	
Ambivalent	(1) 4%			(1) 3%	
Negative	(4)[c] 14%		—	(4) 11%	
	(28) 100%		(7)	(35) 100%	

[a] Two of the authors made these ratings independently.
[b] Four out of six of these persons are from the same family.
[c] Two of these persons are from the same family.

misunderstanding with the hospital bureaucracy over the autopsy and a reported coolness of staff attitude further increased their negative attitudes. The fifth respondent was one of the parents who believed the estranged wife of the cadaver-donor had assumed too much authority in allowing the donation. The fact that an attempt to visit the patient one more time at the University was too late and the fact that the eyes had been removed left the respondent with a generally negative impression. Two other members of the same family felt "primarily positive" toward the donation but were critical of the hospital for the same reasons.

Many of the factors responsible for the above complaints have already been corrected, as indicated earlier, either by changes in the University protocols for communication with cadaver donor families or by the introduction of the preservation machines, which allow the body to remain at the original hospital.

All but four of the respondents whose attitudes were other than "clearly positive" are thus identified above. The four remaining persons were classified as "primarily positive," although they held some reservations. For example, a patient's sibling and his wife were very positive toward the actual donation of their sibling's organs, but were not certain whether they would be willing to donate their own child's organs if an accident were to happen to him.

All in all, the 11 respondents who reported other than "clearly positive" attitudes were from six out of the 14 families.

Several of the respondents who maintained *very* favorable attitudes over the long-run commented on the donation as the one positive aspect of the death. The following remarks were typical:

> The transplant was one of the few bright spots in the whole experience.

> The death was not a total loss. There was something good that came out the whole thing.

> I feel good about the transplant. I'm sure we did the right thing.

> We decided to donate so he could keep living somehow.

> The idea of donation helped; it gave me something tangible to hold on to.

> If we can't save him, we can save someone else.

> I feel good knowing that somebody got some benefit from his death, that there not only was a divine reason for it, but that there was something else, something tangible, that somebody profited some way.

> I feel like part of him lives in somebody else. I really feel that he has done well for himself, that he gave all that he could give in his life and his death.

> Maybe that's why he was here, or something. Maybe the other children [recipients] will do something, make a contribution or something.

For many respondents, then, the donation seemed to give meaning to an otherwise meaningless death.

Long-Term Salience of the Donation

At the time of the interview families varied in the degree to which the donation was still salient in their thoughts or talk. While most family members still thought about the death often, even daily, the donation occupied their thoughts only occasionally; some respondents reported that they didn't think about it at all anymore. In one family, however, the donation was still a relevant part of their thinking. Over 200 people had sent in donor cards because of the death of the child in this family, and the mother often talked about the donation in her contacts with friends—so often, in fact, that the other sons in the family were upset with their mother's preoccupation. The brother said:

> Even when we told her that we didn't think it was necessary she still went on.

> You don't have to go around saying, "Oh, look what we've done." Maybe that's why I didn't say as much to other people about it because I didn't think it was anything that I wanted people to praise us about.

Easing Grief

Did the respondents believe that the donation had played any role in easing their grief? Of the 17 respondents who were asked explicitly whether they felt that the donation had helped them in their own grieving, nine indicated that it had, and two others were not sure whether it had made any difference. Of the six respondents who reported that the donation had not played such a role, two claimed that if they could have had knowledge that the transplant was a long-term success, their grief might have been eased. Without such knowledge, the donation affected their grief very little.

In sum, for various reasons, most respondents remained quite positive in their feelings about the donation. For a significant number of individuals, the donation appears as the one good thing in the death, and for several others, it served to ease their grief. In fact one father believed the donation had actually had a positive impact on the interaction of the family. He explained,

> It [donation] has probably made us more appreciative of his [the son's] memories, and I think that probably all our kids look up to us with a little bit more respect. I think they probably accept us and evaluate us more than the older generation. I think it served to bring us closer together.

For other respondents, however, the donation, while viewed positively, is seen to have little current salience in their lives and little impact on their grief. In the words of one mother who had made an instantaneous decision to donate:

> Donating hasn't made any difference. . .neither easier to accept the death nor more difficult. Nothing one way or the other. If I had not donated. . .I don't know how to say it. . .as long as she was dead I'm glad that medical science has advanced to the point where some use can be made of the organs, but that's all.

Thoughts about the Transplant Recipients

At sometime or another the thoughts of virtually all the survivors turned to questions about the recipients of the donated organs. Fifteen family members specifically indicated that currently or previously they wanted more information about the recipients than they had received. In fact for many relatives, this desire for more information was quite strong. The current policy of the University Transplant Services is to send a letter to the family of the cadaver-patient shortly after the surgery thanking them for their donation and telling them something about the operation(s). Although the recipients are not named, the letter generally mentions which organs were used, the sex and age and some other basic information about the persons who received them, and some statement about the success of the transplants.

The University does not give the name of the recipient so as to protect the recipient from the well-meaning but possibly guilt-provoking concern of the cadaver-patient's family. While many recipients have stated that they would like to thank the donating family, the University staff feels that the stress of being a transplant patient is significant enough without exposing the patient to the grief of the donor's family.

The first families interviewed, however, received no information about the recipients, and because of the concerns expressed in our interviews basic information was added to the letter. As one mother said, "If you want people to do it, they have to be told more. . .they've given so much and they want something back." Without some information, the gift appears unreciprocated.

Sometimes this information is enough to give the families pleasure as well as concern. There seems to be a sense of satisfaction that one person can help the lives of more than one other person (in that two kidneys can be used and sometimes other organs as well). The information as to the sex and age of the recipients, however, was cause for momentary concern among a few respondents. One mother of an adolescent whose kidney had been transplanted to a 26-year-old man, said, "I was hoping it would be a younger person." Another respondent, a father, made the remark that he thought it was funny that a woman instead of a man would receive his son's kidney.

The letter from the transplant services was usually the only information that the family received following their donation, and however inadequate the information may seem in the light of their questions, the letter was eagerly received. One wife said:

> When I received the letter, it was about a month and a half after. In my case I was just feeling so terribly down and I've never been a down person in my whole life. But I would say that was one of the most rewarding things, to hear that something good came out of his death. Just the way it was written and everything. It really pleased me. You don't get very many rewards out of something like this.

Many family members took pleasure in sharing this letter with friends, especially if the letter implied that the transplants were successful. One mother reported, "I got a letter from the University stating that two people in their thirties had received them, and I took it to a wedding and I let 'em all read it and they thought it was just great that you could do something like that in the circumstances where he was, to help two people." Obviously, the praise and support of other people may be a significant ancillary gain of having made the decision to donate organs.

Many respondents at a year or more after the death still wanted to know how well the recipients were doing. One woman, for example, felt that following the transplant, in fairness to the cadaver-patient's family, as well as to encourage others to donate, the transplant service should send the family periodic reports on the recipients' progress.

Another mother mused over whether, and how much, the donor's relatives should be told about the recipients:

> Maybe they've got their reasons why they don't want us to know who his kidneys went to. I don't know why. We wouldn't do anything to 'em or anything but, oh, you just sometimes sit and wonder how they are. And maybe if there was a way of people checking up, maybe they'd feel freer to give parts because you could always maybe send a card and say, "How do you feel?" and then the person could write back and say, "I'm feeling great." And then you know that you've done something.

One reason that families are not always informed about the success of the operations is that not all of the organs are tolerated by the body of the recipient. One-half of all recipients of cadaver kidneys return sooner or later to the hospital with irreversible kidney rejection. This fact means that if one donor contributed two kidneys, the probability is that one recipient did well and the other did not. Seven family members were asked whether they would like to know about the recipient's health if the transplant had not been successful. Upon reflection, six out of the seven realized that they only wanted information if the operations had been a success.

One woman remarked:

> I have mixed emotions about knowing who the recipients have been. I would like to know only if it was successful. If there were some complications or if it was rejected or didn't work, then I wouldn't feel as satisfied as I do right now just from having that first letter that gave me just a little bit of information.

And another mother concurred:

> If the patients weren't doing well, we [the parents] wouldn't want to know. It still gives you a little bit of hope that he didn't die for nothing, and maybe somebody is getting some help from this. Maybe somebody else has a child that is alive on account of my son and they can live a normal life.

One father had originally been notified that one of his son's kidneys was donated to a boy his own son's age, the other to a married man with several small children. Although he would be able to tolerate the failure of the kidney to function in the adult, the success in the child-recipient was of great emotional importance to him.

Even at a year after the transplant, many cadaver-donor families feel a need to know whether the donation was successful or, in other words, whether the death had any meaning. Such positive information would serve as reciprocation to the families that gave this major gift. Yet, the hospital staff has not instituted any such long-term feedback because they are uncertain how to handle the cases in which the transplant has failed.

The Reaction of Others

There is information about others' reaction to the donation for 12 families. In all of these cases the family received some positive reaction to the donation, and this praise may have functioned as an additional reward for them. One mother said:

> It made me feel good that other people knew. I didn't know how other people would react. Everybody thought it was marvelous. They thought it was big of me. . . .Some of them didn't know if *they* could do it but they thought it was wonderful.

Others commented:

> For the most part people said "Well great." They thought it was a tremendous thing to do.

> The priest thought it was a fine idea. He assured us there was no conflict with the church. As a matter of fact, he thought it was a wonderful thing to do.

Yet not all comments of outsiders were completely favorable. Many families reported some less positive feedback as well. After one mother noted a lot of positive support from friends we asked:

INTERVIEWER. Did anyone say anything the other way?

MOTHER. Only one. . .a friend of ours. . .he doesn't believe in playing God, and if someone is sick, "let 'em die". . .he feels very strongly that we shouldn't be messing around with lives. . . .

INTERVIEWER. How did you feel when he said [this]?

MOTHER. Hurt. I felt real bad. But then I know him well enough to think, "Well that's him, no matter what we would have done he would have found something [to criticize]."

In one case a family received unpleasant crank phone calls when some persons read the news about the transplant in the paper and checked the obituary column to find a child the age of the reported cadaver donor. These calls generated much unnecessary stress.

In some cases outsiders were uninformed about the donation. Among the young siblings of a cadaver-patient, for instance, the donation did not seem a salient enough issue to discuss with their friends. And a few of the adults avoided telling others because of an anticipated negative reaction or because those they did tell did not react very positively. "You tell someone that your child had a transplant and they look at you as if, you know. It's nothing that's said. It's just the look you get."

Friends not only expressed positive or negative opinions about the donation, they also reacted with a curiosity that sometimes caused difficulty. A few respondents mentioned that the questions they received from friends were hard for them to handle because the families lacked the necessary information with which to answer them. One woman, who was not certain which, if any, organs were used, stated:

> It made me feel uncomfortable because people would say something and I thought it was very dishonest to be taking credit for something that I didn't even know. . .maybe they didn't take anything [from the patient]. This bothered me quite a bit those first few weeks. Finally I called the hospital because I had to know.*

The curiosity on the part of the friends of one family was so extreme that the mother felt she had to serve a fielding function between the transplant recipient and her friends. She said:

> Some of our friends have expressed concern about what happened to the children, and they wanted us to come over and visit the children that the transplants were made to. They were quite upset that we didn't. Some friends

* This was an early case. Better information now is transmitted earlier by letter to the families.

wanted to come with us too, to reassure themselves that everything would be all right. We don't want to bother these people.

CONCLUSION AND SUMMARY

Relatives of potential cadaver-donors are confronted with a major decision. The type of decision is similar in many ways to the one faced by potential *living related* kidney donors. In both cases the decision once implemented will be irreversible, and its consequences will be highly significant. In both situations, the decision has to be made in the context of a major stress or crisis involving the decision-maker's family. For both, it is an important, unique, and nonrepetitive decision, rather than a choice which is likely to confront the decision-maker again.

There are, however, several differences between the decision facing the cadaver-donor family and the potential living related donors. First, the time deadline for the cadaver-donor family is considerably shorter. The decision to donate cadaver organs must be made in the space of a few days at most, and usually within several hours; whereas the living donors have weeks, months, and even sometimes years to deliberate if they so desire. Similarly the time between the resolution and implementation of the decision is much shorter in the cadaver-donor case, leaving effectively little or no time for the family to change its mind.

In addition, the decision is presented to the cadaver-donor family as one whose outcome entails no direct risk and no direct benefit for the donor himself. The donor is defined as effectively dead, unable to be harmed, and the person to benefit from the act will be a stranger. In contrast, the related living donor assumes a definite known risk himself, and presumably also benefits directly from the fact that a close relative will continue to live because of his efforts. In reality, families of the cadaver-donors sometimes still hope for a miraculous return of consciousness while the machines are artificially maintaining their brain-dead relative's respiration. Thus they view donation as ending the very small possibility that their relative might revive. In this sense donation is perceived by them as a real risk.

Finally, a major distinction between the living and cadaver-donor decisions is that the latter is more likely to be made at the family level. When there is a search for a living related donor, any one family member can solve the problem alone by volunteering to donate and by relieving other family members of the decision. However, in most cadaver-donor cases all key family members believe they must reach consensus before the donation can be allowed.

Yet the family definition of which members are key is important to note. In most of the 14 families studied there were strong normative feelings defining the family members who had a right to help make the decision. Consensus was fairly easily achieved because relatives who were likely to oppose the decision (i.e., the older generation of grandparents) were excluded as legitimate participants. Parents and sometimes older, but not younger, siblings were seen as the proper decision-makers.

When the cadaver-donor was married, the spouse was defined as the legitimate decision-maker. However, as in the case of living related donors, conflict and stress occurred where there were two families instead of one, where there were parents and a spouse who could participate in the decision.

Frequent factors motivating the key family members toward donation were their empathy with the ill kidney recipients, their desire for some type of physical immortality for their own relative, and their relief at not having to decide when to turn off the artificial respirator. At the same time the decision and the period following the decision were sometimes made more stressful because the relatives had difficulty in accepting the concept of brain death when the cadaver appeared to be breathing and when his heart was still beating. They experienced uncertainty when no exact moment of death could be identified in other than an arbitrary way. Despite the fact they had been told the patient was dead, some relatives felt guilty at having to sign the papers that guaranteed his removal from the machinery maintaining his heartbeat.

Initial reaction to the idea of donation seemed to be dependent upon the relatives' full realization of the fact that the patient was dead. In some cases the physician's first mention of donation served as the announcement of death or the announcement that the situation was hopeless. At that moment, as the relatives reacted emotionally to the announcement that there was no longer hope, any plans for the future seemed inappropriate. In the stages of grieving there seemed to be a need for a time lapse, even a short one, between the period of desperate hope when the dying patient was still defined as alive and the period of time when plans for handling the death could be made. During this transitional time period the situation was redefined as hopeless or the patient as dead. Once the redefinition appeared to have occurred and the associated shock absorbed, the relatives were able to react decisively to the idea of donation.*

* For further discussion of the stages of grief, see Glick et al. (1974) and Lindemann (1944).

We have noted earlier that the act of donation appeared to enhance the living related donor's feelings of self-worth and happiness over the long-term. Because the cadaver-donor family still had to confront the tragedy of their young relative's death, no such substantial effect was expected. Rather, the question was whether the donation mitigated or intensified the family's grief over the long-run. Although at a year or more after the death the donation was not salient to all relatives, most felt positively about the fact that they had donated. Several relatives indicated that the grieving process had been made easier by the transplant, because the donation gave some meaning to an otherwise meaningless death and their relative had achieved a type of immortality through the donation.

However, the need to feel that their relative had attained a type of immortality was somewhat frustrated by the lack of long-term information about the recipients. Many family members indicated a desire to have continuing knowledge about the health of the recipients as well as some detail about their lives. They wished to know that the gift was a successful and valuable one. Yet, they did not wish to know if the transplant had been unsuccessful.

While most members of cadaver-donor families were generally positive about the donation despite complaints such as these, five of the 35 family members interviewed held negative feelings toward the donation a year later. Some of their reaction was attributable to guilt and some to the probably inevitable displacement of anger about the tragic death onto the University Hospital personnel, who were the ones to actually remove the donor from the machines that had maintained the heartbeat. But other complaints seemed to be due to the hospital's insensitivities to the family's feelings, particularly in the early days of the program. Even the more "positive" relatives sometimes voiced such complaints toward the hospital and toward the University physician who secured their signatures.

Expensive medical innovation is likely to be instituted at large bureaucratic University hospitals. And these bureaucracies, particularly at the beginning of a new program, are likely to be unresponsive to unique needs of special groups. In addition, physicians are untrained in methods of aiding grieving families, especially in situations in which they are not offering medical help to these families.

A major cause of many of the difficulties that we have discussed in this chapter may emanate from the term *cadaver-donor* itself. While the "cadaver-patient" is labelled as the "donor," in reality it is the family who makes the donation. This mislabelling seems to have given rise to a misperception of the crucial role that the family actually plays in the donation proceedings and subsequently to the failure of the staff to be attentive to many of the psychological and social needs of the donor families. The family gives the gift of the organ and they expect information, recognition or gratitude in return. Because the family tends to perceive the entire hospital as benefiting from the donation, they can be angered by any seeming lack of consideration even when it originates from hospital officials who have little association with the transplant service.

In conclusion, donation, whether it originates from living related donors or from the families of cadaver-patients, has many long-term psychological benefits and therefore appears to be positively regarded by the majority of donors. Yet neither type of donation is free of stress, and in a minority of cases the stress has been severe. Although there is no quantitative method to weigh the comparative psychological costs and benefits of related and cadaver donation, these data do not establish a clear comparative advantage for cadaver donation. Katz and Capron (1975) and Brewer (1970) and many others suggest curtailing donation from living related donors. The increased reliance on cadaver donors, were there no cadaver donor shortage, would not necessarily reduce the overall level of stress or the ethical dilemmas.

IV

HEALTH CARE DELIVERY ISSUES AND CONCLUSION

11

HEALTH CARE DELIVERY: THE FINANCING OF TRANSPLANTATION

Organ transplantation, as a new medical technology, has clearly raised significant socioethical questions. For the individuals who are most intimately involved—the patients, the donors, and their families—the new technology has developed faster than the ethical questions could be resolved. The concept of "cultural lag" appears appropriate to describe this gap between development of the new technology and the resolution of related ethical problems.

Cultural lag is also evident in the hiatus between the advancement of transplantation technology and the development of a health care delivery system necessary for its optimal use. The technological changes required social adjustments; and until such adjustments could be made, unanticipated stress occurred for the government, the medical system, and the patients requiring treatment. Originally there was a severe problem of adequate access of patients to treatment because of financial shortages, the nature of the organization of medical care, and the referral and communication systems among physicians.

THE ORGANIZATION OF MEDICAL CARE AND ACCESS TO TREATMENT

Technological advances in medicine have significant consequences for the organization of medical care and its availability to the public. (See Simmons and Simmons, 1971). Therapies such as organ transplantation, open-heart surgery, and cancer chemotherapy move medicine one step further toward the bureaucratization, organization, and specialization that is characteristic of almost every sphere in modern industrial society, particularly those influenced by technological advances. Medicine is becoming more of a specialized team operation and less of a relationship between an individual family physician and his patient. As Rosenblatt and Suchman (1964) point out:

> During the twentieth century, medicine has become increasingly specialized and highly organized. We have witnessed the creation of enormous hospital complexes, highly technical research, specialization, and the trend toward group practice. The private family physician has often been replaced with a much more imposing bureaucracy of aides, nurses, ancillary therapists, technicians, and highly qualified specialists.

To the metropolitan working-class patient who is accustomed to visiting hospital clinics, treatment in a kidney transplant or a cancer chemotherapy center may be just another step in the customary pattern. To the middle-class or small-town patient who is used to more personal contact with a family practitioner, however, the mode of treatment may seem very new. He is accustomed to being referred to individual specialists for specific ailments, but here he is referred to a hospital and a large, somewhat impersonal, and constantly shifting medical team. Table 11-1 shows the organization of the renal transplant team at the University of Minnesota. The patient in the hospital may be under the care of six or seven physicians at once, who are aided by a variety of special nurses, technicians, and therapists. The central therapeutic event, the transplantation operation itself, requires 12 people. After discharge, when the successful transplant patient returns to the hospital clinic for routine tests, he does not usually engage in one-to-one interaction with a physician at the University of Minnesota. Rather, he talks in the morning to the nurse coordinator and then in the afternoon waits for his turn to enter a roomful of the members of the transplant team—that is, a faculty surgeon, one or two members of the surgical house staff, the nurse coordinator, her assistant, the clinic nurse, the psychiatrist, the social worker, the dietician, and the assistant dietician. Such a roomful of staff can be overwhelming for the patient who has minor questions or

TABLE 11-1 PERSONNEL OF A TRANSPLANT CENTER PERFORMING 100 TO 200 TRANSPLANTS PER YEAR AND MAINTAINING FOLLOW-UP FACILITIES FOR 500 POSTTRANSPLANT RECIPIENTS [a]

	Director Transplantation Center (surgeon)	
Administrative assistant (nurse)	Director Transplantation (surgeon)	Director Hemodialysis (nephrologist)
1 nurse in charge of patient education 2 secretaries	Recipient Service: 1 surgical fellow 2 full-time residents 2 full-time interns Donor Service: 1 part-time surgical staff 1 surgical fellow 3 part-time residents Nursing Service: Head nurse 44 nurses, practical nurses, and student nurses	1 adult nephrologist 1 pediatric nephrologist 1 resident 1 head nurse 11 nurses 8 technicians
Special laboratories:	Assigned consultants:	Consultant services:
Histocompatibility testing Director 3 technicians Antilympocyte globulin manufacture and quality control 1 immunochemist (Ph.D.) 3 technicians Organ preservation: 1 full-time technician	Psychiatrist Social worker Dietician Pediatrician Neurologist Otolaryngologist Orthopedist Ophthalmologist Urologist	Nuclear medicine Diagnostic radiology Radiotherapy Pharmacy Vocational rehabilitation Physical medicine Occupational therapy Blood bank Hematology Microbiology Laboratory medicine Infectious diseases

[a] University of Minnesota Clinical Transplantation Center (Chart excludes personnel engaged primarily in research.)

"private" problems to raise. Reinhard (1970) indicates that in the early days heart transplant teams were even larger. For one particular heart transplant performed at the Texas Heart Institute, Reinhard estimated that over a five-day period 141 persons were involved in one official capacity or another; 21 were physicians.

In addition to the personnel, special facilities must be immediately available at a kidney transplant center: the artificial kidney to support patients with inadequate kidney function; a preservation machine and the technical assistance to maintain it so that kidneys from cadavers can be preserved until they are transplanted; specially collected and stored blood for transfusion because whole blood transfusions may immunize patients against future organ transplants; tissue typing and cross-matching services; a mobile team of surgeons to travel to outlying community hospitals to remove and preserve kidneys from cadavers.

Only relatively large hospitals can support so many personnel and special facilities. Transplantation, therefore, like other advanced medical technologies, tends to be concentrated in a number of large centers throughout the country. Large cities and university areas are more likely to have such centers than are smaller cities and towns. Patients must adjust to the new experience of traveling away from their communities to these centers for medical treatment. Furthermore, this restriction of transplant centers is extraordinarily important when the availability of medical resources to patients is considered. What type of patient is likely to be cared for there? How do patients from various social strata and from communities all over the United States flow to these centers? How does the individual uremic patient come to be treated at one of these transplant centers?

LAG IN MEDICAL ORGANIZATION AND COMMUNICATION

The optimal flow of patients to the centers of transplantation seems to have been affected by a communication barrier between these centers and local referring physicians, as well as by a scarcity of facilities. Originally, prior to the federal funding of kidney transplantation which was implemented in 1973, many patients who were suitable for treatment were dying of kidney disease. By 1972 it was estimated that 10,000 to 13,000 new patients a year could be treated by transplantation or dialysis (Altman, 1973; National Kidney Foundation, 1973). At that point, without federal funding, approximately 6000 people a year were dying because they could not afford the new technology.

These statistics suggest that an overload of applicants forced kidney transplant centers to reject many candidates. There is also some evidence, however, that the flow of suitable patients to centers was blocked at certain points and may still be so. In Minnesota, for example, despite the fact that many patients with primary renal disease who would respond to dialysis or transplantation continued to die, the renal failure centers were not overcrowded with applications. Medically eligible candidates were not being denied treatment because of shortages of facilities. Surgeons at another center reported that they had virtually no applicants from one entire area of the state they serviced. Furthermore, a study published by the Comptroller-General, reports that 33 out of 53 transplant and dialysis physicians queried perceived lack of patient referrals to be a problem, and several reported cases in which patients had sought dialysis treatment despite the opinion of their local physician that their disease was terminal (GAO, 1975). At the University of Minnesota 50 patients or approximately one-quarter of all patients followed from 1970 to 1972 told us that the physician they first consulted indicated that there was no help for them.

Referring physicians apparently have not sent all possible candidates to renal failure centers. The reasons for this have not been systematically investigated, but several channels of speculation are open. Without question, the technological potential seems to have outstripped the communication networks in medicine, as well as the resources (Coleman et al., 1959). The diagnosis of uremia traditionally evoked a feeling of hopelessness in most physicians. Palliative treatment was all physicians had to offer until recently, and such attitudes are not easily cast off. In addition, many physicians have probably been unaware of the success of kidney transplantation and dialysis, the categories of patients who can benefit, and even the presence of the nearest center. They may believe that the patient is too old, or that children cannot be dialyzed, or that the sacrifices in travel and expense are too great for the family.

The centralization of these specialized resources may act as a further deterrent to the referral process. A recent report indicates that in 12 states the proportion of the population being treated for kidney disease was much greater within 20 miles of a major treatment center than between 20 and 40 miles (GAO, 1975). It is always difficult for physicians to refer patients to centers and hospitals where they have no personal acquaintances among the professional staff. In general physicians have developed ingrained patterns of referral that are seldom varied. For most medical problems, the physician's local mutual referral network is adequate (Freidson, 1963). Most specialists can be found within a reasonable distance to participate in this network. Yet the physicians within the centralized university center form their own networks and do not usually refer patients to local nonuniversity physicians (Kendall, 1965). University physicians tend not to participate in local medical society activities. Thus the local physicians, even within easy distance of the large medical center, may be unacquainted with many university physicians. As distance from the university center increases, personal contacts naturally decrease. Paradoxically, although originally there were not enough facilities for all uremic patients, in some areas of the country there is underutilization of such facilities because the patient and his physician are effectively unaware of the availability.

The effect of a patient's class background upon his chances to be referred for transplantation is another point for investigation. People from the lower-class utilize medical services less than middle- or upper-class members (Rosenblatt and Suchman, 1964). Yet if the lower-class patient seeks medical care in a large city, he is likely to attend the large hospital, clinic, or veteran's hospital where referral to a transplantation center is probable. Perhaps investigation would show that the lower-class patient from outside of the metropolis, from the smaller towns and cities, will be the last to benefit from this type of medical advance. The role of the local physician's conscious or unconscious racial or social class bias in referring patients to this type of medical facility requires study.

Social factors governing the dissemination of accurate information concerning medical innovation, and social factors affecting the interrelationships between centralized medical centers and referring physicians play a large role in whether a patient will live or die.

Communication Lag and the Cadaver-Donor Resource

At present in the United States the mobilization of the cadaver-donor resource is also restricted by many of the same factors that have prevented a uremic patient from being referred to a transplant center. Lags in medical organization and communication affect the availability of organs for transplantation, because a high percentage of such organs must come from cadavers. The role of the local referring physician is again crucial; the family physician cares for a high percentage of potential cadaver-donors, and he is usually the one who first approaches the family with the suggestion of donation (see chapter 10). However, the possibility of donation may not even occur to him; or he may find approaching the family difficult; and he may not be well enough acquainted with a transplant center for referral to be psychologically easy. The limitation in number of centers means that many potential donors will be excluded because of distance.

Furthermore, even when local physicians are aware of referral mechanisms, organizational and logistical problems make the procedure of cadaver donation difficult. When the transplant service sends a team to the local hospital to remove the kidneys and transport them back to the transplant center, the local physicians and hospital authorities must be willing to undergo considerable inconvenience. The frequently overtaxed community doctor must await the transplant surgeons and then help them mobilize the hospital facilities. The hospital must be willing to clean and set up a surgical suite, reserve some personnel to help, and sometimes disrupt schedules and rules to satisfy the necessary procedures and time pressures. Until the implementation of federal funding, payment for the use of these hospital facilities and personnel was uncertain, adding a further barrier to the ready availability of cadaver kidneys.

LAG IN ALLOCATION OF FINANCIAL RESOURCES: HISTORY PRIOR TO 1972

The best known and most significant way the society lagged behind the technological potential of transplantation involved the allocation of adequate financial support. The scarcity of resources for transplantation and dialysis involved not only personnel and available hospital beds, but in the decade prior to July 1973 there were not adequate funds to pay the patient's hospital bill. Technological advances in medicine are extremely expensive and appear to require government decision on reallocation of resources. John Knowles (1969), analyzing manpower shortages in radiology, writes:

> New technologies create new options and opportunities. . . .The decision must be made whether the benefit of the new technology will ultimately justify the cost of establishing it and the diversion of scarce resources away from other critical areas of development.

Federal experts have estimated a first-year cost of $135 million rising to $1 billion in a decade to treat medically-eligible terminal kidney patients (Lyons, 1973). If transplantation of other organs also achieves success, these costs will skyrocket. If an artificial heart becomes technologically feasible, the annual costs have been estimated at $250 million to $1 billion, figuring $15,000 to $25,000 for each heart, for 16,750 to 50,300 patients a year (Artificial Heart Assessment Panel, 1973). As additional medical technologies develop, the government will be increasingly confronted with a fundamental decision: can this society allocate major sums of money to saving the lives of the previously incurable?

Most patients themselves could not be expected to pay for the costs of expensive new technologies like transplantation and dialysis—costs that usually run into the \$10,000 to \$30,000 range. Even less controversial technologies are very expensive—for example, a course of treatment for childhood leukemia costs approximately \$9000; a coronary bypass surgery, \$8000. Without a comprehensive national program, the collection of such funds has in the past caused major difficulties for government agencies, the hospital, and the patient. Before the new federal legislation (which we discuss below), some of the cost for kidney transplantation was paid by federal research grants to the institution, but these grants were being withdrawn as the procedure became a therapeutic reality. Insurance paid some of the cost, but policies were limited in the number of days of coverage; it was estimated at one center that they paid less than one-third of the average transplant costs. The Arthur D. Little Report (1969) estimated conservatively that approximately 8% to 10% of the American population were adequately covered by insurance for transplantation (also see Wilkins, 1972). In fact many families of lower socioeconomic status had no hospitalization coverage at all (The Artificial Heart Assessment Panel, 1973, p. 135).

Until July 1973 the sources of funding for kidney transplants and dialysis could not begin to cover the actual need, although some public funds were available through Regional Medical Programs and other sources (see Table 11-2 for representation of these sources of funding; also see Wilkins, 1972). Patients in some states were more fortunate, because they could turn to government agencies for major help in paying their bills under Title 19 of Medicaid. However, many states had interpreted Title 19 in such a way that (a) dialysis and transplant patients were excluded completely; (b) patients could receive benefits only if they were already on welfare; (c) it was difficult to obtain benefits if patients were treated out-of-state, despite lack of facilities in their home state; or (d) very few days of coverage were permitted.

Even if Medicaid was available in the home state, the cost of transplantation could threaten whatever financial security a patient had. To qualify for Medicaid in Minnesota during the years before the 1973 "kidney amendment" was passed, a patient had to pass a means test. He must have been earning less than \$2200 a year plus \$500 for each child; his cash assets must not have been greater than \$1000; and his property assets must not have exceeded \$15,000. If he had greater assets, he had to contribute a significant amount toward the transplant, and the hospital could put a lien on all property except his home in an attempt to collect the bills. The lower-middle and middle-class patients probably suffered most from such requirements.

TABLE 11-2 PUBLIC SOURCES OF FUNDING FOR DIALYSIS AND KIDNEY TRANSPLANTATION IN 1969[a]

National Institutes of Health Research Grants to Medical Centers
U.S. Public Health Service Grants and Contracts to Medical Centers
Title 19 Medicaid
Title 18 Medicare
Vocational Rehabilitation Program
Regional Medical Program
Special State Legislation for financial support of renal patients
State Crippled Children's Services
Public Law 89–749 (Section 314d and e)—Support given directly to kidney disease programs
Veterans Administration Hospital Funds and Benefits—primarily for veterans and family

[a] From *Kidney Disease Services, Facilities and Programs in the United States*, Washington, D.C.: United States Government Printing Office. Public Health Service Publication No. 1942. May, 1969.

The tendency for transplant centers like other new medical technologies to be concentrated in relatively few medical facilities had many important, unanticipated consequences in connection with the scarcity of of funding. As in the case of the University of Minnesota, the limited number of transplant centers that existed had to service many nearby states. Yet these hospitals could not continually afford to absorb the costs of patients from states with less liberal interpretation of Title 19. The losses from unpaid bills on the transplant service would have been a severe financial strain for the hospital. Some centers were forced to reject all but wealthy out-of-state applicants. Doctors were forced to tell dying out-of-state patients that only if they could bring $20,000 to the center would they be accepted for treatment.

While national financial planning was out of pace with the available technology, patients were denied treatment on arbitrary bases, such as their state of origin or their financial status. These geographic discrepancies were further widened by the fact that there were a few states that had set aside state funds in addition to Medicaid to pay for residents' transplantation and dialysis expenses (Little, 1969). Prior to 1973 it appeared to be much better to be suffering from terminal kidney disease in Illinois than in Idaho or Wyoming, where few public funds were available. In Illinois Medicaid and Medicare moneys could be used, and the state had appropriated an additional $1,000,000 for the care and treatment of persons suffering from chronic kidney disease who were unable to pay for life-saving treatment (Kidney Disease Services, Facilities, and Programs in the United States, 1969).

Even the county of origin became important. In Minnesota, for example, the county decided on the patient's eligibility for Medicaid funds, and the county contributed to the benefits along with the state and federal government. One expensive transplant could exhaust a rural county's entire annual medical welfare budget, so subsequent patients from that county would be denied.

Our goal in this section is not to review all the past sources of transplantation funding. Instead, it is an attempt to illustrate how technological potential outstripped the allocation of financial resources until 1973, with the result that patients were denied treatment for arbitrary geographical and social reasons; and hospitals, patients, and local agencies were subject to great financial strain. Most of the existing dialysis and transplantation facilities were financed originally in large part by federal research funds, yet they did not appear to be used to the equal benefit of all citizens. Kidney patients able to pay for treatment appeared to have an advantage. Without a national catastrophic health insurance plan, such inequities would operate for any new expensive technology. However, to assume a middle-class bias on the part of physicians as the major cause of this situation would be an oversimplification. Although class bias may exist, the organizational and societal pressures will be much more powerful factors in the overselection of patients able to pay.

This analysis has also indicated that the concentration of new medical technologies in a few large hospital complexes penalizes those patients who are geographically removed from such centers. Not only do local physicians appear less likely to refer such patients but funding has been more difficult to obtain.

CLOSING THE FINANCIAL GAP: REDUCING THE LAG

Should society reallocate its resources to correct these imbalances and inequities? This question has sparked a political controversy of values and priorities. A Chronic Kidney Disease Amendment to the Social Security Act of 1972 was passed which now pays for almost all transplantation and dialysis expenses as of July 1973 (PL 92–603, popularly known as the HR–1 amendment), and the federal government seems to be on the way to establishing some form of catastrophic or national health insurance. Thus the society has attempted to make major financial reallocations and, as we discuss later, major changes in the health care delivery system, to solve the problem emanating from technological progress.

HISTORY OF MEDICARE AND THE KIDNEY AMENDMENT

Medicare

Acceptance of government funding of medical payments did not occur suddenly, and the history of the movement toward this goal is an interesting example of the process of social and political change, and it enhances our understanding of federal funding for kidney disease. The first major step was the creation of Medicare and Medicaid. Theodore Marmor's excellent review of the politics of Medicare (1973) identifies important characteristics of this type of change. The process of change can be described as "incremental" rather than sudden. Although the result produces major changes in the health delivery system, the movement in that direction is gradual and slow, so that each step seems a small one.*

It has taken 40 years since the question of national health insurance was seriously raised by Roosevelt and more than 20 years since Truman tried to resurrect it for the United States to be as close as it is to health insurance for catastrophic disease. In the early 1950s, when the proponents of a national health insurance realized that the United States Congress would not follow the example of Britain and create a major national health insurance program or even a program to insure the poor, they decided to create a narrow less controversial bill that would cover far fewer medical costs but would "get a foot in the door." The target of the bill first presented in 1952 was narrowed to include only the aged and only their hospital costs rather than physician's bills. Thus the bill looked less like an attempt to alter the medical system fundamentally. It took supporters of the Medicare bill six years to create enough congressional interest in the bill to hold annual hearings, and it took until 1965 for the bill to pass.

In 1964 it looked as if the politics of incrementalism, a process of narrowing the issue and gradually building up support, would finally be successful and the narrow bill would be at least voted on, if not passed, the next session. A landslide victory in 1964 for Lyndon Johnson hastened the politics of incrementalism and made Congress feel that there was a mandate to pass Medicare. With this mandate everyone, including prior opponents such as the Republicans and the AMA, attempted to get on the

* See Etzioni's (1968) discussion of incremental and mixed scanning policy-making.

bandwagon and produce bills of their own. The compromise bill turned out therefore to be a broader one than expected or hoped for under the politics of gradualism.

Two amendments to the Social Security Bill were passed: Title 18 and 19. Part A of Title 18 was the old narrow bill paying hospital costs for the aged, financed by Social Security payments. Part B was a voluntary doctors insurance for which each elderly person had to pay a premium. Title 19 of Medicaid enabled a state at its option to elect to cover lower-income individuals *of any age* with state and federal funds, and this part of the bill has paid for kidney patients in many states. The bills were broader than hoped for but narrower than originally conceived in the New Deal and Fair Deal periods. Yet the precedent was there for Social Security to be expanded once more to cover catastrophic disease such as end-stage kidney disease. The establishment of a small program as a precedent that can later be expanded is the hallmark of incrementalism.

A second characteristic of change in this area involves pressure-group politics; the opposition pressure groups, of course, slow down change and help to maintain the cultural lag between technological advance and whatever reorganization of the health care delivery system might be necessary to ensure its distribution. According to Marmor (1973, p. 107) Medicare was a case of a policy of "redistribution of resources." In general, as postulated by Lowi (1964) such policies of redistribution frequently reveal basic social-class cleavages in the society and therefore foster polarized enduring conflict among large national pressure groups. The Medicare bills certainly revealed basic class cleavages in the society, with political conservatives and liberals at loggerheads on the issue. The large national pressure groups in conflict over the decade were the labor unions (AFL–CIO) as proponents of the bill and the American Medical Association (AMA) in opposition.

The underlying issues on which they fought were not only basic differences in liberal-conservative ideology or the fear that physicians' economic interest was threatened. The major underlying issues are still problematic in terms of the federal policies concerning kidney disease. A major issue from the point of view of the AMA then and now involves potential threats to the *independent professional status* of the physician, an independence they believe is necessary for adequate patient care (Taylor, 1968, chapter 5). Many professionals in a variety of fields believe that their own commitment to service and to their discipline is motivation enough to ensure that they will regulate themselves. They place high value on autonomy in carrying out their tasks. As experts in medicine or in other professions, they tend to be very resistant to the idea of having their behavior dictated by nonprofessionals, who are less knowledgeable than they (Freidson and Rhea, 1965). The AMA and most physicians have felt strongly that the government should not dictate what treatment they may prescribe for patients.

At the time of the Medicare controversy the argument was made that once the government pays the bills, the next step would be the regulation of permissible medical treatment. *From the point of view of the physician*, the danger is bureaucratic inefficient regulation of medical treatment by those who lack expertise and the bases for judgment. The physician sees innovation as being suppressed and patient care suffering.

From the point of view of the government proponents of Medicare, even in the 1960s there *was* felt to be a need for some regulation of patient care. However, they termed such regulation "quality control"—that is, regulation of the physicians for the *benefit* of the patient. Wolkstein, one of the chief HEW participants, complained that a weakness of the Medicare bill was the "absence of quality standards" (Marmor, 1973, p. 65). But this weakness in Medicare was necessary, at least temporarily, in terms of the politics of incrementalism, for a bill regulating quality could not have been passed at that time.

The independent professionalism of the physician appeared to be threatened still further by the government paying the fees. The physicians were afraid that the next step would involve the government deciding on the size of the fees, as well as destroying the traditional "fee for service" relationship between the patient and his doctor. AMA policy was that it was important that the physician collect from the patient rather than from the government or from the hospital.

Again, in fact the AMA was not wrong about the intentions of government proponents of Medicare; such proponents were *not* averse to some regulation in terms of the size of fees. Certain officials believed that the potential for overcharging was a weakness of this bill (Marmor, 1973, p. 65). However, the politics of incrementalism led to a law (1) that avoided prescribing fee schedules but directed instead that doctors be paid their "usual and customary fee," and (2) allowed the physician to bill the patient who would be reimbursed by insurance. Therefore, the physician had the option of charging the patient more than the Medicare fee.

Thus, many of the proponents of Medicare would have desired some "cost" and "quality" control, but their tactic was to eliminate such features temporarily and to get a program started that could later be expanded if public support was forthcoming. The program was designed to mitigate controversy and to be so narrow that opposition would seem politically unpopular. Both the proponents and opponents viewed the bill as a first step to be followed by further government regulation of treatment and of size of medical charges. However, from the supporters' view, the beginning was a positive one to be improved by later cost and quality control. To the opponents it was a dangerous precedent to future programs that would threaten responsible autonomous professionalism.

These issues of cost and quality control have continued to remain major points of controversy between proponents of expanded health insurance and a large segment of physicians in private practice represented by the AMA. Before proceeding to the more modern history of the HR–1 amendment funding kidney transplantation, we should note one more important variable affecting this type of political and societal change—that is, the larger political setting or context. In the 1950s when the Medicare bills were first presented, fear of communism seemed to be the overriding issue. While the liberals were attempting massive social reform under New Deal and Fair Deal policies, the conservatives were frightened of an internal move toward communistic or socialistic policies. Thus the AMA was able to capture much sympathy from many non-medical quarters when they pointed to the dangers of socialized medicine and government control of the free professional.

In the 1970s the larger political context has changed. Consumer protection is a major issue, and in that light medical cost and quality control seem very different. And as expensive new medical technologies threaten to impoverish middle-class patients as well as members of the working class, the issue of federal funding for catastrophic disease seems much less a fundamental social class controversy.

*The History of the HR–1 Kidney Amendment: 1972**

The answer to the problem of overwhelming costs for expensive new medical technologies has seemed for a number of years to be either catastrophic or national health insurance. In line with the policy of incremental social change, experts expected that it would be some time before enough support could be mustered for such a program but that it would eventually become an actuality. Many members of the National Kidney Foundation (a major voluntary association) believed that a general catastrophic health insurance bill or another form of national insurance would be the solution for kidney transplantation and dialysis. †

However, to the surprise of many, the kidney patient did not have to wait for such a general bill. In September 1972 the following amendment

* This section is based on interviews with members of various physicians' groups such as the National Kidney Foundation and the Renal Physicians Association, as well as with many key officials in various government offices, particularly within the HEW.

† See Tomkins (1974) and Somers and Somers (1972) for a review of 15 bills pending and the issues involved in national health insurance.

to the 1972 Social Security bill (PL 92–603) was passed, along with its parent bill:

> (e) Notwithstanding the foregoing provisions of this section, every individual who—
>
> (1) has not attained the age of 65;
>
> (2) (A) is fully or currently insured (as such terms are defined in section 214 of this Act), or (B) is entitled to monthly insurance benefits under Title II of this Act, or (C) is the spouse or dependent child (as defined in regulations) of an individual who is fully or currently insured, or (D) is the spouse or dependent child (as defined in regulations) of an individual entitled to monthly insurance benefits under Title II of this Act; and
>
> (3) is medically determined to have chronic renal disease and who requires hemodialysis or renal transplantation for such disease; shall be deemed to be disabled for purposes of coverage under parts A and B of Medicare subject to the deductible, premium, and copayment provisions of Title XVIII.
>
> (f) Medical eligibility on the basis of chronic kidney failure shall begin with the third month after the month in which a course of renal dialysis is initiated and would end with the twelfth month after the month in which the person has a renal transplant or such course of dialysis is terminated.
>
> (g) The Secretary is authorized to limit reimbursement under Medicare for kidney transplant and dialysis to kidney disease treatment centers which meet such requirements as he may by regulation prescribe: Provided, that such requirements must include at least requirements for a minimal utilization rate for covered procedures and for a medical review board to screen the appropriateness of patients for the proposed treatment procedures.

Like Medicare this amendment can be seen as the result of incremental legislative change. More than 100 bills to aid the kidney patient preceded this amendment over a four- to five-year period ("The Kidney Care Issue," 1973). Some of these were successful small programs such as the $15 million allocated to the Regional Medical Program for several regional kidney centers (see Table 11-2 for a list of Federal programs that help fund kidney patients). Others had not been passed. In the course of hearings and hundreds of hours of testimony for these kidney bills and for catastrophic and national health insurance, much congressional sympathy had gradually developed for kidney transplantation and dialysis. However, the final output was not a bill in its own right that would be debated and voted on directly in both House and Senate, but a floor amendment, a rider that was introduced in the Senate by Senators Vance Hartke and Russell B. Long.*

The amendment can be viewed as the narrowing down of Senator Long's original more general catastrophic insurance proposal, which failed to be incorporated into the 1972 Social Security Act. While pending, this general proposal seemed a potential vehicle for helping kidney patients; and when the Finance Committee omitted it from the final act, Senators Hartke and Long were sympathetic to funding kidney disease alone through a floor amendment ("The Kidney Care Issue," 1973). The kidney amendment also was a stepwise expansion of still another stepwise extension of Medicare. In the 1972 Social Security Act, Medicare benefits were to be extended to the 1.7 million permanently disabled persons of any age in the Social Security system. Yet without an amendment, dialysis patients who were able to work would not be classified as disabled under this act and therefore would not secure medical coverage. Thus the amendment simply classified patients with end-stage kidney disease as disabled, whether or not they could work, thereby making them eligible for benefits.

In sum, the Medicare mechanism could be easily expanded to include permanently disabled persons of any age and to cover one catastrophic disease. By narrowing the bill to one health problem rather than all major diseases, the expansion of coverage seemed small rather than major. Yet although it was not deliberately planned that way, once one particular catastrophic illness had been covered, a new bill to fund all catastrophic disease looked somehow less revolutionary. This pattern is the trademark of incrementalism. Stepwise alterations make major change appear minimal. In fact, however, the social changes in health care delivery encompassed by the HR–1 amendment are potentially quite far-reaching.

Although both the original Medicare bill and the HR–1 amendment share a history of legislative incrementalism, the pressure-group politics were different. Instead of a case of intense polarization and conflict, this amendment was produced by a special-interest group, the National Kidney Foundation, working closely and *quietly* with congressional and senate staffs, with no organized opposition.

Although the Kidney Foundation leaders saw the implications for larger catastrophic funding, they chose to work for their own special-interest group as is customary, rather than to ally themselves with other voluntary health agencies. The chances for rapid success and lesser controversy seemed more likely in this way. In fact, the lack of publicity

* For other analyses of the history of this amendment, see Rettig (1976) and Zeckhauser (1975).

was probably crucial to the easy passage of the amendment. However, the Kidney Foundation had to supply some justification to congressional and senate leaders for funding this disease as a separate category. The Kidney Foundation and the government characterized kidney disease as more manageable and controllable than other diseases in terms of accounting. The population affected each year was definable and relatively small—approximately 13,000 patients suitable for dialysis or transplantation each year.* The therapy is also definable, and the success or failure is easily measured in terms of patient survival and kidney survival. To try coverage of such a disease before full catastrophic insurance was passed seemed sensible. According to Senator Long, the kidney provision was not a step toward costly piecemeal catastrophic health insurance with each disease covered by a separate bill. The next step was to be a more general national health insurance or catastrophic health insurance bill.

Members of the senate staff working on the more comprehensive health insurance bills do not see the fate of their bill to be dependent on the successful implementation of the HR–1 kidney amendment, but they do see themselves learning from the problems that are emerging as it goes into effect. Thus HR–1 can be considered a pioneer venture into funding catastrophic disease. It is a major breakthrough, and may be used as a pilot or model for future broader bills. In Senator Hartke's words:

> Mr. President, one of the proudest achievements of my 15 years in the U.S. Senate was the passage of the kidney disease amendment on September 28, 1972. That amendment inaugurated the first national catastrophic health insurance program in the history of the United States (Hartke, 1974).

And the Final Policy Statement of April 1974 dealing with the implementation of the kidney amendment notes:

> Our policies will undoubtedly be carefully scrutinized as possible forerunners for future federal health care legislation and programs.

HR–1: ORGANIZATIONAL INNOVATION AND CONTROVERSY

Although there was little controversy involved in the passage of the HR–1 amendment, controversy erupted once the bill was passed. The *New York Times* (Lyons, 1973) criticized the bill, saying that in the 1980s

* If, however, treatment is extended to new groups, particularly the elderly, these figures would be increased (see Kerr, 1973).

the cost would be $1 billion a year to save only 5000 lives at a time when government resources could be better allocated.

The Kidney Foundation refuted the *New York Times* article on several fronts. First, they claimed that with improvements in technology and experience, the costs would decline over time and that therefore projections beyond the first five years were impossible. Second, they noted that the 130,000 people saved during the decade would be rehabilitated and capable of paying tax dollars. Third, they reminded the public that death from kidney disease itself is very expensive in money and medical resources (Altman, 1973). Finally, they said that the governments of Western Europe were able to pay for national health insurance programs without becoming bankrupt.

Larger issues were also raised in controversy. Proponents question whether the preservation of human life was not worth even large outlays of funds. If it was not, the national expenditure of research funds appeared to be irrational. Why, asked some writers, should researchers be allowed to spend tax money to find new cures if these therapies cannot be implemented? In particular, Altman (1973) wrote:

> Americans, for example are spending hundreds of millions of dollars to combat. . .cancer. Now is the time for Americans to ask if they are willing to spend the money to deliver such a cure. . .to tens of millions of victims, because the existing body of medical knowledge suggests that a cancer cure will not be in the form of 10-cent pills but therapies costing each patient thousands of dollars.

The immediate outcome of this controversy was two-fold: (1) concerned Congressmen and HEW officials were reinforced in their belief that the next step should not be a piecemeal series of "special-interest" legislation benefiting victims of one disease after another, but rather enactment of a broader national health insurance program; (2) HEW officials and the Kidney Foundation were even more intensely motivated to keep the costs of this therapy in line with careful cost accounting, lest the entire program be threatened. As one of the Kidney Foundation officials stated, "I have a responsibility to the Long and Mills' committees for what they did for the patients—in terms of quality and cost control."

Issues of cost control and quality control have played major roles in subsequent controversy over the implementation of the HR–1 legislation just as they did in the Medicare controversy. The attempts to create cost and quality control involve significant innovation in health care delivery and organizational arrangements. Such prospective changes would be *expected* to produce conflict, and indeed they have.

PARTIES TO THE CONTROVERSIES

There have been several groups that have played major parts in these conflicts and controversies. First of all, the *federal government* has of course played a major continuing role through interested senators and representatives and through several offices in HEW: the Office of the Assistant Secretary of Health, the Social Security Administration, and the Bureau of Quality Assurance. Many government officials wished to develop policies to implement the kidney disease amendment that would have had implications for future national health insurance programs.

Staff in the Assistant Secretary's office felt that the amendment to HR–1 provided an unprecedented opportunity for major change and improvement of health care delivery. In the words of one such man:

> We have the authority here to do things and affect health care delivery in a way unprecedented. . . .This is not only an important thing to do but we have the authority. We've been bombarded from within government. . .because we're not doing things the way they've been done. . . .We said, "Whoa! There are problems here, we're not just going to run the same way. We must rethink policy."

In July 1973 HEW promulgated Interim Guidelines setting some temporary policy to cover the year July 1973 to June 1974. These guidelines established some highly controversial temporary policies but left undecided a number of other sensitive matters. Several opposing interest groups were then consulted by the government and drafts of final policy regulations circulated and published (HEW, 1975). In June 1976 the actual final regulations were published (HEW, 1976).

In addition to the government, there are a number of different groups of concerned *physicians*, "each with their own channels into HEW and Congress" ("Medicare Dialysis Score," 1974), that are also involved in the controversy. First of all the *National Kidney Foundation* (NKF) has been particularly important at every stage in the process. Prior to the passage of HR–1, it was the only organized group interested specifically in the politics of renal disease. Immediately after the HR–1 amendment was passed, an Ad Hoc Committee was set up to write a document suggesting policy for the government to implement. Many of the members of this committee could be considered "academic elite."*

* The 12 members of this Ad Hoc Sub-committee on Dialysis and Transplantation tended to be university affiliated rather than in private practice. Of the 12, 11 had academic affiliations. Only one was in traditional private practice, although three were involved in proprietary dialysis—that is, in dialysis centers that are owned and run for profit. The committee members were also primarily nephrologists, although two transplant surgeons from very

The document produced by this committee was digested by the relevant administration policy groups and served as one major influence. It advocates much innovation in cost and quality control and the organization of health care (see "Dialysis Patients Get a New Deal," 1973). One could hypothesize that a group of physicians actively involved in radical *technological change*, whose members constantly experiment with patient care regimes in university settings, would be more receptive than others to social change in health care delivery. Individuals who are dependent in part on academic salaries rather than solely on patient fees might also be less concerned with changes in the methods of payments.

After the government's Interim Guidelines were published, the Kidney Foundation ceased to be the sole organization speaking for the physicians. Other groups were organized in reaction and opposition to the new policies. While the Kidney Foundation had been primarily concerned with major alterations of the health care delivery system for this one type of patient, the new groups, such as the Renal Physicians Association and the American Society of Transplant Surgeons, were more analogous to professional unions in their desire to make certain the physicians' interests and view were represented and protected.

A primary emphasis of the Renal Physicians Association was to represent physicians treating renal disease more broadly than the Kidney Foundation. Several types of physicians deal with end-stage renal disease. First, there are transplant surgeons and dialysis nephrologists. Second, among nephrologists are (a) those in solo private practice who work at community hospitals; (b) those who are on the full-time staff of large nonprofit kidney centers, universities, or veteran's hospitals; (c) proprietors who own and operate dialysis centers for profit; and (d) some hybrid types. Finally, a distinction can also be made between physicians closely involved in the day-to-day patient care and higher level administrators who, in the past, have been leading spokesmen for the field. These groups differ in their financial base, with the private practitioners relying traditionally on fee-for-service, those attached to large centers and university hospitals frequently receiving partial or total salary payments from the facility, and the dialysis proprietors dependent also upon organizational profit.

While the membership and leadership of the Renal Physicians Association and the Kidney Foundation committees overlap, the Renal Physicians Association's leadership appears to have a higher proportion of

---

large university centers were on the list. Consultants to the committee, however, did include additional private practitioners and individuals involved in proprietary dialysis.

private practitioners and fewer "university elite" and prior leading spokesmen.

Although approving the Kidney Foundation Guidelines, this group differed in ideology and viewpoint in a more conservative direction. Leaders of the group appear to be less trusting of the ability of large-scale federal programs to make efficient, economical, and rational changes in the best interest of the patients and health care. At various stages they have seen this particular program as being implemented in a "bureaucratic" and unresponsive manner:

> Decisions are not being made according to the criteria the people involved in services recognize, but according to someone's idea of health care delivery in an autocratic and unresponsive fashion.

The underlying issue appears to be a sensitivity to encroachments on local professional judgment by the inexpert bureaucrat.

> The more government we see, the less we like it. I am a devoted proponent of local programs. The government cannot dictate everything centrally. They can't control it. They are thoroughly bureaucratic. . . .There is a complete lack of understanding in the government about what makes a professional. The local professional's judgment is being ignored.

In addition to a general distrust of federal bureaucracy, some of the leaders see inefficiencies in this particular program emerging from the larger health care delivery context. On the one hand, the Kidney Amendment is tied to Medicare and to *past* policies suitable for the aged, but not the young, chronically ill. On the other hand, the administration's major interest is in the *future* national health care bill. One leader believes that the administration regards the "kidney amendment" as an obstacle to future programs rather than as a model for them. The administration's main concern, in his view, is to prevent policy from setting precedent:

> The decisions are made. . .that can be easily erased. . . .What we have been dealing with are appendages to Medicare which were originally set up for old people. It is hard to change. It is a morass. . . .A lot of people don't want this program to go because it is one disease. They think National Health Insurance will take care of it. . .they are trying to keep it from becoming a pattern. . . .People who had to administer it were not in favor of it. It has been encumbered by a bureaucracy and inappropriate regulations. People who could change policy don't care.

In this view the politics of incrementalism have produced a stepping-stone bill that does not efficiently fund the particular disease for which it was created because of the past and future programs to which it is wedded.

The Renal Physicians Association group has attempted, through organizing, to modify new regulations that are not in the specific interest of renal physicians, renal patients, or the overall cost-efficiency of the program. Their leaders have consulted with various key officials in HEW and with major senators and congressmen and have had significant input. A main focus of its concern, like that of the American Society of Transplant Surgeons, originally involved the level and form of reimbursement. Many of the major controversies have been settled in the final government policies in a way acceptable to these new interest groups.

While the renal physicians have been interested in the policy outcomes for their particular programs, the AMA, like the government, has been concerned with the larger precedents for future comprehensive health insurance. Although less opposed to sociomedical innovation than at the time of the original Medicare–Medicaid debates (Bullough, 1973), the AMA has certainly been more conservative than the Kidney Foundation and the government on the issues discussed below.

ISSUES AND INNOVATION

The issues of controversy, for the most part, involved major innovation in health care policy. However, the first issue we will discuss is not one of policy, but rather the delay in setting and implementing policy. There was a long delay between the initial date of coverage (July 1, 1973) and the start of any payment. A second delay occurred between the beginning of coverage and the date by which the final policy could be formulated. To cover this period, the government promulgated a document with interim guidelines as stopgap measure (HEW, 1973a). Some of these temporary policies as well as the delay in payment resulted in much anger and concern. The delay seemed to give time and motivation for the opposition to mobilize—particularly time for the California Association of Physicians and Surgeons to call a meeting and organize what was to become Renal Physicians Association to make their views known to the administration.

Cost Control

Issues of greatest controversy involved cost and quality control—in particular the government's cost-control policies as originally outlined in the Interim Guidelines (HEW, 1973a). Both the government and the Kidney Foundation officials were concerned about keeping costs for this program in line with initial estimates, lest the entire program and future programs be threatened. Through cost control the government has attempted to alter the health care delivery system significantly.

Setting Maximum Fees. In the early Medicare controversy organized physicians feared that government payment of the bills would lead to federal determination of the *size of the fee* the physician could receive. Local conditions would be ignored, and a national system of fees would be created similar to those in nations with "socialized medicine." To mitigate this controversy the government under Medicare had developed a mechanism by which it paid the equivalent of the customary and usual *regional* physician fee for Medicare and Medicaid patients. Medicaid and Medicare insurance carriers were able to develop a list of customary and usual regional charges based on the bills of *non-Medicare* patients for the year or two preceding.

From the point of view of the government, such a policy failed to control costs. Each year the charges to the program increased as physicians raised their prices along with inflation, and health costs in general skyrocketed. In implementing the kidney amendment, therefore, the government came much closer to determining the *size of the fee or charge* the physician and facilities could receive than ever before, particularly under the interim policies.

To control upward spiraling of health costs *maximum fees* (or so-called "screens") were set for the major procedures for the first time. However, physicians and facilities were not allowed to raise their existing prices to these maxima. According to Medicare rules, the government was to pay 80% of the maximum allowable charges.

For some programs, such as kidney transplant surgery, the interim maximum fees were well below the customary and usual charge (GAO, 1975, p. 40), and protest emerged until particular fees were raised. In line with AMA policy specific charges are adjusted for current regional differences. However, without a facility applying specifically for an "exception" there is a maximum fee that can be charged to the government from any region. (Exceptions are being granted on an individual basis, if they appear justified.)

Given the well-accepted principle of customary and usual charges and the prior antipathy to maximum fees, how was the government able to innovate in this direction? The answer lies in the fact that traditional methods of determining charges were no longer possible. Previously, the Medicare carriers had based their charge-screens on the bills of non-Medicare patients. However, with the national funding of end-stage renal disease, there will be few non-Medicare renal patients whose bills can be so used. Almost all renal patients are covered by the new legislation. The same universal-coverage situation is likely to occur after any comprehensive health care program is instituted. Because accepted methods of computing fees cannot be used, the government is able to innovate in a way that might slow down skyrocketing health costs. Maximum possible charges now can be legislated; and although these ceilings will undoubtedly be increased with time, there is an opportunity to control the rate of increase.

Can the Physician Charge the Patient More? For the first time, according to the Interim Guidelines, some physicians and facilities—for example, those involved in routine maintenance dialysis—were not allowed to bill the patient for more than the government was willing to pay (aside from the deductible and coinsurance portion of the bill). Traditionally in the Medicare situation the facility and the physician had been able to bill the patient, and the patient collected from Medicare whatever portion Medicare approved. If the physician felt Medicare charge-screens were too low, he could charge the patient a higher fee. Thus the government could not determine the size of the physician's fee, despite the fact that federal money constituted an important part of it. In implementing the kidney amendment the government wanted to protect the patient from large excess charges and insisted at first that dialysis facilities and doctors accept the Medicare-allowed fee (or not participate—i.e., not practice in their specialty).

However, this policy of forcing the physicians to "accept assignment" generated a great amount of opposition, particularly from the American Medical Association which considered this directive an ill-advised precedent. In the final policies this innovation did not survive. Physicians were allowed to bill patients directly. In the words of one policy-maker:

> The AMA influenced this. Most of the physicians in end-stage renal disease don't feel strongly about this. It's mostly not to provoke a battle with the AMA—they do feel so strongly.

Despite the formal concession, however, physicians and surgeons were told informally that billing the patient in excess of Medicare allowances would be unwise. With the program already under attack for its single-disease approach and its great expense, proponents did not wish to place it in further jeopardy. As one nephrologist said:

> Assignment is not mandatory, but it is expected. We were told in no uncertain terms that if the MDs charged more, mandatory assignment would come. I don't think they can do this legally, but they said they would.

The draft of the final policy issues in April 1974 states:

> Mandating assignment. . .may simply not be necessary since physicians have generally been more willing to voluntarily accept assignment in cases of prolonged illness, particularly when patient resources are low. *At this time,* we will retain the voluntary approach to assignment [emphasis ours].

For the most part physicians seem to be accepting Medicare assignment without additional billing.

Maximum fees seem to be an important cost-control innovation that will establish a precedent for national health insurance and will put some limits on the federal expenditure. However, the inability of the government to couple this innovation with a formal policy of requiring physicians and facilities to "accept assignment" means that costs to the patients themselves could continue to rise with time. Whether local practices will protect the patient without alienating the physicians remains to be seen.

Regulating the Process of Care and Quality Control. The two major fears of organized medicine at the time of the Medicare controversy were that the government would first "set fees" and then regulate care. The implementation of the HR–1 amendment originally seemed to reinforce not only the former but also the latter fear. Originally as part of cost-control the government appeared to be proceeding in the direction of detailed *regulation of care.*

To prevent the sudden proliferation of services the early policy of the Social Security Administration (HEW Intermediary Letters 73–25; 73–22, July 1973c), set the number and type of routine tests a patient could have and how frequently he could have each. Additional tests required special justification. This policy covering the interim period also *specified the number of visits a physician could make* to his dialysis patients without special justification—that is, one office visit per month and two in-depth evaluations per year. Originally to keep costs in line the government was attempting to limit the number of "routine" visits a physician could make to a stabilized patient. Although funding was available when the patient needed more care, the physicians had to complete additional forms.

This government regulation of tests and physician visits was unprecedented and sparked a great deal of anger, particularly among the private practitioners who felt their professional judgment was being by-passed. The anger of one key private practitioner nephrologist is telling:

> It is generally held in the [government paper] that a patient needs to be seen only 5% of the time while he is dialyzed. . . .I would venture to say that today 95% of the prominent physicians in the country would disagree with that. . .they have even threatened the whole practice of nephrology to the point that if the present guidelines were to continue, many people would stop performing dialysis. . . .[They] say I'm supposed to see a patient [only] once a month. I can't do it effectively. Now the government has always replied that you can apply for an exception. . .but if I have to spend all my time applying and reapplying just to be able to see my patients, it's a ridiculous waste of time. . . .You must allow [the physicians] freedom without having to apply for an exception every time they do a test.

To many the original fears voiced by the AMA when the Medicare issue was first raised seemed to be materializing. One could seriously argue that the detailed regulation of allowable tests would function as a damper to continuing experimentation, innovation, and improvement of therapy. Quality of patient care was being defined, not in terms of outcome, but in terms of the detailed process of care established in the past.

The major consequence of these regulations about tests and visits was to provide an additional *spur to the organization of opposition*. However, they proved to be only temporary measures used by the government until the insurance carriers could determine the customary tests at a center and usual charges for them.

Innovative Methods of Reimbursement. In addition to controversy over the government's initial limitation of fees and regulation of care, there has been conflict over the method of reimbursement itself. As part of cost control, the interim policies required that supervisory physician services for the routine stabilized patient be billed *as part of the total* hospital dialysis charge, *not as a separate fee*. Only if the patient needed emergency medical care would a separate fee-for-service be honored. The reasoning was that only a small proportion of patients on routine dialysis (5%) required personal service from the physician.

For the nephrologist on salary, this innovative method of billing was not a problem. However, for the private practice physician, this regulation represented a major change and forced him to negotiate with the hospital for payment. The AMA and the private practitioners as represented by the groups merging into the Renal Physicians Association were hostile to having to negotiate with the hospitals for payment, and some suits were initiated against HEW and its Medicare agents. This controversy between the physicians and hospitals over the directness of payments goes back to Medicare days (Marmor, 1973).

As one physician in the California opposition group put it, when asked what was the real concern over reimbursement:

> The need to negotiate with the hospital as intermediary. It destroys the whole fee-for-service concept. Medicare doesn't use this kind of payment for any other disease—why should kidney disease be different? Fee-for-service is the way medicine has been. . . .It destroys the traditional options.

The argument for fee-for-service was made in terms of upholding tradition. Yet the underlying motivation was probably the professional's desire to maintain his autonomy and freedom *as* a professional. To the government and to many other leaders in the kidney field, tradition in payment mechanisms was not what was needed; rather innovation was needed to keep pace with changing technology and the requirements of cost control.

The controversy became muted when the government added a different innovative reimbursement mechanism, one orginally suggested by the National Kidney Foundation Position Paper (1973). A physician and a facility may elect to have all their patients cared for under a *monthly fee-for-service option* for the physician. That is, a physician can receive a monthly "retainer" or "capitation" fee for each patient under his care. The amount, which originally varied from \$160 to \$240 a month for each outpatient undergoing center dialysis, covers all outpatient services. The range was \$112 to \$168 for home dialysis patients. The National Kidney Foundation and the opposition groups, were in favor of the monthly patients, particularly home dialysis patients, spends and should spend considerable time and energy in telephone conversation and in reviewing charts and laboratory values even when there is no personal visit with the patient. There should be some compensation for this time.

Originally the American Medical Association objected to the idea of a "retainer" as a *precedent*, because it challenged the traditional "fee-for-service" idea and resembled the broadly based single national capitation of "socialized medicine" as implemented in Great Britain and the Scandinavian nations. However, many nephrologists, within both the Kidney Foundation and the opposition groups, were in favour of the monthly payment and were able to neutralize AMA opposition. The payment was labelled a "comprehensive reimbursement" or comprehensive monthly fee rather than a capitation or retainer payment. However, the terminology should not blur the fact that a monthly payment to physicians for supervision of patients with whom they may have little face-to-face contact is a fundamental change in reimbursement methods* and has broad implication for future national health insurance programs.

* Similar to Health Maintenance Organization options for nonrenal patients.

Rather than being paid by the hospital, great numbers of nonsalaried private nephrologists have elected this monthly fee option, and their opposition to reimbursement policy has been reduced. However, during recent congressional hearings the press reported that the new government policies had resulted in some dialysis physicians being paid as much as $100,000 for not seeing their patients ("U.S. Plan Pays," 1975). Whether such publicity will threaten the retainer concept or will lead to modifications to prevent abuse remains to be seen.

Incentives for Least Expensive Therapies. In addition to instituting changes in reimbursement mechanisms and setting maximum fees for cost-control reasons, the government hopes to be able to establish incentives so that the least expensive therapies will expand and the more expensive will contract. Both the government and the Kidney Foundation favor transplantation over dialysis, home dialysis over center dialysis, and limited-care facilities (where ambulatory patients can dialyze themselves with a minimum of supervisory help) over hospital dialysis. For the government to attempt to alter the distribution of available medical therapies for the purpose of saving money, is very new. There are many arguments whether the government incentives in this direction are adequate or appropriate.

Whether government policies can reverse the proportions of patients treated at various facilities remains an open question. By placing a maximum on the price a facility may charge the government for routine dialysis, the administration gradually may force the more costly operations to economize and encourage the expansion of limited-care facilities. Incentives and pressures have to be aimed not only at the *patient* who will select the therapy and at the *facilities* that make more or less expensive therapies available, but also at the *physicians* whose recommendations have tremendous impact on the patients. In fact, there *are* direct incentives to encourage physicians to recommend home dialysis for their patients. There is a flat fee, currently $500 (subject to the deductible and coinsurance), for the physician supervising the training of each home dialysis patient. The monthly fee for every home dialysis patient is also designed as an incentive to physicians. Furthermore, a bill introduced by Senator Long in April 1975 would establish incentives for the patient by allowing coverage for home dialysis to begin three months earlier than coverage for center dialysis and to be broader in extent (See Rettig and Webster, 1975 for a discussion of the current lack of financial incentives for patients to choose home dialysis).

Yet there appear to be unexpected counterincentives to the selection of the least expensive therapies. These counterincentives are emerging in part simply because the government is paying the bill. For example, at one time there seemed to be a consensus that home dialysis and limited-care dialysis gave the patient a better quality of life and a greater sense of dignity, as well as being less expensive (see Chapter 3). The patient on home dialysis was seen as having more freedom in time scheduling, more opportunity to dialyze during nonworking hours, and more independence. However, this consensus concerning the advantage of home dialysis appears to be dissipating rapidly now that patients have a financial alternative (GAO, 1975, p. 20). Some social workers and physicians believe that the appeal of home dialysis for many patients may vanish with the government paying for dialysis. An article in *Hospital Practice* ("Medical Dialysis Score," 1974) reports that the proportion of patients on home dialysis has decreased from 30% to 20%. (Also see Iglehart, 1976). The security of being in expert hands in case of an emergency may outweigh the added independence for some patients once the personal financial advantage of home dialysis is removed. Family members may be less willing to accept the great stress of aiding the patient on dialysis at home (Bailey et al., 1972; Shambaugh, et al., 1967). Physicians may also feel more secure if their patients are under skilled supervision in an environment they know meets sanitary standards.

In this program and any broader national health insurance program, attempts to economize by reducing medical supervisory personnel will have to be based on the recognition of the unwillingness of many patients to take *any* added risks, unless there are strong incentives to do so.*

One controversial suggestion for such an incentive is for a congressional amendment to allow a fee to be paid to the home dialysis aide (a relative or outside helper). While serving as an incentive to home dialysis, it would increase the total cost significantly. Experts disagree whether there would still be substantial enough savings in home dialysis therapy to warrant such an amendment.

Not only is the government concerned with maximizing incentives for home dialysis, but also with encouraging movement toward the less costly option of transplantation. With this goal in mind, government regulations allow Medicare to pay patients' bills sooner if they choose transplantation early, instead of selecting center dialysis. There appears to be a consensus among government officials, many physicians, and patients that the quality of life is better after a successful transplant than on dialysis (see Chapter 3 for empirical data). However, Lowrie and associates (1973) have noted that in terms of mortality the issue is not

* The lower proportion of patients in home dialysis may be due less to counterincentives in the program and more to the influx of high-risk patients who are unsuitable for home dialysis and who would not have been treated at all earlier.

clear. Although patients receiving kidneys from related donors do quite well, a dialysis patient has a greater chance of surviving than a patient with a *cadaver* transplant, and the stress of an unsuccessful transplant can be great for the patient and his family.

Thus, the encouragement of a patient to choose between a cadaver transplant and chronic dialysis involves ethical considerations as well as cost considerations. With the government paying the bill for dialysis, an unexpected counterincentive to transplantation may be operative: Physicians may be less willing to take the risk of a cadaver transplant. With the spectre of financial ruin gone, the risk of a cadaver transplant may appear too great. In addition, in some cases the monthly fee physicians receive for their healthy dialysis patients may operate as an incentive toward maintaining patients on dialysis.

The Kidney Foundation document was very pro-transplantation in orientation. They recommended transplantation with a related donor as the best therapy and estimated that 80% of patients with end-stage disease are transplantable. Whether 80% of patients will choose transplantation in the years ahead remains to be seen. Currently, of 9700 new patients a year, only about 3200 are being transplanted (Burton, in press). This low proportion is due both to a failure of the patient and referring physician to select transplantation and to the severe shortage of cadaver organs for those who do wish to be transplanted. The unwillingness of many centers to encourage related donation also plays a considerable role.

Although the government has not established any incentives for related donation, there has been an effort to encourage the cadaver-donor resource. Physician and facility costs related to the *harvesting of cadaver kidneys* are specifically covered as an incentive to donation. Thus the physician and local hospital where a potential cadaver donor is located may now be compensated for their time and inconvenience.

The desire of the government to alter the distribution of health care organizations and facilities to encourage the least expensive modes of dialysis and transplantation has been widely publicized. One related controversy, however, has not been extensively discussed——whether physicians should be allowed to set up organizations that make a profit in delivering technologically expensive care if the government is paying for that care. There have been some basic disagreements between dialysis physicians attached to proprietary profit-making dialysis centers and those involved in nonprofit systems. The disagreement is based on philosophical differences concerning the activities appropriate for a professional, on differences in political-economic viewpoint, and on different attitudes toward home dialysis. In the words of one nephrologist who runs a proprietary center:

> In 1973, there looked like there would be a big conflict. People were saying the government should stop proprietary centers. The government didn't see it that way [because the proprietary centers showed lower costs]. It's a matter of the free enterprise philosophy. They'd say, "You're making a profit. You could do it for lower without profit." But when you take free enterprise away like in the VA hospitals, overhead subtly soars. When you take away the profit incentive, the cost goes up.
>
> People said it's not right to make money at the expense of the sick. But doctors have always made money at the expense of the sick. If we wanted to make money we could make a bundle on home-training. We'd get $140 for each patient we didn't have to see. I don't accept that. I don't think I should get paid for not seeing patients.
>
> The only difference I noted from when I was running a [nonprofit] dialysis unit—I can remember calling the dialysis staff to squeeze a patient in. I'd get complaints. Now the staff gets a salary bonus and an incentive. The more patients they do, the more money they make. It's the same staff. But when I call now, they say, "Fine, bring him in." There are no complaints.

From the proprietor's viewpoint, earning an organizational profit is no more unethical for a professional than the alternatives, and the profit-incentive is a valuable mechanism for keeping costs down. In actuality, proprietary centers have submitted bills in line with government guidelines, and the administration has not challenged the existence of this type of organization, despite the controversy.

* * *

In sum, although attempts to institute cost control generated great controversy among physicians, many of the more sensitive issues have been resolved to the relative satisfaction of both the doctors and HEW. The government has been able to establish new and different control mechanisms that have implications for future comprehensive health programs—maximum allowable fees, monthly physician payments, and financial incentives to encourage patients and doctors to choose the less costly of several medical therapies. These incentives are designed to change the *organization* of health care delivery in the area of kidney disease by encouraging the development of low-cost facilities.

Yet there is room for critics to complain that the potential power of these innovative payment mechanisms has been compromised away by allowing the physicians to bill their patients for more than the Medicare allowances. The liberality of the government in granting exceptions to facilities that wish to charge more than the maximum fees may in the future warrant similar criticism. The cost-control changes could be seen as incremental small steps rather than as fundamental innovation. Other critics believe that the physicians are being heeded too little rather than too much. From their viewpoint, much of the government policy appears to be irrational red tape limiting the likelihood the program can really be run economically. They believe the cost-control incentives are not powerful enough to counteract the reduced willingness of patients and physicians to take the added risk of the less-expensive therapies, now that the government will pay for the more expensive.

We cannot know at this time whether in truth the new policies will alter health care delivery in the desired direction while actually containing the cost. The evidence of the first years indicates that many additional lives are now being saved, but that the price-tag is higher than predicted. The current estimate of $728 million for the fifth year of the program is far above the $252 million estimated originally by the Kidney Foundation before the program went into effect. Even the more realistic estimate by Dr. Ron Klar of HEW will in all likelihood be well-surpassed. Dr. Klar predicted that by 1983, the tenth year, the program would cost the government $1 billion; current estimates indicate that the $1 billion figure will be passed three years earlier in 1980 and for no greater number of patients than originally predicted by the Kidney Foundation.

Quality Control

The government defines its responsibility not only in terms of cost-control, but also in relationship to the quality of care received by patients.

> Since the federal government uses tax dollars to purchase such care, it has the responsibility to insist on quality, efficiency, and economy. It is not surprising, therefore that increased federal funding of health services inevitably leads to increased federal regulation of the health care delivery system. However, this in no sense means that physicians and other health care providers will become mere agents to carry out the dictates of a federal health bureaucracy (Klar, 1973).

The original kidney amendment required "a medical review board to screen the appropriateness of patients for the proposed treatment procedures." It was quite clear from the beginning that a peer review system to oversee quality of care would be established *outside* of the individual renal facilities.

Such a peer review process mandated and planned by the federal government rather than by medical societies and hospitals is a major innovation in the health care area. It also has led to significant controversy. This review requirement has to be seen in the context of another amendment of the same 1972 Social Security Bill, the Amendment establishing Professional Standards Review Organization (PSROs) to approve the admission and continued stay of all hospital patients and eventually to judge the adequacy of each treatment regime, given the usual therapy for the particular disease.

Quality review of patient care is a serious government innovation and would be expected to apply to the catastrophic diseases in general and to end-stage kidney disease in particular. The PSRO system has been criticized for focusing on the details and process of patient care rather than on the outcome, when the relationship of the details to ultimate effectiveness is often unclear (Densen, 1973). Chronic renal failure presents a unique opportunity for quality control in terms of outcome. The population and subpopulations are well-defined, and it is relatively easy to measure quality of outcome in terms of the numbers of patients alive and the number of transplant recipients with functioning kidneys. In any sphere cost control and high quality can be negatively associated. If attempts to cut costs in end-stage renal therapy endanger the patients, there is a possibility that statistical monitoring will alert the medical community.

The original Kidney Foundation Position Paper gave strong support to a peer review system with local, regional, and national levels. Groups other than the Kidney Foundation expressed more opposition to such a hierarchy of review. The Renal Physicians Association, for example, responded to the Kidney Foundation document with a policy statement that "peer review. . .should be performed at the most local level consistent with effective review" (Renal Physicians Association, 1974). Some private nephrologists are against a nonlocal review process, under which they feel they would be evaluated by "academic elite" types who may be one step removed from actual patient care. They resent this notion of an elite evaluation of themselves, although they may not be opposed to peer review in general. The cleavage between university and private practitioners is well known (Kendall, 1965; Nolen, 1970, Chapter 22), and each side expresses some superiority to the other. Although the interconnection between the two types are probably closer in the treatment of end-stage kidney disease than in other spheres, differences are still evident. In this light the distaste with which many physicians regard national and regional review and regulation can be understood.

However, neither the government nor the leaders in these physician groups wished to set up a review procedure in which all parties were so closely associated that review would be impossible. In the final policy all renal units in a given region are organized into a network covering population bases of 3,500,000 or more. In fact, some networks contain 11 to 14 million persons. The so-called local review panels attached to these networks will therefore be *regional* bodies in reality; and the hope is that "mutual back-scratching" will not pervade.

According to the final regulations, each network is to establish a medical review board that will coordinate its work with the closest PSRO and will review the adequacy of patient selection, the appropriateness of treatment plans for patients, the availability of needed services, and the quality of care at each facility. The review board is authorized to provide recommendations for improvement to facilities within the network and to communicate to the Secretary of HEW information about any physicians or facilities that continue to deliver inappropriate or substandard care. Each year the Secretary will review the approval status of every facility eligible for the new funding. *Only certified facilities can collect Medicare payment for their renal patients.*

Critics outside of the medical area have raised the question of whether physicians should be allowed to review themselves (McCleery, 1971). The review boards at issue here are to contain approximately five to seven people. The majority *will* be end-stage renal physicians of various specialties, but a nurse and a social worker will also be members.

Because a formal hierarchy-of-review concept proved controversial, no national component is mentioned in the final regulations. However, government officials have suggested informally that the National PSRO Council will consult with end-stage renal disease professionals in an advisory capacity. *Information* collected at the national level will also create the potential for a federal input to quality control. Along with the monthly or regular bill to Medicare, all renal facilities must contribute data about the health of each patient to a national system. The collected outcome data may be computerized and fed back regularly to each network and facility so that the review boards can compare the success of local facilities to national averages, probably for various subgroups of patients (e.g., diabetics vs. others, different age categories, etc.).

In addition to local review, the relationship between facility cost and quality can be investigated at a national level. Physicians involved in designing the information system perceive this merging of cost and quality information to be unlikely because the data about facility charges will be handled by one federal office (the Bureau of Health Insurance) and the outcome data by another (the Bureau of Quality Assurance). Whether these bureaucratic arrangements will actually constrain the government from obtaining a systematic overview remains to be seen. A published comment from HEW indicates an intention by some government officials to obtain just such an overview:

> The Health Services Administration through its Bureau of Quality Assurance (BQA) has developed specifications. . .for the the implementation of a national ESRD* medical information system. . . .Data concerning cost effectiveness as it relates to quality of treatment will also be provided by the system (GAO, 1975, p. 63).

The actual impact of this review system is a question for the future. Certainly there is a mechanism to counteract significant abuse or obvious substandard care. Any grossly inadequate facility can be denied annual certification by the Secretary of HEW and then would be unable to receive Medicare funding for its kidney patients. It *is* unclear whether pressure will also be applied to units or regions in which cost is too high, given the quality of care, or in which patients are failing to select home dialysis or transplantation. The words of one little-known HEW statement indicate that such pressure to allocate patients to less costly therapies is seen at least as a possibility that might result from the national computerized system:

> Additionally, through the use of data generated by the National ESRD medical information system; criteria, norms and standards concerning the desired ratio of percentages of patients to be home trained will be developed (GAO, 1975, p. 67).†

At this point we cannot know whether government officials will actually become involved in the review procedure, above and beyond denying certification to grossly substandard units. However, it is the involvement of the non-physician policy-maker that raises the potential for conflict. While some critics believe it is important that review of medical care not be placed primarily in the purview of the physicians themselves, most doctors are very antagonistic to any system other than peer review.

Organizational Innovation: A Network Delivery System

In the past fragmentation, duplication, and lack of organization have characterized much of the country's health care delivery. Under the kidney program, the government, following the advice of the original Kidney Foundation Position Paper, is attempting to implement an innovative "network" concept whereby different facilities in a geographical region will be reorganized into a more integral entity. All needed

* End-stage renal disease.

† Senator Vanik has proposed a bill which would require regional kidney networks to establish a goal of training 50 percent of all patients to use home dialysis. It is currently considered unlikely that this provision will pass (Iglehart, 1976).

treatment modalities will be represented in the network, including transplantation, inpatient dialysis, chronic maintenance dialysis, and training for home dialysis. Necessary ancillary services will also be available—organ procurement and laboratory testing services.

The purpose of the network is to avoid costly duplication of services and equipment, to assure the patient's freedom of choice of treatment modality, and to encourage excellence through specialization. All facilities related to the treatment of end-stage renal failure would be interconnected in a geographical region. No unit that received Medicare funding could be independent of a network.

Assistant Secretary of Health Edwards of HEW (1974) explained the rationale for the policy as follows:

> If we merely undertook to pay for treatment without also working toward developing the most effective system of providing such care, we could not only open an economic flood gate, but we would also pass up a real opportunity to improve the quality of care, to make it more readily available, and to be sure that these extremely costly services were properly distributed and effectively utilized. . . .
>
> Dialysis, transplantation, and all the ancillary medical services will be provided through networks of facilities. . .if an area to be served. . .has more facilities performing kidney transplants than it can effectively use, then some of these services will be discontinued.

As indicated above, most networks will serve a population base of at least 3,500,000 and will contain two or more transplant centers. Most important and most innovative are two principles: the principle of "coupled certification" and the concept of "minimal utilization." To be certified as an end-stage renal disease facility eligible for Medicare funds, each unit must be approved in its own right by the federal government; it must establish official connection with a network; and the network organization as a whole must also be certified as part of the "coupled certification." In consultation with local professionals, the geographic boundaries of the networks have been drawn by HEW. However, the local or regional groups are expected to organize themselves, approve or disapprove local facilities, and present the product to the Social Security Administration for certification.

For a particular facility to be certified in its own right, it must, for the first time, meet definite "minimal utilization" standards. To avoid expensive unnecessary duplication of technology, a transplant center is required to perform a certain number of transplants a year, and a dialysis facility is required to have a minimum number of dialysis stations utilized with a definite minimum frequency. Expansions of services also must be approved by HEW. For both a facility and an expansion to receive approval, evidence must be shown that there are patients in the area who could utilize the facility, who would not be expected to receive care from another treatment unit in the network area.

The "minimal utilization principle" was in fact stimulated by the original congressional amendment and thus cannot be completely compromised away, although movement in this direction has occurred.

Although highly innovative, the network concept has not generated the level of controversy sparked by the cost-control issues. This is not to say there has been no controversy about these issues—there has been some. The greatest difficulty concerns the minimal utilization rate, because some centers have had to be or will have to be phased out. In the interim period from July 1, 1973 until the end of 1973, all facilities in operation as of July 1, 1973 that met minimal standards could be funded. However, within a year after the Final Regulations become effective, those not meeting minimal utilization standards will have to be eliminated. This could mean a reduction from approximately 167 to 130 transplant hospitals. Some congressional staff were angry at the delay in implementing minimal utilization rules. They felt that unnecessary conflict would be produced by first paying units for a time period and then terminating their support. In addition, the details of calculating dialysis and transplant utilization rates are still causing some difficulties at this time. Small transplant centers have objected strenuously to the initial minimal rates. Therefore, in the final regulations the government has compromised from its initial stand by reducing minimal utilization for transplant centers from 25 transplants per year to 15.

In some cases nephrologists have also been upset with the network boundaries and the failure of the government to heed local advice concerning them. One physician-leader felt that boundaries were being set up more with an eye to a future health insurance system than with a sensitivity to customary referral patterns for kidney patients. In any national-health system, organizational criteria created for the health needs of one population might conflict with those of another group. The administrative policy-makers attempted to be responsive to this criticism by stating that patients were free to cross network lines for treatment. Yet some physicians still react negatively to the possibility that another network will have control over what has traditionally been part of their service area.

There *has* been a government attempt to coordinate network boundaries with other regional entities rather than to simply consider kidney disease referral patterns. But in the words of one HEW administrator, the coordination task "boggles the mind." There has been an attempt to make network boundaries congruent with Standard Metropolitan Statistical Areas, PSRO districts, and the new regional health planning areas that are being established and are known as Health Service Areas (HSAs).* But these different regional health care entities have been created by different portions of the federal law; their boundaries have been recommended and reacted to by different local groups. As a result, while there are rough approximations in boundaries, in many cases the boundary lines of one type of health district may cut across the territory of another type district, making any functional coordination difficult.

Another source of disagreement involves the tension between transplant and dialysis physicians. One of the purposes of the network system is to give patients a full choice of therapeutic options. Patients, however, are highly influenced by the recommendations of the physicians they see first. Transplant surgeons feel that some dialysis physicians have not considered the suitability of transplantation for eligible patients. Therefore, the Kidney Foundation guidelines suggested that each patient referred to a center was to have a consultation with both a nephrologist and a member of the transplant team. The Final Government Regulations have insisted that a written plan for each patient's long-term care be established and periodically reviewed by a team consisting in part of representatives of the three major options—that is, a dialysis physician, a physician-director of a self-care dialysis unit, and a transplant surgeon (*Federal Register*, 1976).

Other Sources of Controversy

One major type of complaint about the HR–1 amendment is due to limitations present in the parent Medicare Bill. Although officials in the administration have received criticism about certain policies, the bill itself, rather than the administration, is responsible for these policies. According to the Social Security Bill: (1) The patient must pay 20% of the cost of the treatment; (2) the dialysis patient is not eligible for coverage until the third calender month after dialysis is begun; and (3) coverage is extended only to persons who are eligible for Social Security benefits because they, their spouses, or their parents have enough working experience. About 90% of Americans are eligible for Social Security benefits ("Dialysis Patients Get a New Deal," 1973). There are also some other sources of funding for the first three months of dialysis (e.g., see Vocational Rehabilitation Act of 1973).

* See Public Law 93–341.

Where patients do pay the uncovered 20% themselves, dialysis costs still represent a significant sacrifice, perhaps $4000 to $5000 a year. The same statewide inequities in coverage that existed before the passage of the kidney amendment still persist on a smaller scale. In some states the patient will receive help for the amounts uncovered by the amendment; in others he will not.

A final source of controversy involves the entire catastrophic disease insurance approach, rather than the HR–1 amendment specifically. Some proponents of a more general national insurance bill rather than a catastrophic health insurance bill, believe that the allocation of resources should not be directed to the development of expensive new medical technologies, but rather to primary and preventative care (Somers, 1971, p. 213–214; Thomas, 1973; Rettig, 1976).

According to this view, open-ended payment for catastrophic disease will lead to the intensive development by superspecialists of ever-more costly equipment and to the encouragement of hospital care for select and small groups of patients. Resources will be diverted from the development of less-expensive preventative and routine treatment that could benefit a much larger segment of the population.

CONCLUSION

In this chapter we have examined the impact of one costly new medical technology upon the health care delivery system. Kidney transplantation and dialysis can be seen as a prototype of other expensive technological advances in medicine, both present and future. The social history of kidney transplantation, like that of other technologies appears to be one of "cultural lag"—that is, the technology changed faster than the resources and social organization necessary for its optimal use. Transplantation placed stress on the larger social and medical delivery systems as well as on the individual hospitals and patients, a stress that could be relieved only by major alterations of the medical delivery system. Partially because this new technology received unprecedented publicity and caught the public imagination (Fox, 1970), social and government changes were instituted to help alleviate the stress, and these changes have far-reaching ramifications for the care of all catastrophic diseases and perhaps for all medical health care.

First of all, we indicated that there appeared to be a communication lag between transplant centers and referring physicians. Because expensive new technological advances tend to be centralized in a relatively few facilities, many physicians are probably unaware for a considerable period of time of the success of the new therapy and therefore fail to refer patients. In the case of organ transplantation, many such physicians also appear somewhat reluctant to approach the families of dying patients with the idea of donating their relatives' organs for transplantation.

The new bill, the HR–1 amendment to the Social Security Law (Section 2991 of PL 92–603), may have some effect on closing these communication gaps. First, the publicity the law has received may lead to greater awareness of transplantation's success rate for all physicians. Second, many physicians may have failed to refer patients in the past because they were afraid the patient would be turned away due to scarcity of resources. Now that the government is paying the bill for almost all patients and now that resources will be expanded, such reasons for nonreferral are likely to disappear. And finally, the bill may provide some incentives to the physician to seek cadaver donor organs because the government is willing to pay for costs incurred in acquiring the cadaver organ, including surgeon's and anesthetist's fees, operating room expenses, telephone, consultation charges, intensive care costs, and so on. Thus the referring physician can be paid a consultation cost and the referring hospital can easily be reimbursed for all its expenses. These changes should provide some incentive to those who are in a position to help transplant services gain access to cadaver organs, or at least they should remove some barrier to referral (see Chapter 2 for further suggestions in innovation in this area).

However, the implementation of the new bill will limit the number of transplant centers to avoid costly duplication of services. In July 1974 there were 167 transplant centers, some of which will be phased out. Thus there still will be a problem of the flow of patients from communities all over the United States to these few centers—that is, a problem of ensuring equal access of all to the new treatment. Patients who are geographically removed from such centers may still be less likely to receive treatment. The role of the referring physician will remain central. However, whereas the number of hospitals performing transplants will be very limited, dialysis facilities will be more dispersed geographically. Once a patient is accepted for treatment by a center, travel to a local limited-care dialysis facility is likely to be less of a major problem.

Thus the communication lag between referring physicians and technological centers is likely to be reduced by the new law, although some problems will remain. However, the most important reason technological change was impeded in the past involved the inadequacy of funding rather than the communication lag. Resources were scarce and there were not enough facilities to treat all patients needing care. Many suitable patients did not receive treatment and died—perhaps more than 6000 a year. With the centralization of facilities and the extant channels of funding, patients clearly did not have equal access to the scarce facilities. Patients were denied treatment on arbitrary bases, such as their state of origin or their economic resources.

The plight of such patients attracted much sympathy, and 13 years after the first successful transplant with a non-twin as a donor and five years after a government report noting the severe shortages of resources (Gottschalk, 1967), the major bill described above was passed to remove this financial lag. This amendment to the Social Security law represents a dramatic turning point in the American health legislation history and may portend significant social changes in the health care delivery system. One of the physicians active in the Kidney Foundation termed it "one of the major pieces of legislation to occur in the entire century."

The passage of such a bill for one disease makes a more comprehensive national or catastrophic health insurance bill appear less revolutionary. This is not to claim that a more comprehensive program will pass soon because of the kidney amendment or that it could not have passed anyway without the kidney bill, but at the least it may make passage seem somewhat less difficult, provided the kidney program is defined as moderately successful. More important, the implementation of this bill serves as an important test case: Problems created and solved in the course of implementing the bill may help administration officials avoid some difficulties in establishing a more general program. If such a general bill is passed, new medical technologies may not have to confront the same lags in funding faced by kidney transplantation.

In addition, the new bill is seen by the government as a chance to innovate in the area of health care delivery. As one HEW memorandum (1973b) stated:

> The legislation. . .constitutes an initial experiment in a form of catastrophic illness health insurance. . . .The Department will have a significantly better opportunity than under other aspects of Medicare to develop a program with strong quality and cost control.

Changes are being instituted that may serve as precedents for later more general legislation.

These changes have been both significant and controversial. In terms of cost control the government has for the first time established maximum allowable charges for physicians and facilities, created an innovative monthly retainer payment mechanism, and set up incentives to encourage physicians and patients to choose the less expensive of several alternative therapies in the hope that less costly facilities will expand while the others contract. To assure better quality control, peer review boards covering a large regional area have been mandated and planned, along with a national data system that may feed outcome data back to the review boards and facilities on a regular basis. This review system is supposed to coordinate with the PSRO systems regionally and nationally. Finally, all renal facilities in a region are to be organized into a closely cooperating network. For a facility to be eligible for Medicare funding, it will have to align itself with the network and demonstrate that it fulfills a need. To avoid expensive duplication of services all centers have to show minimum utilization rates, and new or expanded services will be certified only if patients cannot obtain the needed care at another appropriate facility in the network.

After reviewing the case histories of nine programs that were set up to produce innovation in health care delivery in New York City, Herbert Hyman (1973) concluded that major change was difficult and unlikely:

> The nature of our political society with its pluralistic self-interest groups, operating to protect their varied interests. . .encourages only incremental or marginal changes. . . .Too many individual careers and organizational power sources are at stake to permit large-scale innovative changes from taking place that they could not control. . . .
>
> Changes in health care come about only incrementally and with minimum interruption to the established way of doing things (pp. 197–198).

All the dramatic changes formulated on paper may in practice fail to produce significant innovation, due either to the opposition of established medical groups or to the program's own internal flaws. Many physicians question the ability of the federal bureaucracy to create cost-effective, efficient, high-quality systems for local health care.

It could be predicted that the opportunity for social change is greatest in a sphere of technological change, because of the lower value placed on tradition and the experience of a constantly changing clinical environment. Yet only the future can tell us whether the actual implementation of policy will result in significant change or merely in elaborate mechanisms to conform in letter, but not in principle, to the mandated policy and whether the unanticipated consequences of the program will enhance or decrease program cost and quality.

Whatever the results of this bill may be in practice, significant controversy remains on the larger issue of whether the society should move in the direction of funding expensive new medical technology, given other societal needs.

12

SUMMARY AND CONCLUSION

Organ transplantation as one of the most dramatic of the new medical technologies has intrigued the public to an unprecedented extent. Due to the extensive publicity and inherent drama social processes that seem generalizable to other situations stand out in high relief. In addition to describing the social impact of transplantation itself, a major object of this study has been to analyze the aspects of this new technology that have general implications for public policy and for sociological theory. In the summary we focus first on policy-related issues and second on the findings that yield theoretically relevant insights.

TRANSPLANTATION AND POLICY

A repeated question throughout this work is whether the transplantation of kidneys is worth the enormous expenditure of money and effort being applied to it. From this viewpoint, we have discussed the impact of transplantation upon the health care delivery system and upon the patients themselves, their families, and their donors. Future new medical advances will be expensive, and the question arises whether the society can afford the reallocation of resources necessary to deliver costly cures for previously fatal diseases. Analysts have questioned the sense of the federal government funding the research designed to produce these cures if they cannot actually be delivered. The fact that these issues have even been raised in a society that places such a strong value on individual life and on progress through science points to the magnitude of the health care delivery issues involved.

Health Care Delivery

Inaccessibility of Treatment. The social history of kidney transplantation, like that of other technologies has been described in this monograph as one of "cultural lag"—that is, the technology changed faster than the resources and social organization necessary for its optimal use. Stress was placed on the medical delivery system as well as on the individual hospitals and patients, and this stress could be relieved only by major alterations of the health delivery system. Before appropriate changes took place, the major social defect involved insufficient funds to provide treatment for all who needed it. There were simply not enough facilities to treat all patients requiring care. Furthermore, even when facilities were available, many patients could not afford treatment, particularly if they came from states or localities without public programs to help defray the enormous cost. Every year more than 6000 patients who were eligible for kidney transplantation or dialysis died. Ability to secure treatment was affected by arbitrary considerations such as the individual's economic resources or public programs within the region in which he lived.

These problems were compounded by communication lags within the medical community and by the centralization of facilities. Because technological advances in medicine have tended to be centralized in a relatively few facilities, many potential referring physicians were probably unaware for a considerable time of the success of the new therapy, and therefore they failed to refer patients. Travel costs added to all other costs also made the therapy inaccessable for many.

Without major change in the health care delivery system, such inaccessability is likely to be a problem for the development of many, expensive new technologies.

A Step Toward Catastrophic Health Insurance. Federal changes were instituted to help alleviate this stressful situation for patients with kidney disease, partly because of the unprecedented publicity given to transplantation and partly because of the long and gradual movement toward national or catastrophic health insurance. In 1972 an amendment to the Social Security Bill was passed (Section 2991 of PL 92–603) which legislated that all individuals, their spouses, and dependants insured under Social Security were eligible for Medicare coverage if they needed long-term dialysis or transplantation. For almost all patients the major expenses would now be paid by the government and therefore facilities could afford to expand. This amendment, as the first national catastrophic health insurance program in the history of the United States, represented a dramatic turning point and may portend significant social changes in the health care delivery system.

This amendment is one more step in the 40-year incremental process from the first discussions of a national health insurance program under Franklin D. Roosevelt, to the original Medicare legislation in 1965 and then to the present period in which a national health insurance or comprehensive catastrophic health insurance bill appears more possible. Yet it is a significant step. Although no one wishes to develop future national programs for only one disease at a time, we have postulated that the passage of this bill for kidney disease has made a more comprehensive national or catastrophic health insurance bill appear less revolutionary. More important, the implementation of this bill can serve as an important test case for the development of new policies that may have wider applicability later.

The Federal administration has viewed the implementation of the kidney amendment as an opportunity to innovate in three areas: cost control, quality control, and the coordination of health care facilities. The changes made have been both significant and controversial. The government and program supporters have been concerned that costs for this program be kept in line with initial estimates, lest the entire program and future programs be threatened. They have attempted in this one area to institute policies that will retard soaring medical costs. For the first time the government has established maximum allowable charges for physicians and facilities, created an innovative monthly retainer payment mechanism, and set up incentives to encourage physicians and patients to choose the less expensive of several alternate therapies.

However, it is too early to tell whether all the significant changes formulated on paper will produce actual innovation. One could predict that the opportunity for social change might be greatest in a sphere dominated by technological change, because of the lower value placed on tradition in a constantly changing environment of clinical experimentation. Yet, even in the area of kidney disease, interest groups of physicians have emerged and influenced significant compromises in policy

Exceptions have been granted to certain centers on individual bases. The full impact of opposing medical groups remains to be seen.

Critics within such physician groups claim that there are unintended counterincentives to true cost control and that the overbureaucratization of the federal government renders it incapable of creating cost-effective, efficient, high-quality systems for local health care. In fact the actual costs of the program for the first year ($300 million) were more than double the original estimate ($135 million). Clearly the $1 billion price tag estimated for 1985 will be significantly exceeded, and what this means for the cost of a more general national or catastrophic insurance program is an important question.

Meanwhile, proponents of a general national insurance bill (rather than a catastrophic insurance) believe that allocation of resources should not be directed as extensively to the development of expensive new medical technologies but instead should be concentrated on improving primary and preventive care.

Ambiguity and Changing Norms

As difficult as the larger health care delivery issues are, the ethical questions related to transplantation are even more complex. For the physicians, ethical ambiguity is focused around two domains: selection of patients and use of organ donors. In both cases physicians find themselves in uncharted territory, and the issues involved make the establishment of clear norms and policies difficult.

Selection of Patients. Originally the shortage of money and facilities meant that many patients had to be denied treatment. The criteria to be used in condemning kidney patients to certain death were unclear and controversial. Whether centers should use factors such as apparent psychological strength, social worth, intelligence level, or predicted ability to cooperate with the treatment regimen were significant matters of controversy. With the government now paying for the treatment of kidney disease, and facilities therefore expanding, the ordinary patient no longer has to worry about being turned away and many of these arguments have become moot for this therapy. For transplantation of other organs and for future new technologies, such issues remain highly relevant.

The expansion of facilities for kidney transplantation and dialysis has made treatment available for high-risk groups who would not have been eligible for treatment before—the elderly, the diabetic, those with other physical diseases. The question still remains whether such an expensive treatment should be allocated to those for whom success is doubtful. The issue of quality of life has been raised. If the elderly patient on dialysis becomes senile and incapable of caring for himself or if the physically ill patient is severely restricted by his other diseases, is the quality of life so poor that maintaining physical existence is contraindicated? Physicians and policy advocates alike are concerned that if the federal costs of this program skyrocket because of such patients, this and other future catastrophic disease programs will be threatened.

There are three alternatives for such high-risk patients, all of which have their proponents: not to accept them for treatment, to accept them but withdraw treatment if quality of life becomes exceedingly poor, or to accept and treat them as long as they can maintain life. The entire issue of removing a patient from treatment, either at his own suggestion or that of the physician, has been difficult to resolve. Does the patient have the *right* to withdraw from treatment? Does he have the ability to make such a decision rationally? How much should the staff attempt to intervene against this type of suicide?

The patient at high physical risk is not the only individual who poses selection problems. Should patients apparently at psychological risk prior to treatment be accepted for treatment? What policy should apply to social deviants? Should the patients who have revealed a strong tendency to violate medical orders be allowed this expensive therapy? On the basis of a dying person's behavior, can a psychologist or psychiatrist predict his reaction to a medical regime that will restore him to partial or full health?

In addition, the overriding issue that has been raised is whether the quality of life for all transplant patients, not only those at particular risk, is high enough to warrant allocating such extensive resources to this therapeutic modality.

Use of Organ Donors. The normative issues concerning the use of organ donors have proved even more ambiguous than those concerned with selection of patients. For the first time physicians are placed in a position where they may cause harm to one individual to save the life of another. Where the donor is living, either related or unrelated to the patient, the issue is especially difficult. Here is a healthy person who is being exposed to a small but definite risk to his life; and even if all goes well, he will sacrifice one of his normal organs.

Recipients are much more likely to do well if they receive kidneys from living relatives than from cadavers: Nationally the two-year success rate has been 74% if the kidney comes from a sibling, as opposed to 43% if the kidney comes from a cadaver. The waiting lists for cadaver organs are extraordinarily long. Yet centers vary dramatically in their willingness to use kidneys from related donors: Only 2% of the kidneys transplanted in Australia and only 15% in Europe are from related donors, in contrast to 35% in the United States and 66% at the University of Minnesota. The reluctance to use related donors at many centers is in part due to a widespread feeling that family members are unable to make such a decision willingly, that they will respond to family pressure and will later regret their sacrifice.

Each center must decide whether to encourage or even allow related donation. If they do allow relatives to donate, should only the most aggressively willing be accepted—those who persist in their offers despite initial hospital refusal? How much psychological screening should there be? If the staff senses ambivalence or family conflict, how quickly and how firmly should they intervene to prevent donation? If there are problems of willingness, the recipient is usually told the donor is medically ineligible, but ethically, can a donor be refused without informing him that the reasons for refusal are psychological? Are there special groups, such as adolescents, who definitely should not be allowed to donate? Is there a "right to give" that must not be violated?

The utilization of *cadaver* organs has not appeared as distressing or normatively ambiguous to the transplant physicians. Yet among the lay and medical public, fundamental questions have been raised about the definitions of life and death. A new concept of death—brain death—has emerged, and the details and legality of its application have been challenged. The use of cadaver organs for transplantation has highlighted a larger concurrent ethical issue: How long should any apparently hopeless patient be kept "alive" with the use of extraordinary and expensive medical care?

Many of these normative and ethical problems appear insolvable; others could benefit from empirical data about the effects of transplantation and donation on those involved. One major purpose of this work is to provide empirical data where possible—first, in terms of the quality of life, rehabilitation, and adjustment of the recipients of this expensive therapy; and second, in terms of the social-psychological consequences of being a related donor or a family member of either a related or cadaver-donor.

Impact of Transplantation on the Recipient

In 1969 an editorial in the *American Journal of Public Health*, "Should We Transplant Organs or Efforts?" indicated that money allocated to kidney transplantation could be better allocated to preventative health care, in part because of psychological problems and poor rehabilitation among transplant recipients. In actuality the purpose of kidney transplantation as a therapy is to remove the patient from the role of social invalid. There would be little sense in such a large expenditure of money and energy on this therapy if the patient were to remain a social-psychological invalid.

There is no doubt that this therapy meets the standards of a *physical* cure. At Minnesota 70% of patients receiving related kidneys still have functioning kidneys five years later, as do 50% of those with cadaver kidneys. The policy question then is whether the therapy is "worth it" from the point of view of "quality of life." Furthermore, is it worth it for the high-risk patients? Many hospitals do not accept diabetics or children for kidney transplantation on the grounds that their adjustment and rehabilitation will be poor. The University of Minnesota is one of the few centers that accepts large numbers of both types of patients.

In this set of studies a series of quantitative sociopsychological measurements were administered to all adults transplanted at the University of Minnesota between 1970 and 1973 prior to their transplant ($N = 178$) and, if the transplant was successful, again at three weeks and a year after the transplant. In addition, essentially the first 100 children transplanted at the University were followed over time by a child psychiatrist; and in 1972–1973 those who were 8 to 20 years old and had maintained their new kidney for at least a year were measured with quantitative social-psychological scales ($N = 52$). As is obvious, the focus here was on the successful posttransplant patient. Our impression is that the psychological stress of an unsuccessful transplant is extreme and clearly not "worth" the immense effort*. Our question was whether the psychological cost was also too great for a successful transplant.

The overall results point to a high quality of life both for the adults and the children at a year or more posttransplant. The adults, both the nondiabetic and diabetic, showed *marked improvement* after the transplant along all dimensions of adjustment that were measured: (1) feelings of physical well-being including the ability to perform daily activities well and the absence of significant symptoms; (2) social-psychological adjustment including high levels of happiness, favorable self-images, high feelings of independence, control over one's destiny, and low levels of anxiety and preoccupation with the self and one's illness; and (3) satisfaction with major role-relationships including marital and sexual relationships, general social life, and job situation.

In fact there was some evidence that although the adults were considerably less happy before the transplants than normal controls, restoration to health and life rendered them *more* happy than normal adults at a

* However, the reactions to an unsuccessful transplant should be studied in future research.

year after the transplant. Severe psychopathology—that is, psychosis or suicidal behavior—was rare among successfully transplanted healthy adults. Furthermore, 88% of the nondiabetic men and 44% of the nondiabetic women were working or in school at a year posttransplant, and 73% of the women reported no difficulty with their housework. However, the one area where problems remained significant, despite improvement, was the sexual one. Although the frequency of sexual impotence was reduced after the transplant almost to half of the pretransplant level, it still remained as somewhat of a problem for half of the men.

The posttransplant children also showed high levels of adjustment. Like the adults posttransplant, they demonstrated a great increase in physical vigor and energy. For preschool children these changes were dramatic: Children who could not walk before the transplant began to run in a few weeks' time. Cognitive growth appeared to follow suit. Children aged 10 and over rated as favorably as normal control groups in levels of happiness, anxiety, self-esteem, self-image stability, self-consciousness, distinctiveness, and in ability to reveal their true feelings to others. The vast majority did not show major psychosocial problems at any time, especially when kidney function was adequate. Only three out of 100 children demonstrated major psychosocial problems at a time when the new kidney was functioning satisfactorily.

The only dimension where dissatisfaction was evident among children involved the physical appearance. About 20% of transplanted adolescents were extremely short due to their prior disease, and 40% of the children demonstrated the abnormal Cushingoid appearance that results from the steroid medication they must take if they are to retain the kidney. The Cushingoid full moon-face and rotund figure can be unattractive and abnormal-looking in severe cases. Thus it is not surprising to find that a higher proportion of transplanted children than normal youngsters were dissatisfied with their appearance.

Patients at Risk. Although both adults and children appeared to react well to transplantation, the subgroups listed in Table 12-1 were at greater risk than others and might benefit from greater psychological support. The greater inability of these particular subgroups to cope with the stress of this illness and major therapeutic intervention could be expected to generalize to similar illnesses and crises.

Among those at risk are the controversial diabetic patients. Although they showed significant improvements, they frequently started and ended at a less high level of adjustment than other patients. For the blind diabetic whose disease may have created neuropathy, that is numbness in his limbs, vocational rehabilitation remained a problem. Only 44% of

TABLE 12-1 PATIENTS AT GREATER RISK

Adults at greater risk—studies of transplanted adults

- Male patients
- Patients with lower socioeconomic status
- Patients with other medical problems (e.g., diabetics)
- Patients with impaired physical appearance
- Patients rejected by spouses or family
- Patients with problems with kidney donor
- Low psychological adjustment previously
- (Low staff optimism—hypothesis)

Children at greater risk—studies of chronically ill and transplanted children

- Those with more severe illness or children threatening to reject new kidneys
- Adolescents
- (Females)
- Children from rural, lower-class, large families
- Children dissatisfied with body-image
- Children who take less self-responsibility for their illness
- Children whose mothers are confused by the sick role

the men had returned to work at a year after the transplant. Rehabilitating the blind diabetic appears to involve the same problem as rehabilitating the blind in general.

Some writers (Abram and Buchanan, 1975) have suggested that recipients of related kidneys are at greater risk than recipients of cadaver kidneys because of the inherent difficulty of the donor–recipient relationship. Our data do not support this view, however. In general patients who received related and cadaver kidneys did equally well psychologically. In most cases the gift of a relative's kidney did not appear to be so stressful for the patient that his overall level of adjustment was affected. However, the few recipients who reported problems with their donors posttransplant did react less favorably in terms of their own emotional adjustment (Table 12-1).

Several subgroups of children seem to be at greater risk than other children. Our associated studies of chronically ill youngsters (Chapter 4) revealed that children were at greater psychological risk if they assumed less responsibility for their own care and if their mothers were confused about the proper method of handling their illness. Because this particular study of chronically ill children involves measurements at only one point in time, however, we cannot be certain of the direction of causality. Children who started out at higher levels of adjustment may have been the ones to assume more self-care and their mothers, as a result, may have been more able to deal with the child's illness. In any case there appears to be no contraindication to encouraging the child to assume a good deal of responsibility for his own care. Physician-time in making certain that the mother is clear about the proper method of handling the serious illness of a child may also be very beneficial for the mental health of that child.

One additional hypothesis for which we have no data involves differences among transplant centers. We have predicted that where the staff is more optimistic about the patient's long-term chances of survival posttransplant, the patients will react more positively on a psychosocial level. The staff at the University of Minnesota is perhaps more optimistic than staff at other centers, particularly centers with higher proportions of cadaver kidneys and therefore higher failure rates. Our hypothesis is that staff optimism is contagious, particularly in new technological areas because the true long-term survival chances for new therapies remain unknown for many years.

This study has not compared the adjustment of long-term dialysis and transplant patients to see which group is at greater risk, although pretransplant patients on dialysis are shown to be considerably less well adjusted than posttransplant patients. However, some comparative data presented in Chapter 3 indicates a higher level of vocational rehabilitation and a higher income for transplant patients than for those on long-term dialysis even when age is controlled. Yet the two groups probably were not equivalent before institution of the therapy. The group selecting dialysis may be quite different from the group who deliberately rejected or were advised to discard dialysis or choose transplantation.

If, as we and many others would hypothesize, future comparisons of *equivalent* groups do demonstrate that quality of life is higher posttransplant than on long-term dialysis, the choice posed in many physicians' minds, will continue to be between quality of life and risk to life. If the patient considering transplantation must have a cadaver donor or if the center discourages related donation, the risk to the patient's life will probably be less if he remains on dialysis than if he undergoes transplantation.* No such conflict occurs if a related donor is used. Yet the reluctance of many physicians to use related donors is a central issue

* There are, of course, many patients for whom there is no choice, who are suitable for dialysis but would not at this time be considered good risks for transplantation—particularly older patients without related donors, patients especially prone to infection, and patients with shortened life expectancies due to certain additional diseases.

here, and it is in part for this reason we have examined the impact of the donation experience upon the related donor.

Impact of Transplantation on the Related Donor

There is a widespread skepticism about the ability of an individual to make the major sacrifice of a kidney willingly and without significant regret later on. The perception is that family blackmail and pressure will be pervasive and will be the major factor motivating the potential donor. Posttransplant the loss of a body-part will engender long-term regret and depression. Thus at many centers the policy of using related donors is regarded as a major ethical problem.

To explore the impact of donation on the related donor and his family, we collected the following data: (1) Between 1970 and 1973 we administered questionnaires to all 130 related donors pretransplant, at five days posttransplant, and at one year posttransplant if the transplanted kidney was still functioning; (2) between 1970 and 1972 we followed 205 families intensively through the donor search, interviewing all possible members repeatedly over time; and (3) between 1970 and 1972 we administered questionnaires to 186 nondonors at a month posttransplant when the transplanted kidney was still functioning.

Our findings point to a much greater willingness to donate an organ than is assumed by the lay or medical public. Family members are surprisingly willing to make this major sacrifice to save the life of a loved one. Out of all eligible family members, 57% volunteered to donate and took the definite preliminary step of having their blood tested. Furthermore, the vast majority of those who do donate reported little or no ambivalence related to the basic decision to donate, although concerns about the surgery were not infrequent. In the majority of cases the decision to donate was an immediate, instantaneous one, made with no deliberation and usually with no later regret.

Unwelcome direct family pressure occurred for only 11% of the donors. However, more subtle pressures appear inevitable. The donor frequently learned of the need for donation in the presence of his dying relative, and volunteering at such an instant would probably appear highly desirable, especially to a relative who was already positively oriented. Feelings of family obligation were common but appeared to make the decision easier rather than more difficult. The obligation to sacrifice for one's family was widely accepted as legitimate among these donors, and those who felt more obligated were also likely to be the more willing donors.

Posttransplant the vast majority of donors indicated they were without regret, and in fact were extremely happy that they had donated and that the recipient was alive and healthier. They felt closer to the patient, an emotion that was warmly reciprocated. Most donors received a great deal of family praise and gratitude both before and after. Most interesting is the finding that donors' global self-esteem and level of happiness rose after the transplant, and these improved feelings of well-being persisted to a year posttransplant. Although the level of happiness of the donor pretransplant was similar to that of normal control groups, the level at a year posttransplant exceeded that of these groups.

These measures were collected following an interview about the donation and the transplant, and these improvements in the self-image might have been less evident if the questionnaire were administered in a situation unrelated to the donation. Nevertheless, when the transplant is made salient, there is evidence that the donors think more highly of themselves and are happier than they were pretransplant. In-depth interviews also demonstrate a great exhilaration on the part of many donors when they speak of the gift a year later. Thus far from pointing to a major psychological cost of donation, these results suggest that donation may in fact have sizeable social-emotional benefits. The donor thinks more highly of himself after having saved the life of a loved one.

Despite this benign picture for the majority of donors, at all points in time there appeared to be a small group of donors who were extremely ambivalent or regretful of their decision (5% to 8%). Although no one factor is highly predictive of later regret (see Table 12-2), psychological screening and exclusion of highly ambivalent donors would appear to be advisable, as would counselling help for other relatives who wish to donate despite normal fears.

One of the major ethical controversies has involved the use of teenaged donors. The question is whether such young people are capable of informed consent. At the University of Minnesota, 18 donors from age 16 to 21 were used and evaluated. There was no more evidence of blatant family pressure in this group than in the other age groups, and there was only one donor who showed long-term ambivalence about the donation. In general the adolescent donors indicated highly positive attitudes toward the donation and improvement in the self-picture afterward. In particular they were likely to view the donation as a sign that they had mastered the maturational task of adolescence; they had demonstrated maturity by their ability to make this sacrifice. Younger donors were also less likely to complain of pain in the days immediately following the transplant.

Because the younger donors were unmarried, they were not confronted with one of the primary conflicts facing other potential donors. Frequently the potential donors regarded donation as a conflict between

TABLE 12-2 DONORS REACTING MORE NEGATIVELY TO DONATION

Status
Males
Nonparents
Among siblings and children, those who are married
Emotional relationship
Persons less close to the patient
"Black sheep" donors
Persons who do not receive gratitude from family and patient
Personality
Less-happy persons
Persons with lower self-esteem
Less-obligated donors
Not "only possible" donors
Not A-match donors
Prior attitude
Persons with high ambivalence to donation pretransplant

the dying recipient and their own spouse and children. Often spouses of family members were opposed, at least initially, to the donation.

To investigators who are suspicious of the donor's motives, the donor is seen as making this sacrifice to assuage prior family guilt, or to alleviate feelings of low self-esteem and unhappiness, or because of family pressure. A comparison of the donors to relatives who did not volunteer to donate—that is, the nondonors—indicates that donors were not more likely than other family members to be motivated by such factors. Although family "black sheep" sometimes did donate in part to regain the good grace of their families, nondonors were as likely as donors to be family "black sheep" and were also as likely as donors to be subject to family pressure to donate. In addition, nondonors were slightly more likely than donors to suffer from a low self-picture and feelings of unhappiness and therefore were more likely to be in need of a boost in the self-picture.

The major psychological differences between donors and nondonors appeared to involve a greater closeness to the recipient on the part of the donor, as well as a greater feeling of family obligation to help, a more positive view of the risks and benefits of the medical procedures, and a lesser likelihood of defining the choice as a conflict between one's obligations to the recipient and to one's own family of procreation. Although due to the timing of the measurement we cannot be certain that these differences preceded the donor search, they suggest, as do the in-depth interviews, that the major motivation to donate came from the desire to keep a loved one alive and to fulfill important family obligations rather than from more ethically problematic sources.

For some donors, the major worry was not whether they wished to donate but whether after the physical examination they would be allowed to:

INTERVIEWER. When you found out about the need for a donor, was there a period of time when you thought about various aspects of your donating, things that concerned you?

DONOR. Yes, I was worried if I qualified. Wouldn't you if you had someone you loved in trouble?

At the family level the successful transplant experience seemed to have the unintended consequence of increasing family cohesion. The majority of both donors and nondonors reported that the family had become closer as a result of this shared crisis.*

Family Conflict. Despite this positive picture for the majority of donors and their families, we also found a sizeable minority of families (25%) in which the donor search generated significant conflict and stress. Although the level of stress in these families was extreme, only rarely did this stress involve the actual donor. The primary sources of difficulty were the hurt and anger directed toward the nondonors because of their failure to volunteer and the nondonors' own anger at the percieved pressure to do so. Other causes of stress involved only a few families each: donor-ambivalence, nondonor guilt, recipient guilt at accepting a kidney, recipient fear there would be no donor forthcoming, relatives' fear for the lives of recipient and donor, difficulties in requesting a kidney, problems of gratitude between recipient and donor, conflict between volunteers and their own spouses who were opposed to the donation.

In the policy evaluation of related donation, such high levels of family stress in even this minority of cases cannot be ignored. Yet neither can

* A future study of the impact of the unsuccessful transplant would be of interest in the light of many of the issues raised here.

their context. By and large the anger felt at or by the nondonor was not expressed directly to the other party involved. Thus after the transplant, family wounds could be more easily healed. In fact the stress of the donor search appeared temporary in all but a few cases. Once the crisis was over and the transplant successful, a process of denial and forgiveness of past conflict and nondonation was evident. Although there was a long-term cost in terms of lesser closeness to nondonors, these feelings were not openly expressed.

It should also be noted that the families in which the donor search generated significant stress were more likely than other families to have had a history of significant family conflict. In general we cannot assume that overall family stress would have been less had there been no donor search. If related donation were not allowed and the failure rate increased with more extensive use of cadaver organs, more families would have been faced with the traumatic rejection of the kidney, long periods of uncertain prognosis, and death of a loved one. The source of the stress would have been different, but whether there would be a reduction in amount is unknown.

Whether these results apply to cultures and subcultures other than that of the midwestern United States is unknown, but there is collaborating evidence from other large centers.

Reaction of Policy-Makers. Resolution of issues involving social policy can be only partially responsive to empirical data. Our data show that the majority of donors, families, and patients react exceedingly positively to the experience of related donation and that the recipient is much more likely to have a successful posttransplant course because of it. But, a few deaths occur (2 out of 2000) over the short or long term by donation, another few donors experience regret and distress at their gift, and a sizeable minority of families find the period of the donor search extremely stressful at least temporarily. Whether the costs to the minority should be absorbed for the benefit of the majority is not an empirical question, but one of values.

The drama of the families undergoing stress and conflict should not blind the policy-maker to the experience of the majority of donor-recipient pairs whose course is more benign and therefore less colorful. Still, actual decision-making will of necessity be based on value-positions, not simply data. Nowhere is this dichotomy between final evaluation and empiricism more evident than in a recent series of articles and editorials in the *British Medical Journal* ("Adolescent Kidney Donors," 1975; "The Shortage of Organs," 1975). Because related donation is frowned upon at many centers in Britain, the shortage of cadaver organs there, as in the United States, has resulted in long waiting lists and placing more patients on the more expensive therapy of dialysis. One solution to the problem would be to increase the use of related donors ("Kidneys from Living Donors," 1974). Yet this suggestion does not appear an acceptable one to many physicians. Recently an editorial in the *British Medical Journal* ("Adolescent Kidney Donors," 1975) reviewed an article of ours (Bernstein and Simmons, 1974) that showed that most older adolescent donors had little ambivalence and reacted positively to donation to the point of demonstrating a boost in the self-picture. The editorial reported the results correctly and for the most part did not question their accuracy. Yet the conclusion was:

> In British centers, discussion of the question of transplantation has always been seen as an extremely responsible and onerous task even with adults fully competent to decide their actions. Most transplant surgeons would hesitate before recommending nephrectomy in a healthy minor to obtain a kidney for transplantation even after the most careful psychiatric screening.

One interpretation of the fact that most donors, including teen-agers, decide instantaneously to donate without deliberation has been the one emphasized here: The decision is usually an easy one because donors are so strongly motivated to keep their loved relative alive. Yet to censure the program and the donors, as does the British journal, for not encouraging more deliberation about such an important life-decision is equally possible:

> One wonders how a school child can understand the procedures involved in renal transplantation and their consequences, and whether there was adequate communication between him, other members of the family, and the transplant team. . .they often decided to donate without much deliberation. . . .Perhaps there should be more stringent legal protection before such an irrevocable step is allowed.

The ethical conflict is likely to persist between those who champion the right of the individual to make a sacrifice if he wishes to save the life of a valued family member and those who consider even a slight risk to a healthy life too great and the risk of family coercion too abhorent. In one view the individual is deemed capable of making such a decision; in the other, true informed consent is prejudged as impossible.

Titmuss (1971) in his study of blood-donation has emphasized the importance of allowing the individual freedom to enter gift relationships:

> The notion of social rights—a product of the twentieth century—should thus embrace the "Right to Give.". . ."Gift Relationships". . .have to be seen in their totality. . .; in modern societies they signify the notion of "fellowship.". . .If it is accepted that man has a social and biological need to help, then to deny him opportunies to express this need is to deny him the freedom to enter into gift relationships (pp. 242–243).

All of these policy issues are interrelated. If related donors are not used, waiting lists for cadaver kidneys will lengthen, transplantation will be less successful and time on dialysis will be prolonged. If the choice is between cadaver donation and dialysis, many patients and physicians will opt for the more conservative and more expensive therapy of dialysis; and costs are likely to soar far above that originally estimated by the government.

New medical technologies are particularly likely to spawn ethical controversy. Yet the uniqueness of the donor resource makes the ethical issue related to transplantation particularly difficult to resolve.

Impact of Transplantation on the Family of the Cadaver-Donor

Thirty-five members of 15 families were interviewed in-depth about their long-term reaction to donating an organ of a brain-dead relative. Most reacted positively to the fact they had donated. Some viewed the donation as making their grieving process easier because the donation gave the tragic unexpected death some meaning or because it symbolized a type of immortality.

Only five relatives were regretful or ambivalent about the donation a year or more after the fact. In some cases these negative feelings were due to early insensitivities within the hospital bureaucracy which have since been corrected. In other cases guilt about making the decision to terminate artificial support was a negative factor; in some families the concept of brain death was a difficult one to accept.

Some family members accused the transplant staff member who contacted them of being insensitive to the feelings of the grieving relatives in his eagerness to obtain the needed organs. The difficulty of this contact between the strange new physician and the grieving family can be substantial.

Most family members desired more long-term information about the recipient and his health than was forthcoming. At a year or more after the donation they wished to know that the donation had been successful, that one or two lives had been saved beause of their gift; and they also wished to know something about those lives. Yet if the gift was unsuccessful, as it is in approximately half the cases, they did not want to be informed.

* * *

For all the policy-relevant findings reported above—whether relevant to recipient, related donor, the recipient's family, or the cadaver donor family—the extent of generalizability to other, very different populations is unclear. In our samples non-white families are particularly rare.

INSIGHTS RELEVANT TO THEORY

Because of the crisis nature and newness of transplantation technology, fundamental social-psychological processes reveal themselves with special clarity. Throughout this work we have regarded the transplantation situation as a research site for exploration into several important areas: the investigation of the consequences of crisis management for the self-image; the analysis of the impact of health status upon social-psychological adjustment; the conceptualization of rehabilitation and quality of life; the study of family roles in illness and help-giving; the investigation of the consequences of interpersonal altruism and gift exchange; the exploration of family communication when help is sought; the analysis of individual and family decision-making processes under stress; and the exploration of family grieving processes. The major conclusion of these explorations are reviewed here.

In some of these areas data analysis is based on careful quantitative measurement; in others upon qualitative case material. We are not claiming a test of preformulated theories or full-fledged theory development, but rather a set of insights, themes, analyses, and hypotheses emanating from the data that are relevant to sociological theory.

The major theme that emerges from this entire analysis concerns the *positive* impact of successfully resolved crises. For the majority of patients and families for whom the transplant was successful, this work is a case study of the positive impact of stress. Not only do the majority of patients, families, and donors cope well with stress, they exhibit some long-term gains from having successfully survived this enormous crisis. Our purpose here is not to minimize the extreme costs for the minority who are not able to withstand the stress nor for those for whom the transplant fails; it is simply to emphasize an often-ignored issue—that the consequences of crisis and stress are not uniformly negative for those involved. If the crisis is one that is overcome, many of its effects may in fact be positive.

ILLNESS AND CRISIS

Restoration to Health

The stress facing the patients with end-stage kidney disease is extreme. The ordeal of a dangerous, debilitating, long-term chronic illness followed by major surgical intervention would appear to place individuals at considerable psychological risk. However, when we distinguish the potential sources of *stress* from the patients' reactions in terms of their actual level of *distress*, we find an amazing resiliency among these patients, both adults and children. Despite the severe challenge to their mental health, the children who have received kidney transplants show levels of adjustment equal to normal controls along most dimensions measured. The transplanted adults not only indicate high levels of adjustment in general, they demonstrate levels of happiness and feelings of exhilaration greater than that in the normal population, according both to quantitative measurement and in-depth interviews.

The transplanted adults and children, as well as some of the chronically ill children, indicate that the crisis experience and the brush with death has given them a greater appreciation of life, a greater maturity, and a clearer sense of values. The "second chance at life" is regarded with deep appreciation.

Most interesting is the importance of the past reference point to the definition of the present self. According to the theory of relative deprivation, an individual's absolute level of satisfaction is dependent upon his point of comparison. To these long-term transplanted patients, the memory of how they felt and how they performed when they were dying of kidney disease or on hemodialysis appears to be a pervasive comparison point. They report constant gratitude and high levels of happiness because they no longer are suffering from the severe symptoms of kidney disease, because they no longer feel ill, because they once again have enough physical vigor to operate normally in their social and personal roles. The definition of the present self is determined by a comparison to the sick self even at a year after the transplant. The escape from such an overwhelming crisis creates high levels of daily satisfaction.

How long these effects can last is a question for future research. How long can the successful emergence from a past crisis shape one's life-picture? Will the heightened pleasure in life and greater maturity erode as the crisis recedes into the background and the problems of daily life become more salient?

Psychosocial Impact of Illness

Although the resolution of a health crisis has beneficial social-psychological consequences, the psychological impact of severe chronic illness itself is quite negative for the adult. The focus of our studies was on the patient's self-image in the face of the serious challenge of illness. For the adult *prior* to the transplant when he was ill with end-stage kidney disease, psychosocial adjustment was low; self-esteem and levels of happiness were considerably lower than those of normal controls within and outside the family and lower than his own scores after health was restored through the transplant. The negative impact of chronic disease is also demonstrated by an examination of the reaction of the diabetic patient whose illness usually has a longer history and is more pervasive. Both before and after the transplant the diabetic patient shows a lower level of social-psychological adjustment than other patients along several, though not all, dimensions.

Many theorists have hypothesized that the need to maintain a high self-esteem is one of the most important motivational components of the personality, and the individual resists challenges to his self-picture through various defense mechanisms (Allport, 1943; Murphy, 1947; Rosenberg, 1965). The individual who is chronically ill has the option of perceiving his illness as temporary, atypical, unreflective of his true ability, and a matter of fate rather than his own "fault." He could reduce his aspirations in the face of reduced energy and thereby protect his self-esteem against the pain of failure. Yet despite these potential defense mechanisms, the experience of severe chronic illness is a powerful enough stimulus to overcome these mechanisms and damage the self-picture, at least for the adult.

On the other hand, *children* with chronic kidney disease illustrate the great resiliency of persons under stress. Chronically ill children score as high as normal control groups on almost all dimensions of psychosocial adjustment. The puzzle is why these children do so well. In part, the reason may be simply a matter of the severity of the illness: The majority of these children were not so ill as the adults who were awaiting a transplant. To counteract the defense mechanisms protecting the self-picture may take a much more severe level of illness. In fact children who were more seriously ill did indicate a less favorable adjustment.

Haggerty and associates (1975), whose studies indicate more negative effects of chronic illness than do ours, also show that along many dimensions, though not all, the difference is only between the severely ill children and the normal controls. On these measures the moderately ill children are little different from the normal controls. Our findings may not generalize beyond the population we have studied; however, relatively high adjustment of samples of ill children have also been reported elsewhere (Collier, 1969; Crain, et al., 1966; Gates, 1946).

Other hypotheses may help to explain the lack of damage to the mental health of chronically ill children. These hypotheses relate to the childhood role in general and to the role of the family in protecting the youngsters. Whereas the dependency of illness conflicts sharply with expectations of independence for the adult, such dependency is more compatible with the role expectations appropriate for the normal child. Also, the child's major functional role—his ability to attend school—may be less disturbed than the adult's ability to perform adequately at work.

Furthermore, there is evidence presented that indicates that families, particularly mothers, focus extra attention and love upon the ill child in the family. Given the overwhelming importance of parental high regard for a favorable self-image, this extra attention may serve to protect the chronically ill child against the potential destructive forces of the illness. The family of the ill adult does not seem to protect him in the same way, especially if he cannot perform in his or her major occupation or functional roles. Classic studies of the unemployed male during the depression indicate that the male without a job lost considerable prestige within his own family (Angell, 1936), despite the widespread recognition that the fault for high unemployment lay outside individuals' control.

The importance of family support in protecting the individual against stress is suggested in other findings both for adults and children. The adult who perceives his family as rejecting him prior to the transplant is less likely to react favorably to the transplant experience later on. Among the ill children, those whose mothers are confused about how to handle their illness are more at risk emotionally.* Posttransplant suicidal children frequently have been rejected emotionally by their families and therefore are unable to cope with medical complications.

Factors Affecting the Impact of Illness and Crisis

Several other factors in addition to family rejection place some ill individuals at greater risk than others (Table 12-1). Those with fewer resources cope less well, whether the resources are socioeconomic or a matter of personality strength (adults whose prior psychological adjustment is low cope less well with the transplant experience). Other important factors of interest to sociological theory involve the visibility of the disease itself and age and sex roles.

* However, see above for discussion of problems in imputing causal direction here.

Both adults and children are much better able to cope with invisible illness than illness that changes their physical appearance and body-image. Dissatisfaction with their looks is the one dimension along which chronically ill and transplanted children score more unfavorably than normal youth. Both adults and children whose physical appearance is more abnormal and who are dissatisfied with that appearance are considerably less well-adjusted than other patients.

Sex is also a factor in overall adjustment. Adult females do better than males both prior to the transplant and after it, a finding compatible with results from other studies of chronic illness (see Litman, 1974). The following hypotheses were formulated to explain these differences. First, just as it is easier for the ill child to continue his prime functional role than the adult, it is easier for the female than the male. She may consider herself rehabilitated if she can perform fairly adequately in caring for a home, whereas a man must maintain a job outside the home and perform well in it. Securing such a job is not totally within his control. Alternately, the adult female is resistant to assuming the sick role even when ill, because her failure to function is more likely to produce chaos for the entire family. The idea that the greater coping ability of the adult female is related to the role demands placed on *adults* of both sexes is supported by the fact that no such sex differences appear among children. In fact female *children* cope slightly less well than their male peers.

In examining the impact of age upon adjustment, we note the special vulnerability of adolescents to the stress of illness and transplantation. Many writers have theorized that adolescence is normally a particularly disturbing time for the self-image (see Simmons, et al., 1973b). During illness severe psychological reactions, though rare, are much more likely to occur among adolescents than in other age groups. Adolescents are more likely to demonstrate suicidal tendencies and to react severely to threatened immunological rejection of the transplanted kidney. Suicidal gestures occurred in three teen-agers, that is, in 13% of the transplanted adolescents posttransplant.

Measurement of Rehabilitation and Quality of Life

Rehabilitation, adjustment, and quality of life are general and imprecisely defined concepts. Yet there is a need to measure the mental health impact of crisis or stress on individuals. Our study begins to specify the dimensions of such concepts so that they can be more precisely measured. This conceptualization, as used in this work, is summarized in Table 12-3. The heavy emphasis on the self-image reflects both of the importance of this

TABLE 12-3 DIMENSIONS OF ADJUSTMENT

- Physical well-being
  - Global feelings of well-being
  - Symptoms of illness—frequency
  - Ability to perform daily activities
- Emotional well-being
  - Happiness level
  - Self-image level
    - Self-esteem
    - Stability of the self-picture
    - Self-consciousness
    - Feelings of independence
    - Feelings of control over one's destiny
    - Sense of distinctiveness
    - Preoccupation with self
    - Satisfaction with body-image
    - Perceived opinion of significant others (perceived popularity)
  - Anxiety level
  - Gross psychopathology and suicidal behavior
- Social well-being in major life roles
  - Social life
    - Satisfaction
    - Participation
  - Vocational or school adjustment
    - Satisfaction
    - Participation
- Adjustment of other family members
  - Family disruption
  - Individual adjustment

dimension to mental health in general and our special interest in the concept.

Overall, although there is an extensive literature on chronic disease, there are few attempts to measure the consequences quantitatively. Even fewer studies utilize normal controls to interpret their results. Although the qualitative insights of the clinician are vital as sources of ideas and hypotheses, these hypotheses must be tested more rigorously, and we have attempted to do so to enhance our understanding of the mental health impact of physical disease.

THE DONATION PHENOMENON: A DECISION-MAKING CRISIS

The issue of organ donation touches on a wider variety of theoretical concerns than do the studies of patient illness. Primarily this unusual phenomenon has provided an opportunity to study major life decision-making under stress and the consequences of this decision-making. Each family member must decide within a limited though variable time period whether he will or will not volunteer to donate a kidney to his dying relative.

Processes at the Level of the Individual

The Altruistic Decision. A question at issue is the extent to which altruism, or help-giving behavior without expectation of external reward, is really possible and the nature of the psychological consequences of such altruism.* Altruism in both the theoretical and lay literature has "fallen into disrepute" (Fellner and Marshall, 1968, 1970). According to exchange and reinforcement theory, individuals "give" to others to obtain certain rewards for themselves. "Merely" saving the life of a loved one is not regarded as strong enough motivation for sacrificing an important body organ at the risk to one's own life. The search is for other rewards the donor expects to receive or the negative consequences he expects to avoid. The emphasis is on the disillusion and regret the donor will feel when rewards do not match the sacrifice.

Our data suggest, however, that altruistic behavior is intrinsically rewarding for great numbers of donors whose self-images and levels of happiness rise after the donation. Because of their ability to undergo self-sacrifice to benefit another individual, the donors feel that they have become better and more worthwhile persons with a greater appreciation of life. The entire experience of having themselves rescued a close relative from death is regarded as a peak life experience; and like the recipients, the donors perceive themselves as consequently more in touch with truly important values. As in the case of the recipient, the successful weathering of a major family and individual crisis appears to have had a positive impact on most donors and an impact that persists at least to a year after the sacrifice was made.

Our findings do not eliminate situational pressures, guilt, family pressure, a low self-picture, or other less positive forces as operative in

* See Chapter 7 (p. 228) for a discussion of the definition of altruism in relation to organ donation.

motivating some donors. Nor are negative reactions unknown after donation, especially when the explicit reward of family gratitude is absent. Donors who may have been motivated originally by guilt or a need to benefit the self-picture are among those more likely to react negatively after the gift is given. "Black sheep" donors who have had major problems with the family in the past and donors who start out with low self-images and low levels of happiness are less likely to be happy with the donation a year later. Yet these donors are not the typical ones. The typical donors appear to be especially close to the recipient prior to the transplant, more likely than nondonors to have a high faith in people in general, and less likely than nondonors to believe that there are obligations to other family members that override their obligations to the recipient.

In summary, the skepticism with which altruistic acts are regarded in the literature should be reexamined. This and other studies of organ donors indicate that individuals find meaningful altruistic acts deeply rewarding intrinsically. The rewards appear to come primarily from pleasure at viewing the benefit received by the recipient and from happiness at realizing they were capable of making a significant sacrifice to help another. One could predict that altruism would have less favorable psychological effects in situations in which the benefactor is less able to perceive the consequences of his gift and when he cares less about the recipient of it. Also, the greater the sacrifice, the more significant the positive impact should be, perhaps up to the point where the long-term cost of the sacrifice to the individual becomes sizeable and apparent in daily life. For these donors, the short-term costs, in terms of pain and time lost from work were substantial and evident—evident enough to convince the donor that his sacrifice was a major one. Yet although the loss of a kidney presents some potential long-term cost, its implications for the daily life of a donor at a year after the event are minimal in most cases. For the most part the earlier stress is successfully overcome. In other situations in which the costs of altruism might persist at high-stress levels over a long period, we would predict less favorable reactions.*

* Theories of cognitive dissonance, however, might make different predictions. The hypothesis might be that the more costly the gift for the donor and the fewer the benefits for the recipient, the more favorably the donor would perceive the donation. However, we are not simply speaking of the specific attitude toward the donation, but the consequences of the gift for an entire life-attitude, the positiveness with which one views oneself as a person, and one's level of life-happiness. Although one might attempt to reduce cognitive dissonance by justifying the unsuccessful donation to oneself, it is difficult to imagine that major long-term costs to the recipient and donor would not render the donor less happy in general.

The Individual Decision-Making Process. A major focus of this study has been on the process of decision-making as perceived by those involved. The decision to donate an organ is one type of decision, and our findings about the process would be expected to generalize more easily to other decisions of a *similar* nature. Organ donation, for example, is a decision made under stress with few established norms to guide the decision-maker. It is an irreversible major life decision with high stakes in which probabilities of success or failure are known. The family context of the decision is important because the individual's central and closest interpersonal relationships are involved. Given this particular type of decision, what was found about the perceived process of decision-making?

To the ordinary individual as well as to many decision-theorists, decision-making implies a period of deliberation followed by a conscious choice of one alternative. Although this decision is one of the most important decisions individuals might ever have to resolve, the majority of potential donors do not perceive that they have made a deliberative choice. The word *decision-making* does not seem to fit many individuals' perceptions of their decision-process, despite the fact that the transplant has occurred and they have either volunteered or not volunteered to donate a kidney.

Models other than the classic deliberative one appear to be more compatible with potential donors' perceived process. The majority of donors and a sizeable proportion of nondonors perceive that their choice to donate or not was an instantaneous one, made at the time they first heard of the donor need, without any period of conscious deliberation. The decision was never reopened later. No pros and cons were weighed consciously either to determine whether any option open to them was minimally satisfactory (a satisficing decision) or to decide which option was optimal (an optimizing decision). Despite the importance of the decision, the choice appeared to be a "gut-level" one without a conscious attempt to evaluate alternatives.

For a few donors and a sizeable proportion of nondonors, an interesting pattern of decision-postponement, evasion, and stepwise decision-making was noted. The individuals fitting this pattern postponed making a definite, final choice until they perceived that events had locked them into donation or nondonation without their ever having come to a final decision. The *nondonors* evaded the issue; when another volunteer emerged or the patient received a cadaver kidney, they seemed to perceive that events precluding their own donation had occurred before they had thought it was time to make their own difficult choice. The *donors* in this category also postponed deciding whether to donate, but agreed to take the first steps toward donation to find out if they were eligible. If they were ineligible after this first step of the blood test or the second step of the extensive physical work-up, they never had to make a final decision. However, if they were still eligible after proceeding so far into the process, they found that others' expectations had locked them into donation without their ever having finally resolved the issue in their own minds. Others had assumed that their willingness to proceed with so many early steps signified willingness to donate.

It was hypothesized that this pattern of stepwise decision-making and decision-evasion is more widely congruent with major life-decisions than is perhaps realized. The applicability to many occupational, delinquency, and even mate-selection decisions was noted. It is proposed that in many situations an individual takes small steps in one direction, postponing final choice, until he finds that the cost of cancelling the commitments already made are too great to withdraw from the course of action initiated.

Although a *deliberative* pattern of decision-making is not the most common mode, it does occur for a sizeable minority of both donors and nondonors who weigh the pros and cons and arrive at a conscious choice. In terms of a continuum in which a satisficing type of decision stands at one extreme and an optimizing decision at the other, these individuals move closer to the optimizing pole. Yet even in this group independent information-seeking was limited, despite the importance of the decision. The majority of these donors relied on the transplant physician for information; many sought no new information other than that provided by the family prior to the blood test; and about one-third of these nondonors sought no information at all. The deliberation that did occur in this situation was less a matter of calculating risks against benefits than of weighing competing normative obligations to the patient and to one's own family.

It has been proposed that the more important the decision, especially in an emotionally charged area, the more uncomfortable the deliberative mode will make many individuals. Where the potential costs of both alternatives are very high, thinking about these costs and taking responsibility for the resultant choice is uncomfortable. If the individual feels his obligations in one direction are overwhelming or if he believes he has become "locked into" one alternative by the course of events, he may more easily be able to justify a course of action.

In some cases at the *family-level* decision-making in this stressful area also appears to be highly unorganized. Although the donation decision is one that has important consequences for all eligible donors as well as for the recipient, in approximately 15% of the cases the selection of the final donor out of the eligible pool of volunteers was made without any concerted or organized communication on the part of the family. The final choice of one donor seemed to occur because of the way situations structured themselves or because of isolated decisions of individual family members, perhaps in concert with the medical staff. Turner (1970) terms such a decision a "*de facto* decision" and notes that this type of evasion of family decision-making is likely to occur when the issue is too emotionally charged for open discussion.

Processes at the Family Level

Family Roles. Family processes, as well as individual processes, become highlighted in the donation situation. The reactions of different family members to the problems of donation suggest more fundamental characteristics of their roles within the family.

1. *Age and Sex Roles.* The differential reactions of male and female donors appear to reflect their differing roles within the family. Males were more likely than females to react dramatically to donation either positively or negatively. To interpret these results, we suggested that donation was a more momentous event for the men, who responded either with regret or with a great boost in the self-picture. The females appeared to take donation more for granted, neither reacting as unfavorably nor seeing donation as indicative of improved worth.

We proposed that donation was a simple extension of the traditional female roles of nurse, of family caretaker in times of illness, and of the woman's accustomed role in childbirth. To enter a hospital to give a family member a second chance at life does not seem symbolically so different from entering it to give an infant his first life-chance. No such life experiences or expectations prepared a male for donation, and he was more likely to perceive that he had performed an exceptional act. The extent to which other types of family sacrifice would evoke similar sex differences remains a research question.

Although the sexes reacted differently *after* the sacrifice was made, comparison of donors to nondonors did not indicate an overall difference between the sexes in the extent to which they volunteered to make this major sacrifice. However, a closer analysis of age and sex roles does suggest that bonds of closeness among siblings in a family are forged on the basis of their age and sex. Siblings of the same sex as the recipient and of closer age were considerably more likely to give this gift to the recipient than were siblings of the opposite sex and dissimilar age.

2. *Role of Geographical Distance.* Ties of closeness within the larger family in this situation appeared to be surprisingly unrelated to geographical distance among family members. Excluding potential donors who shared

a household with the recipients, nondonors were no more likely than donors to live far from the recipient. The key transition appeared to involve family members' leaving the original household, so that potential donors and the recipient no longer were part of the same immediate family. For each type of blood relationship, relatives who no longer shared the same household with the recipient were more likely to be nondonors than were those still in the household.

Once the original family splits into several loosely connected nuclear families, new responsibilities and potential lines of cleavage develop. The spouses who were unrelated to the family member in need of a kidney were the ones likely to oppose their husband's or wife's taking the risk involved in donation. From the potential donor's viewpoint, obligations to his new family were likely to be seen in opposition to obligations to help needy members of his original family.

Among relatives who had left the original home, geographical distance did not appear to further weaken their tendency to give family help, at least in this extreme case where a dying relative was in need of aid. The emotional bonds forged in the family appeared to be able to withstand the challenges of widespread mobility. However, at the family level donor decision-making was less likely to be efficient, coordinated, and stress-free if the family was geographically dispersed.

3. *Role of Parents.* Not only are the ties between parents and children firmer than that between siblings, with parents the most willing donors and children the second most willing, but parents play an important role in all aspects of the illness and donation. The role of the parent seems to be considerable in protecting the adult offspring in trouble, in organizing or preventing family sacrifice, and in promoting family cohesion after the children are grown. The parents, particularly the mother, was sometimes a constant hospital visitor and was frequently a spokesperson for the recipient, informing family members of the need for a donor. In a few cases the parent pressured the recipient's siblings to donate; in a few cases at the other extreme the parents prevented all siblings from volunteering. By and large, however, the donor decision-making was more efficient, the communication more open, the stress-level less, and the rate of volunteering higher if at least one parent was alive and active enough to be part of the donor pool. Parents play an important part in creating cohesion among the loosely connected set of adult nuclear families that constitute the extended family.

Family Communication. Family communication patterns found during the donor search can increase our understanding of family communication processes in general. The most interesting aspect of family communication is the interplay that results when one family member requests a major favor that might be denied. A pattern was identified that probably occurs in many situations in which a favor is requested and the person from whom the favor is sought wishes to deny help without embarrassment or risk to the relationship. The request is made so indirectly that it can be ignored, and the second party does ignore the request. In this situation the potential donor frequently acts as if he had not heard the implied question. He neither says he will donate nor refuses, nor makes excuses, nor indicates he will deliberate on the issue. He simply changes the subject or says nothing. The person making the request does not know whether the question was heard at all.

Some evidence is presented that indicates that over the long-term this type of non-communication is functional for continued family cohesion and for the particular relationship.* However, at the time the favor is needed, uncertainty and stress is intensified because of the inability of the recipient to ascertain whether help will be forthcoming and whether the need has even been communicated.

Impact of Crisis on the Family. Over the long-term, the successful emergence from the crisis of transplantation seemed to have a positive impact on most families as well as on most recipients and donors. The majority of donors and nondonors perceived the family to be closer because of the transplant events and because they had weathered this stress together. In some cases the crisis was consciously perceived as an opportunity to overcome earlier family tension and to institute desired closer relationships.

The crisis period itself, and in particular the donor search, did generate major tensions in a sizeable minority (25%) of families. The following types of extended families were particularly vulnerable to this stress: larger families; families in which the parents were no longer alive or active; families in which the member in need of help was an adult rather than a child; geographically dispersed families; and families with a prior history of major internal conflict.

Yet, once the crisis passed, there was a definite attempt to forgive prior transgressions, to attempt to reintegrate the family, and to cover-up and

* The view that closed communication can be beneficial for interpersonal relationships is controversial (see Coser, 1956, for one contrary view). We are not arguing against the idea that the closest relationships are characterized by open communication. Rather we are suggesting that certain types of negative feelings in the extended family are better not communicated if a moderately close and civil relationship is to continue.

deny prior conflict and unwillingness to help. In very few families did significant conflict or stress persist to a year after the event.

Within the general pattern of increased family closeness and smoothing over of wounds, there was some long-term reshuffling of emotional ties, however. Recipients ended up feeling much closer to donors and volunteers than to nondonors. Yet greater contact and help-giving exchanges were also resumed between nondonors and recipients.

Although a shared crisis successfully resolved can increase family cohesion, the characteristics of the crisis that make this outcome more or less likely are not clear. Future research must specify relevant differences among crisis situations. For example, these family patterns and individual reactions may differ in situations where the crisis was not resolved successfully—in this case where the kidney was rejected or the patient died.*

One hypothesis that does emerge from our data involves the extent to which the communication of negative feelings is inhibited during the period of crisis. On the basis of our findings, it is hypothesized that where conflict or unwillingness to help exists, patterns of *noncommunication* or inhibited communication during the crisis period may aid later family reintegration. Where there is no explicit statement of requests for help, refusals of requests, temporary indecisions, or anger, later reintegration and denial of past conflict may become easier.

Exchange Patterns within the Family. The issues of gift-exchange and gratitude within the family have intrigued most of those who have written about the phenomenon of organ donation. Therefore, although our primary purpose in this chapter has been to summarize conclusions reached throughout the book, at this point we wish to explore some of the implications of this gift for obligations of exchange within the family. Most of those who have written about organ donation have treated it as a problem of unequal exchange, a case of a gift whose value is so great that equivalent reciprocation is impossible. Organ donation is seen as engendering an enormous debt on the part of the recipients, a debt that cannot possibly be repaid. Mauss (1967) in his classic work on the norms of the "gift" notes that there is a normative obligation to reciprocate a gift, and the "gift not yet repaid debases the man who accepts it" (p. 63). Blau (1964) writes that unreciprocated benefactions produce differentiations of status between the gift giver and the recipient, with the recipient in such situations forced to assume a subordinate status.

* For this reason it would be valuable to extend our study to families and patients where the kidney was rejected.

The prediction is that problems of indebtedness will create great tension in the donor-recipient relationship after the transplant. The recipient will resent and avoid the debtor for placing him in this subordinate position; the donor will take advantage of the debt by attempting to exert power over the recipient, particularly in matters related to care of the gift—that is, he will try to make certain the recipient does not engage in behavior that would endanger the kidney.

Such problems between recipient and donor do occur in this and other series of cases. The puzzle is not why they occur, but why they occur so rarely. Only 7% of recipients and an equal proportion of donors in our series indicate that the donation has made their relationship difficult at a year after the transplant.

This infrequency is only one of the puzzles presented by the data. In cases where there *has* been tension over the gift, the nature of the difficulty raises questions. Under certain circumstances mentioned earlier, either the donor or recipient has felt betrayed by other family members. The exact meaning of these betrayals requires interpretation:

1. Despite the enormous value of the gift, many recipients have felt they are justified in being hurt and angry at the *nondonors* who failed to offer the gift.
2. In a few cases recipients have felt betrayed when the *donor* has openly requested gratitude or a material return of the favor, or when the donor's gift was given with reluctance. In fact, in these cases less gratitude is felt; the enormous gift is belittled; and the internal feelings of indebtedness are reduced. Why should the symbolic value of the gift and the recipient's feelings of obligation be decreased when the donor indicates ambivalence or a desire for reciprocation?
3. Similar reactions of anger and betrayal have been experienced by *donors* in those few cases where they receive little explicit gratitude. In this situation they feel as if they have been manipulated and "played for suckers."

In all of these cases one of the parties believes that important obligations due him have been ignored and violated by another family member. The nature of these obligations needs to be explicated, as well as the reasons why the potential problem of indebtedness so rarely causes difficulty in actuality.

One of the most likely reasons that there is so little difficulty between most donors and recipients lies in the rewarding nature of their emotional relationship. An intimate, intense, equal-status relationship serves as a reward in itself. A major gift that cannot be reciprocated threatens to disrupt the closeness and equality of this relationship by subordinating the recipient. However, the donor seems to be strongly motivated to avoid such a disruption of the relationship, for in its maintenance lies his primary compensation for donating. Homans (1961) notes that in social interaction a major reward for helping another may be the increase in social approval obtained from the one helped. Similarly, generous expressions of gratitude that symbolize increased love may be defined as an adequate return by the donor for the gift of a kidney, along with the continued life of the recipient.

The donor frequently expresses anxiety over the possibility that the recipient will feel guilt or indebtedness about the gift and that a barrier will emerge between them. To forestall such feelings of debt the donor frequently will redefine the situation to the recipient:

A son tells us about the way in which he informed his mother he would donate. He indicated he was simply repaying her earlier gift of life to him.

SON. When I told her, I think I said she gave it to me, and she could have it back.

A daughter tells about her offer to her father

INTERVIEWER. How do you think he felt about that then [your offer]?

DONOR. I think he was glad. He wanted to know if I really would want to. [I said yes.] He said what if something would happen to your other one later? Then where are you: I said "that's just a chance I'll have to take." I'm sure if the situation were in reverse, he wouldn't think twice about doing it for me.

A recipient recalls the event in which his sister first volunteered

RECIPIENT. Her attitude was that her husband had died and she couldn't do anything for him and was pleased she could do this for me. Then she turned the question around and asked if I wouldn't do the same for her. I said, "I hope so."

In this type of case the recipient is informed either that the donor is himself reciprocating a prior gift or that the obligation to give help when needed had been a mutual one. In effect, the recipient is told that his debt is reduced, because the donor would have expected to receive this kind of help from him had the situation been reversed. The donor, motivated to maintain the warm regard of the recipient, tries to cancel much of the larger debt.

We have been speaking of one danger to the close equal-status relationship between donor and recipient—the danger that the recipient will be subordinated because of the debt. However, reestablishing this relationship after the gift is given requires the avoidance of another danger as well—the danger that the value of the gift will be ignored and the donor, not the recipient, will thereby lose rank. As Schwartz (in press) notes, a special hazard of altruism is the possibility of exploitation of the altruist. He may be drawn into an extreme sequence of demands in which he becomes in essence "servant" to a demanding "master." In an intimate relationship, according to Blau (1964), the party who values the relationship more and gives more to maintain it will lose power relative to the other. If the recipient expresses no gratitude, not only does the donor fail to achieve the reward of increased closeness to the patient, but he is likely to feel devalued and taken for granted.* He resists suffering the dual sacrifice of loss of a body-part and loss of status by having the value of that gift ignored. While too much gratitude is upsetting to the donor, too little creates feelings of anger, hurt, and betrayal.

Underlying the norms of help-giving exchange within the family are the larger set of norms governing primary or intimate relationships. In these relationships persons must not be regarded as means to an end but as ends in themselves. The goal should not be to obtain anything from the loved one except the continuation of the relationship. Only in a secondary relationship, as in a business contact, is one entitled to think of the person as a means to an end. The greatest sense of betrayal occurs when an individual believes he has been "used" by the other without consideration of his intimate status. The donor who is courted prior to the transplant and ignored afterward feels that the lack of expressed gratitude symbolizes a lack of love. His body-part was needed but he himself was not valued. He has been "used"; he is a "sucker."

Similarly, if the donor expresses a desire for some repayment of the gift, some repayment of favors or an increase in power over the recipient, his motives become suspect. He is using the gift as a means to an end rather than as a way of maintaining the life of a loved one. The relationship is not a reward in itself for him. The gift no longer meets one of the normative standards of the gift—that is, that it be given without thought of a gain (Gouldner, 1960). His sacrifice has lost its meaning. Therefore, he is not entitled to increased love or even the type of sacrifices based on love. He may, however, be entitled to some type of repayment more customary in secondary or instrumental business relationships. By

* This discussion is appropriate primarily for cases in which the recipient is an adult. Parents of small children wish the donation to be taken for granted.

calling for repayment, he has lost most of the good feeling upon which substantial gifts might be made to him in a future time.

The norms about gift-giving, particularly as part of an intimate relationship, have always been described as unique, full of internal contradictions (e.g., see Gouldner, 1960). While the individual is "obligated to give" in certain situations, he should give of his own free will because he desires to, not because he is constrained to do so. He should give without thought of gain; but the gift should be reciprocated and he is entitled to expect reciprocation (if possible, reciprocation in kind; otherwise, expressions of gratitude.) If the norms of gift-giving are violated—that is, if the donor gives with reluctance or out of desire for gain—the gift is tainted and requires less reciprocation. Thus the ambivalent donors, as well as the ones seeking some return benefit, are less eligible for reciprocation.

While many of the puzzles presented initially in this section can be interpreted in the context of the above discussions, the anger of the recipient at the failure of the nondonor to volunteer, remains at issue. The distinction between asking for a loan and requesting credit that has been earned is an apt analogy in this case.

Family relationships and the professions of love that accompany them carry with them an assumption that one has earned great credit. Such relationships are like money in the bank that will be spent if one needs help. A love relationship is in part credit—if one needs help here is a source that will aid. Each party is establishing an account of credit for the other. However, unlike a bank account that one has saved oneself, the amount of credit is ambiguous and unclear. Only in the parent to minor-child relationship and secondarily in the spouse relationship is there clarity. The credit there is normatively defined as almost unlimited—whatever the small child needs, whatever the spouse needs, will be forthcoming if at all within the realm of possibility. Only the life of the potential giver is excepted, and even then considerable risk to one's life is expected in a crisis.

From other relatives the amount of credit one has earned is unknown. Even the potential giver is not always certain ahead of time what he will be willing to give; he is not sure how much credit the other is entitled to. As long as major credit is unneeded, exchanges of love, good feeling, and lesser amounts of aid are transacted based on the assumption that the relationship is backed by great credit on both sides.

Among relatives who are less close, there is an assumption of less credit and fewer exchanges of good feeling and aid. Distant relatives are normatively entitled to less aid than are closer family members, but the amount of actual credit is still unknown.

When a person actually needs to use a good part of the credit is the time when he discovers if it is really there. If not, he reduces the amount of credit the other can expect from him and reduces the lesser exchanges of favors and expressions of love that symbolize the relationship. If he receives the credit that he hoped was there, he increases the credit the other can expect from him and the everyday exchanges of expressed gratitude and love that symbolize that credit. The reward that the giver obtains from these increased exchanges and from aiding the person he loves can even reestablish most of the original credit. Yet if the recipient or donor feels that the donor gave more than the recipient was entitled to—that he lent him money rather than freed up credit—the relationship becomes that of a debtor-lender in which the debtor cannot adequately repay the debt.

Betrayal is what is experienced when either party suspects he has been saving more credit for the other than the other has been reciprocating. Anger is felt at the nondonor who is loved and who does not appear to reciprocate that love. Anger is similarly felt at the ambivalent donor who seems to be giving solely out of compulsion rather than out of accumulated warm feelings. Anger is also directed to the donor who calls for some compensation after the gift is given. In all cases the potential recipient feels in some sense that he has earned the gift, and it is not a loan to be repaid. If the love relationship is what it should be, the relative should wish to save the recipient's life, even if it means sacrifice. One should have earned this much credit in the closest of relationships. If the "gift" is not the result of such earned credit but is treated as a loan that must be repaid or a resource to which one is not entitled, the potential donor has betrayed a trust. One is no longer obligated to maintain a great reserve of credit for him, nor to behave as if one has in terms of expressions of love.

The potential for conflict could be increased by differences among the parties in their interpretation of the value of the gift. Although some potential donors and recipients regard the loss of a kidney as a minor and temporary hardship, others perceive it as a major short and long-term risk. To some the credit earned within the family far exceeds the value of a kidney; to others the loss of a kidney would surpass the credit legitimately established in any close relationship. In general the recipients are motivated to minimize the risk to reduce the guilt they would feel at allowing a loved one to take this chance for them. But the potential donors are not so motivated, and thus the possibility of conflict is increased.

Whether or not the credit-loan analogy is completely compatible with the processes of exchange within the family, the following norms are clearly operative: (1) an individual should out of love wish to help save the life and health of his parents, siblings, and children; (2) if he acts to help save a family member's life, that should be the major reward, because he has avoided the great loss that would be felt without that person. If an individual expects another reward, his motives become suspect—love no longer appears to be the motivating force. Whether the obligation to help family members extends as far as to require kidney donation remains ambiguous.

In *sum*, major gift-giving or help-giving within the family offers the potential for many types of family-conflicts. The donor, the recipient, and the nondonor all stand to lose status in intimate relationships that they value. And there are examples within the data of such outcomes. Yet in the majority of families and the vast majority of donor-recipient pairs, the exchange discussed here has been a highly rewarding one with the dyad emerging much closer emotionally than before. The reason for this result probably lies in the value most donors place on their relationships with the recipient. In truth they are rewarded by the fact they have saved the recipient's life, and they try to structure the situation to minimize the recipient's sense of debt. Whether these positive results would generalize to help-giving of a less dramatic nature is a question still to be answered.

* * *

The conclusion of this work is cautiously optimistic. From the policy viewpoint, the consequences of organ transplantation appear to be largely positive. From a more theoretical view, the emphasis has been on the resiliency of individuals and families confronted with major crisis and stress. Yet in a minority of cases this resiliency is absent. Some recipients are unable to cope well with the stress, and in some cases the donor search produced significant short-term and even sometimes long-term distress for the families of both related and cadaver donors. The weighing of this type of distress in a minority of cases against the significant and even dramatic benefits for most recipients and related donors is an ethical problem that undoubtedly will meet various solutions. The drama of the conflict and stress where it occurs must not blind either the behavioral scientist or the policy-maker to the less colorful but more typical and more positive reactions of individuals and families faced with this significant life-crisis.

APPENDIX **A**

ADULT SELF-IMAGE SCALES

Adult Self-Image Scales are administered to recipients, donors, non-donors, mothers of ill children.

A–1 *Self-Esteem* †

Would you agree or disagree with this statement? I am able to do things as well as most other people. Do you

*(1) strongly agree
*(2) agree

† The responses with an asterisk get scored as "1"; the rest get scored as "0." The total score for all 10 questions in this scale varies from 0 to 10, with a high score standing for high self esteem.

Reliability: Cronbach's Alpha = .79

See Morris Rosenberg (1965) for details concerning validation. In general this scale is dependent upon face validity; upon its association with the theoretically relevant variables of depression and anxiety, reflected both in scale scores and in observations by outside observers; on its association with peer group reputation, assessed by sociometric methods as well as by its association with reports of outside observers; and by other additional evidence (see Wells and Marwell, 1976).

To prevent false consistency, items from the same scale are not placed together, but are spread out in the questionnaire.

(3) disagree, or
(4) strongly disagree

Would you agree or disagree with the following statement? I feel that I have a number of good qualities. Do you

*(1) strongly agree
(2) agree
(3) disagree, or
(4) strongly disagree

Would you agree or disagree with the following statement? I feel I do not have much to be proud of. Do you

(1) strongly agree
(2) agree
(3) disagree, or
*(4) strongly disagree

Do you agree or disagree with this? I take a positive attitude toward myself. Do you

*(1) strongly agree
(2) agree
(3) disagree, or
(4) strongly disagree

Would you agree or disagree with this? I wish I could have more respect for myself. Do you

(1) strongly agree
(2) agree
*(3) disagree
*(4) strongly disagree

Would you agree or disagree with this? At times I think I am no good at all. Do you

(1) strongly agree
(2) agree
*(3) disagree, or
*(4) strongly disagree

Would you agree or disagree with the following statement? I certainly feel useless at times. Do you

(1) strongly agree
(2) agree

*(3) disagree, or
*(4) strongly disagree

I feel that I'm a person of worth, at least on an equal plane with others. Do you

*(1) strongly agree
(2) agree
(3) disagree, or
(4) strongly disagree

All in all I feel that I am a failure. Do you

(1) strongly agree
(2) agree
(3) disagree, or
*(4) strongly disagree

On the whole, I am satisfied with myself. Do you

*(1) strongly agree
(2) agree
(3) disagree, or
(4) strongly disagree

A–2 *Depressive Affect or Happiness* †

Do you agree or disagree with this statement? I wish I could be as happy as others seem to be. At this point in your life do you

(1) agree, or
*(2) disagree

Do you agree or disagree with the following statement? I get a lot of fun out of life. Do you

*(1) agree, or
(2) disagree

On the whole I think I am quite a happy person. Do you

*(1) agree, or
(2) disagree

† The responses with an asterisk get scored as "1"; the rest get scored as "0." The total score for all six questions in this scale varies from 0 to 6, with a high score standing for high happiness.

Reliability: Cronbach's Alpha = .71

How often do you feel downcast and dejected? Do you feel that way

(1) very often
(2) fairly often
(3) occasionally
*(4) rarely, or
*(5) never

In general, how would you say you feel most of the time—in good or low spirits? Are you in

*(1) very good spirits
(2) fairly good spirits
(3) neither good nor low spirits
(4) fairly low spirits, or
(5) very low spirits

Right now, on the whole, how happy would you say you are? Are you

*(1) very happy
(2) fairly happy
(3) not very happy, or
(4) not at all happy

A–3 *Control over Destiny* †

Do you feel that most of the things that happen to you are

*(1) the result of your own decision, or
(2) things over which you have no control

Since you've been ill, how difficult is it for you to make and carry out plans? Would you say it's been

(1) very difficult
(2) a little difficult, or
*(3) not at all difficult

Everytime I try to get ahead, something or somebody stops me. Do you feel like this?

(1) Yes
*(2) No

† The responses with an asterisk get scored as "1"; the rest get scored as "0." The total score for all five questions in this scale varies from 0 to 5, with a high score standing for high control over destiny.

Reliability: Cronbach's Alpha = .51

How much control do you feel you have over your life these days since you've been sick? Do you feel you have

*(1) a great amount of control
(2) a moderate amount of control,
(3) little control, or
(4) no control over your life

It's hard for me to do what I really want in life. Do you feel like this ever?

(1) Yes
*(2) No

A–4 *Anxiety* †

How often do you feel uneasy about something without knowing why? Would you tell me whether it happens

(1) always
(2) frequently
(3) sometimes
*(4) rarely, or
*(5) never

How often do you find you can't get rid of some thought or idea that keeps running through your mind? Would you tell me whether it happens

(1) always
(2) frequently
(3) sometimes
*(4) rarely, or
*(5) never

How often do you feel so restless that you cannot sit still? Would you tell me whether it happens

(1) always
(2) frequently
(3) sometimes
*(4) rarely, or
*(5) never

† The responses with an asterisk get scored as "1"; the rest get scored as "0." The total score for all five questions in this scale varies from 0 to 5, with a high score standing for low anxiety.

Reliability: Cronbach's Alpha = .62

How often do you go to pieces? Would you tell me whether it happens

(1) always
(2) frequently
(3) sometimes
(4) rarely, or
*(5) never

How often do you find yourself anxious and worrying about something? Would you tell me whether it happens

(1) always
(2) frequently
(3) sometimes
*(4) rarely, or
*(5) never

A–5 *Preoccupation with Self* †

Since you have been sick in the past few months, would you say that you think about yourself

(1) almost always
(2) often
*(3) sometimes, or
*(4) hardly ever

Would you say that you think about yourself and your illness

(1) all the time
(2) a great deal
*(3) a little bit, or
*(4) not at all

Since you have been sick enough to need a transplant, do you think about yourself

(1) more than before
*(2) less than before, or
*(3) the same as before

† The responses with an asterisk get scored as "1"; the rest get scored as "0." The total score for all three questions in this scale varies from 0 to 3, with a high score standing for low preoccupation with self.

Reliability: Cronbach's Alpha = .64

A–6 *Identity Stability* †

Do you think the experience of being sick has caused your opinions of yourself to change a good deal, or do your opinions of yourself always continue to remain the same? Would you say your opinions of yourself

(1) change a great deal
(2) change somewhat
*(3) change very little, or
*(4) do not change at all

Do you agree with this? Since I have been sick I have found that my ideas of who I am and what I am like seem to change quickly. Do you

(1) agree, or
*(2) disagree

How sure are you that you know what kind of a person you really are these days? Are you

*(1) very sure
*(2) pretty sure
(3) not very sure, or
(4) not at all sure about what kind of person you are

Since you have been sick, how often do you feel mixed up about yourself, about what you are really like? Does it happen

(1) often
(2) sometimes, or
*(3) never

Someone told me: "Some days I am happy with the kind of person I am, other days I am not happy with the kind of person I am." Since you have been sick, do your feelings change like this?

(1) Yes
*(2) No

† The responses with an asterisk get scored as "1"; the rest get scored as "0." The total score for all five questions in this scale varies from 0 to 5, with a high score standing for high identity stability.

Reliability: Cronbach's Alpha = .62

A–7 *Independence–Dependence* †

Since you've been sick, do you feel you

(1) are more dependent on others for help than you'd like to be, or do you feel
*(2) that you'd like to have someone on whom you could depend more, or
*(3) neither

How much of a problem is your dependence upon others since you've been ill with kidney disease? Is your dependence upon others

(1) a great problem
(2) somewhat of a problem
*(3) a small problem, or
*(4) no problem

How *independent* do you feel you are now with regard to managing your life? Are you

*(1) very independent
*(2) pretty independent
(3) not very independent, or
(4) not at all independent

† The responses with an asterisk get scored as "1"; the rest get scored as "0." The total score for all three questions in this scale varies from 0 to 3, with a high score standing for high independence.

Reliability: Cronbach's Alpha = .56

APPENDIX B

CHILDREN'S SELF-IMAGE SCALES

B–1 *Self-Esteem* †

Everybody has some things about him which are good and some things about him which are bad. Are more of the things about you. . .

(1) good
*(2) bad or
*(3) both about the same

† The responses *without* an asterisk get scored as "1"; the rest get scored as "0." The total score for all six questions in this scale varies from 0 to 6, with a low score standing for low self-esteem.

Reliability: Guttman Scale

90.2% coefficient of reproducibility
67.6% coefficient of scalability

This scale has undergone extensive validation tests in Rosenberg and Simmons (1972, Ch. 2) for both whites and blacks. *First*, it has been validated against another measure of the same concept—that is, it appears to have trait validity. It is satisfactorily correlated with adolescents' scores on the Rosenberg measure of self-esteem which had been validated in

Another kid said, "I am no good." Do you ever feel like this? (*If yes, ask*): Do you feel like this a lot or a little? "I am no good?"

(1) no
*(2) a lot
*(3) a little

A kid told me: "There's a lot wrong with me." Do you ever feel like this? (*If yes, ask*): Do you feel like this a lot or a little? "There's a lot wrong with me."

(1) no
*(2) a lot
*(3) a little

Another kid said: "I'm not much good at anything." Do you ever feel like this? (*If yes, ask*): Do you feel like this a lot or a little? "I'm not much good at anything."

(1) no
*(2) a lot
*(3) a little

Another kid said, "I think I am no good at all." Do you ever feel like this? (*If yes, ask*): Do you feel like this a lot or a little? "I think I am no good at all."

(1) no
*(2) a lot
*(3) a little

How happy are you with the kind of person you are? Are you

(1) very happy with the kind of person you are
(2) pretty happy
*(3) a little happy
*(4) not at all happy

---

previous research (Rosenberg, 1965). It was not possible to use the Rosenberg measure for younger children because of its adult language so this scale was constructed in Rosenberg and Simmons (1972) for young school-aged children. *Second*, this scale seems to have construct validity—10 theoretical predictions were made concerning self-esteem and in all cases these predictions were confirmed using the scale. Self-esteem was shown to correlate positively with measures of depression and anxiety, with marks in school, with indicators of school leadership, and with the opinions of several significant others including parents, teachers and friends, for all age groups. *Third*, the scale appears to satisfy the interchangeability criterion: it "behaves" the same way as the Rosenberg measure of self-esteem in relation to other variables. *Finally*, it appears to have face validity as a measure of the individual's global feelings about his own self-worth.

B–2 *Self-Consciousness* †

Let's say some grownup or adult visitors came into class and the teacher wanted them to know who you were, so she asked you to stand up and tell them a little about yourself. . .

(1) would you like that
*(2) would you not like it
(3) wouldn't you care

If the teacher asked you to get up in front of the class and talk a little bit about your summer, would you be. . .

*(1) very nervous
(2) a little nervous
(3) not at all nervous

If you did get up in front of the class and tell them about your summer. . .

*(1) would you think a lot about how all the kids were looking at you
(2) would you think a little bit about how all the kids were looking at you
(3) wouldn't you think at all about the kids looking at you

If you were to wear the wrong kind of clothes to a party, would that bother you. . .

*(1) a lot
(2) a little
(3) not at all

† Responses marked by an asterisk get scored as "1"; the rest get scored as "0." The total score for all seven questions in this scale varies from 0 to 7, with a high score standing for high self-consciousness.

Reliability: Guttman Scale

89.4% coefficient of reproducibility
62.5% coefficient of scalability

To validate the self-consciousness scale, Simmons et al. (1973) asked the interviewers to rate the child as "very nervous, somewhat nervous, or not nervous." Forty-three percent of those students categorized as "very nervous" scored high on the self-consciousness scale in contrast to 24 percent of those rated as "not nervous" ($X^2 = 27.6769$, 4 *df*, $p < .01$).

If you went to a party where you did not know most of the kids, would you wonder what they were thinking about you?

*(1) yes
(2) no

Do you get nervous when someone watches you work?

*(1) yes
(2) no

A young person told me: "When I'm with people I get nervous because I worry about how much they like me." Do you feel like this. . .

*(1) often
(2) sometimes
(3) never

B–3 *Stability of Self Scale*†

How sure are you that you know what kind of person you really are? Are you . . .

*(1) very sure
*(2) pretty sure
(3) not very sure
(4) not at all sure

How often do you feel mixed up about yourself, about what you are really like?

(1) often
(2) sometimes
*(3) never

† Responses marked by an asterisk get scored as "1"; the rest get scored as "0." The total score for all 7 questions in this scale varies from 0 to 7, with a high score standing for high stability.

Reliability: Guttman Scale

89.1% coefficient of reproducibility
64.8% coefficient of scalability

Do you feel like this: "I know just what I'm like. I'm really sure about it."

*(1) yes
(2) no

A kid told me: "Some days I like the way I am. Some days I do not like the way I am." Do your feelings *change* like this?

(1) yes
*(2) no

A kid told me: "Some days I am happy with the kind of person I am, other days I am not happy with the kind of person I am." Do your feelings change like this?

(1) yes
*(2) no

Do you. . .

*(1) know for sure how nice a person you are
(2) do your ideas about how nice you are change a lot

A kid told me: "Some days I think I am one kind of a person, other days a different kind of person." Do your feelings *change* like this?

(1) yes
*(2) no

B–4 *Sense of Distinctiveness*†

How different are you from most other kids you know?

*(1) very different
*(2) somewhat different
(3) not different at all

How much are you the same as most other kids you know?

(1) very much the same
*(2) somewhat the same
*(3) not at all the same as other kids

† Responses marked by an asterisk get scored as "1"; the rest get scored as "0." The total score for both questions in this scale varies from 0 to 2, with a high score standing for high sense of distinctiveness.

Reliability: Cronbach's Alpha = .40

B–5 *Body-Image, Satisfaction with Looks* †

How do you feel about your looks? Are you. . .

*(1) very happy with the way you look
*(2) pretty happy with the way you look
(3) not very happy with the way you look
(4) not at all happy with the way you look

Do you think you are. . .

(1) too fat
*(2) just right
(3) too thin

Do you think you are. . .

(1) too tall
*(2) just right
(3) too short

B–6 *Show True Feelings* ‡

Do you . . .

(1) usually tell people what things you really like
*(2) do you usually *not* tell people what things you really like

A kid told me: "I usually show other people how I really feel." How about you? Do you. . .

(1) usually show people how you really feel
(2) sometimes show people how you really feel
*(3) never show people how you really feel

A person who keeps his feelings to himself usually doesn't tell others what he really thinks and feels inside. How much do you keep your feelings to yourself?

*(1) very much

† Responses marked by an asterisk get scored as "1"; the rest get scored as "0." The total score for all three questions in this scale varies from 0 to 3, with a high score standing for high satisfaction with looks.

‡ Responses marked by an asterisk get scored as "1"; the rest get scored as "0." The total score for all three questions in this scale varies from 0 to 3, with a high score standing for a tendency to conceal true feelings.

Reliability: Cronbach's Alpha = .43

*(2) pretty much
(3) not very much

B–7 *Happiness* †

How happy would you say you are most of the time? Would you say you are. . .

(1) very happy
(2) pretty happy
*(3) not very happy
*(4) not at all happy

Would you say this? "I get a lot of fun out of life."

(1) yes
*(2) no

Would you say this: "Mostly, I think I am quite a happy person."

(1) yes
*(2) no

How happy are you today? Are you. . .

(1) very happy
(2) pretty happy
*(3) not very happy
*(4) not at all happy

A kid told me: "Other kids seem happier than I." Is this. . .

*(1) true for you
(2) not true for you

† Responses marked by an asterisk get scored as "1"; the rest get scored as "0." The total score for all six questions in this scale varies from 0 to 6, with a high score standing for low happiness.

This scale derived from the Baltimore study was revised to improve the scaling coefficients for the ill children. For more detail, see Klein (1975).

Reliability: Guttman Scale

94.4% coefficient of reproducibility
60.0% coefficient of scalability

Would you say that most of the time you are. . .

(1) very cheerful
*(2) pretty cheerful
*(3) not very cheerful
*(4) not cheerful at all

B–8 *Anxiety*†

We want to ask you about being nervous. Are you nervous. . .

(1) often
(2) sometimes
*(3) almost never
*(4) never

I am secretly afraid of a lot of things.

(1) yes
*(2) no

Are you afraid of being laughed at by other kids?

(1) yes
*(2) no

Do you worry about what other people think of you?

(1) yes
*(2) no

Do you think you worry more than other boys and girls do?

(1) yes
*(2) no

Do you worry when the teacher says she's going to ask you questions to find out how much you know?

(1) yes
*(2) no

† Responses *without* an asterisk get scored as "1"; the rest get scored as "0." The total score for all six questions in this scale varies from 0 to 6, with a high score standing for high anxiety.

This scale was created from items in the Baltimore study but scaled on the ill children. For more detail, see Klein (1975).

Reliability: Cronbach's Alpha for ill children = .52

B–9 *Estimate of Popularity* †

How much do *boys* like you? Do boys like you. . .

(1) very much
(2) pretty much
*(3) not much
*(4) not at all

How much do *girls* like you? Do girls like you. . .

(1) very much
(2) pretty much
*(3) not much
*(4) not at all

Would you say that the kids in your class think of you as. . .

(1) a wonderful person
(2) a pretty nice person
*(3) a little bit of a nice person
*(4) not such a nice person

B–10 *Level of Disruption Scale* ‡

Factor 1—General Impact

Some people feel that their child's illness is very demanding of their family's time and energy, while others don't feel this way. Would you say your child's illness has taken. . .

(1) a lot of your family's time and energy
(2) some of their time and energy, or
(3) a little of their time and energy

† Responses marked with an asterisk get scored as "1"; the rest get scored as "0." The total score for all three questions in this scale varies from 0 to 3, with a high score standing for low estimate of popularity.

‡ On each of these questions, the individual was given the number of points indicated in parentheses next to the multiple-choice alternative chosen. For each of the three scales, the number of points for the relevant question were summed. Thus General Impact Scale has a range from 4 to 11, with 11 indicating low impact, Financial and Emotional Impact each have a range of 2 to 5, with 5 indicating low impact. These scales were derived from a factor analysis (see Klein, 1975).

Has your child's being sick interfered with the family routine?

(1) often
(2) sometimes
(3) hardly ever, or
(4) never

Has your child's disease changed your life in any way?

(1) yes
(2) no

Has your child's disease caused any other problems for your family? Has the sickness ever caused your family to change plans?

(1) yes
(2) no

Factor 2—Financial Impact

Have the medical bills been. . .

(1) a great concern
(2) somewhat of a concern, or
(3) no concern for your family

Do you feel the cost of the disease has been one of the major worries caused by the disease?

(1) yes
(2) no

Factor 3—Emotional Impact

Has anyone in the family been particularly worried about the child and the kidney disease?

(1) yes
(2) no

Do you think your parents worry about your sickness. . .

(1) very often
(2) sometimes, or
(3) not very often

B–11 *Child Taking Responsibility for Self Scale*†

The child was given a point if he or she was mentioned in the answers to the following questions:

Who helps you the most to see that you do all the things the doctor tells you to do?

(When you were last home sick) who took care of you?

When your mother has to do something else, who usually takes care of you if you're home sick?

Has the child assumed responsibility for his own care. . .

*(1) a lot
*(2) somewhat
(3) very little, or
(4) not at all

† Items marked by asterisk scored as indicating responsibility.

APPENDIX C

DONOR ATTITUDE SCALES

C–1 *Ambivalence Scale*†

Did you. . .

(1) know right away you would definitely do it or,
*(2) did you think it over

How would you have felt if you had found out that you couldn't donate for some reason? Do you think you would have felt. . .

(1) very disappointed
(2) a little disappointed,
*(3) a little relieved, or
*(4) very relieved that you couldn't donate

† Responses marked by an asterisk get scored as "1"; the rest get scored as "0." The total score for all seven questions in this scale varies from 0 to 7, with a high score standing for high level of ambivalence.

Reliability: Cronbach's Alpha = .78

How hard a decision was it for you to decide to donate? Would you say it was. . .

*(1) very hard
*(2) somewhat hard
*(3) a little hard, or
(4) not at all hard to decide
(5) it was no decision at all [offered spontaneously]

I'm going to read you a list of ways some people feel about donating a kidney and I'd like you to tell me if you agree a lot, agree a little, disagree a lot, or disagree a little:

I sometimes wish the transplant patient were getting a cadaver kidney instead of one from me. Do you. . .

*(1) agree a lot
*(2) agree a little
*(3) disagree a little, or
(4) disagree a lot

I would really *want* to donate myself even if someone else could do it. Do you. . .

(1) agree a lot
*(2) agree a little
*(3) disagree a little
*(4) disagree a lot

I sometimes feel unsure about donating. Do you. . .

*(1) agree a lot
*(2) agree a little
(3) disagree a little
(4) disagree a lot

Many donors have doubts and worries going into the transplant operation even though they go through with it. Did you ever have any doubts about donating?

*(1) yes
(2) no

C–2 *Negative Feelings at 5 Days and 1 Year Posttransplant* †

Would you say you are. . .

*(1) very worried about your own health now
*(2) somewhat worried
*(3) a little worried, or
(4) not at all worried about your own health now

How often do you worry about having only one kidney left? Do you worry about it. . .

*(1) often
*(2) sometimes, or
(3) almost never

I am going to read you a list of ways some people feel after having donated organs for transplantation and I'd like you to tell me if you agree a lot, agree a little, disagree a little, or disagree a lot with these ideas:

I've given up something that is part of me for nothing in return.

*(1) agree a lot
*(2) agree a little
*(3) disagree a little
(4) disagree a lot

Would you say you are generally. . .

(1) very happy
*(2) a little happy
*(3) a little unhappy, or
*(4) very unhappy about having donated

Interviewer Comments:

Would you describe the patient's general spirits as. . .

(1) ecstatic
(2) very cheerful

† Responses marked by an asterisk get scored as "1"; the rest get scored as "0." The total score for all six questions in this scale varies from 0 to 6, with a high score standing for a higher level of negative feelings.

Reliability: Cronbach's Alpha = .73

(3) somewhat cheerful
*(4) a little cheerful, or
*(5) not at all cheerful

How would you judge the patient's general feelings about the transplant? As. . .

(1) very positive
*(2) somewhat positive
*(3) a little positive
*(4) neither positive or negative
*(5) a little negative
*(6) somewhat negative, or
*(7) very negative

C–3 *Perception of Oneself as a Better Person at 5 Days and 1 Year Post-transplant* †

Do you somehow feel like a better person after having donated a kidney?

*(1) yes
(2) no

I am going to read you a list of ways some people feel after having donated organs for transplantation and I'd like you to tell me if you agree a lot, agree a little, disagree a little, or disagree a lot with these ideas:

Donating an organ makes one feel that he (she) is somehow a bigger and more worthwhile person. Do you. . .

*(1) agree a lot
*(2) agree a little
(3) disagree a little, or
(4) disagree a lot

† Responses marked by an asterisk get scored as "1"; the rest get scored as "0." The total score for all 10 questions in this scale varies from 0 to 10, with a high score standing for a greater perception of one's self as a better person.

Reliability: Cronbach's Alpha = .72

A person willing to donate a kidney is almost a hero. Do you. . .

*(1) agree a lot
*(2) agree a little
(3) disagree a little, or
(4) disagree a lot

Donating a kidney was really sort of a high point in my life, making everything seem more meaningful. Do you. . .

*(1) agree a lot
*(2) agree a little
(3) disagree a little, or
(4) disagree a lot

Here is a card listing the ways some people feel about those who donate a kidney. I'd like you to tell me which is the closest to the way you would describe a living kidney donor.

*(1) anyone who donated a kidney could be called a hero
*(2) a person who donates a kidney makes an exceptional sacrifice
(3) anyone who donates a kidney makes a sacrifice somewhat out of the ordinary
(4) it is generous to give a kidney but anyone should do as much

Since the transplant, would you say you think. . .

*(1) more highly of yourself—that you're a better person than you were before the transplant
(2) do you think less highly of yourself, or
(3) would you say there is no change in the way you think of yourself since the transplant

I'm going to read you a list of ways some donors feel and I'd like you to tell me if you've felt this way very much, a little, or not at all recently:

When you think about the transplant, have you felt. . .

*(1) very worthwhile
(2) a little worthwhile
(3) or not at all worthwhile

When you think about the transplant, have you felt. . .

*(1) very proud

(2) a little proud
(3) or not at all proud

When you think about the transplant, have you felt. . .

*(1) very brave
(2) a little brave
(3) or not at all brave

When you think about the transplant, have you felt. . .

*(1) very heroic
(2) a little heroic
(3) or not at all heroic

C–4 *Black-Sheep Scale*†

Has there ever been any period of time in the past, before the transplant came up, in which you and the recipient did not get along well together?

*(1) yes
(2) no

Do you think your parents (and brothers and sisters) during recent years have been. . .

(1) generally approving and accepting of you and your life, or
*(2) not generally approving
(3) don't know

Have you done anything major in your life that your family didn't approve of?

*(1) yes
(2) no

† Responses marked by an asterisk get scored as "1"; the rest get scored as "0." The total score for all three questions in this scale varies from 0 to 3, with a high score standing for a high level of black-sheep motivation.

BIBLIOGRAPHY

"Adolescent Kidney Donors." *British Medical Journal*, June 28, p. 710 (1975).

"AMA Grams." *Journal of American Medical Association*, **227**(7) (1974).

"Bar Assn. Urges States Adopt Brain-based Definition of Death." *Hospital Tribune*, April 7, p. 3 (1975).

"Dearth of Donor Organs is Traced to Doubt About Definition of Death." *Medical World News*, March 22, pp. 14–15 (1974).

"Dialysis Patients Get a New Deal." *Medical World News*, August 10, p. 21 (1973).

"Eleventh Report of the Human Renal Transplant Registry." *Journal of American Medical Association*, **226**(10), 1197–1210 (1973).

"A Fair Deal for Patients with Renal Failure." *British Medical Journal*, February 1, pp. 230–231 (1975a).

"Home Dialysis Study—Results Better Than Center's in 5-Year Tests." *Medical Tribune*, **11**(22) (1970).

"I Can't Take It Any More." *Newsweek*, July 26, pp. 51–52 (1971).

"In the Matter of Karen Quinlan: An Alleged Incompetent." *Atlantic Reporter*, 2nd Series, **355**(3), pp. 647–672 (1976).

"A Kidney in Time." *Newsweek*, August 2, p. 45 (1971).

"The Kidney Care Issue: A Test for National Health Insurance." *Hospital Practice*, **8**(4), 49–59 (1973).

"Kidney Grafting in Sweden is Snagged by Delay in Accepting Death Criteria." *Hospital Tribune*, April 2, p. 2 (1973).

"Kidneys from Living Donors." *British Medical Journal*, May 18, **2**(5915), p. 344 (1974).

"Medicare Dialysis Score: More Plus Than Minus After Year's Functioning." *Hospital Practice*, **9**(10), 214 (1974).

"Medicarelessness" (editorial). *New York Times*, January 14 (1973).

"New Dimensions in Legal and Ethical Concepts for Human Research." *Sciences*, **9**(10) (1969).

"Racism is Charged in Row Over Transplant." *Minneapolis Star*, July 28, p. 17B (1971).

"Rare Kidney Disease Claims 3 Sons." *Minneapolis Tribune*, March 31, p. 10B (1974).

"Should We Transplant Organs or Efforts?" (editorial), *American Journal of Public Health*, **59**(9), 1567–1568 (1969).

Federal Register. "Conditions for Coverage of Suppliers of End-Stage Renal Disease (ESRD) Services." *Federal Register*, **41**(108), June 3, pp. 22502–22522 (1976).

Federal Register: Part II. "Medical Assistance Programs, Review of Utilization of Care and Services," January 9 (1974).

"The Cost of Life" (editorial). *Journal of American Medical Association*, **204**(10), 923–924 (1968).

"The Sale of Human Body Parts." *Michigan Law Review*, **72**(6), 1182–1264 (1974).

"The Shortage of Organs for Clinical Transplantation: Document for Discussion." *British Medical Journal*, February 1, pp. 251–255 (1975b).

"Transplant of Human Organs." *The Lancet*, **1**(7863), 943 (1974).

"Transplant Pioneer Faces Murder Charge." Reuters News Service, *Minneapolis Star*, October 29, p. 1Y (1968).

"Twelfth Report of the Human Renal Transplant Registry." *Journal of American Medical Association*, **233**(7), 787–796 (1975).

"U.S. Plan Pays Some Doctors Over $100,000." *Minneapolis Tribune*, September 10, p. 4B (1975).

"Virginia Jury Rules that Death Occurs When Brain Dies." *New York Times*, May 27, p. 15 (1972).

"Widow: Transplant Wasn't Approved." *Minneapolis Tribune*, July 27, p. 1 (1971).

Abram, Harry S. "The Psychiatrist, the Treatment of Chronic Renal Failure, and the Prolongation of Life: I." *American Journal of Psychiatry*, **124**(10), 1351–1358 (1968).

——— "The Psychiatrist, The Treatment of Chronic Renal Failure, and the Prolongation of Life: II." *American Journal of Psychiatry*, **126**(2), 157–167 (1969).

——— "The Psychiatrist, the Treatment of Chronic Renal Failure, and the Prolongation of Life: III." *American Journal of Psychiatry*, **128**(12), 1534–1539 (1972).

——— "The Uncooperative Hemodialysis Patient: A Psychiatrist's Viewpoint and a Patient's Commentary." In Norman B. Levy, Ed., *Living or Dying: Adaptation to Hemodialysis*. Springfield, Ill.: Charles C. Thomas, 1974. Pp. 50–61.

——— and Denton C. Buchanan. "The Psychology of Renal Transplantation." Presented at Harbor General Hospital, University of California, Torrance, 1975.

——— Gordon L. Moore, Frederick B. Westervelt. "Suicidal Behavior in Chronic Dialysis Patients." *American Journal of Psychiatry*, **127**(2), 1199–1203 (1971).

——— and Walter Wadlington. "Selection of Patients for Artificial and Transplanted Organs." *Annals of Internal Medicine*, **69**(3), 615–620 (1968).

Aldous, Joan, Thomas Condon, Reuben Hill, Murray Straus, and Irving Tallman, Eds., *Family Problem Solving: A Symposium on Theoretical, Methodological, and Substantive Concerns*. Hinsdale, Ill.: Dryden, 1971.

Alexander, Shana. "They Decide Who Lives, Who Dies." *Life*, **53**(19), 102–125 (1962).

Allgower, M. and U. F. Gruber. "Ethical Problems of Organ Transplantation." *Progress in Surgery*, **8**, 1–13 (1970).

Allison, Graham T. *Essence of Decision: Explaining the Cuban Missile Crisis.* Boston: Little, Brown, 1971.

Allport, Gordon W. "The Ego in Contemporary Psychology." *Psychological Review*, **50**(5), 451–478 (1943).

Altman, Lawrence K. "Kidney Foundation Criticizes Articles on Care Costs." *New York Times*, January 18, p. 30 (1973).

Angell, R. C. *The Family Encounters the Depression.* New York: Scribners, 1936.

Anthony, E. James and Cyrille Koupernik, Eds., *The Child In His Family: Children at Psychiatric Risk*, New York: Wiley, 1974.

Appel, J. Z. "Ethical and Legal Questions Posed by Recent Advances in Medicine." *Journal of American Medical Association*, **205**(7), 513–516 (1968).

Arnet, William. "Comments: The Criteria for Determining Death in Vital Organ Transplants—A Medico-Legal Dilemma." *Missouri Law Review*, **38**(2), 220–234 (1973).

Artificial Heart Assessment Panel of the National Heart and Lung Institute. "The Totally Implantable Artificial Heart." DHEW Publication (NIH) 74–191 (1973).

Bachrach, Peter and Morton S. Baratz. "Decisions and Nondecisions: An Analytical Framework." In Michael Aiken and Paul E. Mott, Eds., *The Structure of Community Power*. New York: Random House, 1970. Pp. 308–320.

Bailey, George L. "Psychosocial Aspects of Hemodialysis." In George L. Bailey, Ed., *Hemodialysis: Principles and Practice.* New York: Academic, 1972. Pp. 424–439.

——— A. Mocelin, and C. Hampers. "Adaptation of Spouse Pairs to Home Dialysis." *Dialysis and Transplantation*, **1**(4), 28–37 (1972).

Baker, A. B. and J. Knutson. "Psychiatric Aspects of Uremia." *American Journal of Psychiatry*, **102**(4), 683–687 (1946).

Bamber, James H. "Adolescent Marginality—A Further Study." *Genetic Psychology Monographs*, **88**(1), 3–21 (1973).

Banik, Sambhu, R. B. Baltzan, and M. A. Baltzan. "Psychological Study of Patients Undergoing Chronic Haemodialysis and Kidney Transplants." *Dialysis and Transplantation*, **3**(6), 20–24 (1974).

Basch, Samuel H. "The Intrapsychic Integration of a New Organ: A Clinical Study of Kidney Transplantation." *The Psychoanalytic Quarterly*, **42**(3), 364–384 (1973).

Bavelas, Alex. "Communication Patterns in Task-Oriented Groups." *Acoustical Society of America Journal*, **22**(6), 725–730 (1950).

Beard, B. H. "Fear of Death and Fear of Life: The Dilemma in Chronic Renal Failure, Hemodialysis and Kidney Transplantation." *Archives of General Psychiatry*, **21**(3), 373–380 (1969).

——— "The Quality of Life Before and After Renal Transplantation." *Diseases of the Nervous System*, **32**(1), 24–31 (1971).

Becker, Howard S. "Notes on the Concept of Commitment." *American Journal of Sociology*, **66**(1), 32–40 (1960).

Beecher, H. "Ethical Problems Created by the Hopelessly Unconscious Patient." *New England Journal of Medicine*, **278**(26), 1425–1430 (1968).

Bennett, Alan and J. Harrison. "Experience with Living Familial Renal Donors." *Surgery, Gynocology and Obstetrics*, **139**(6), 894–898 (1974).

Bergan, John J. "The Risk of the Donor." Presented at an International Symposium on the Human Aspects of Clinical Transplantation, September 30, 1972, San Francisco.

Berman, Josephine. "The Machine Gives Me life, and I Live It." In Felix T. Rapaport, Ed., *A Second Look at Life: Transplantation and Dialysis Patients: Their Own Stories.* New York: Grune & Stratton, 1973. Pp. 42–43.

Bernstein, Dorothy M. "After Transplantation—The Child's Emotional Reactions." *American Journal of Psychiatry*, **127**(9), 1189–1193 (1971).

——— "Emotional Reactions of Children and Adolescents to Renal Transplantation." *Child Psychiatry and Human Development*, **1**(2), 102–111 (1970).

——— and Roberta G. Simmons. "The Adolescent Kidney Donor: The Right to Give." *American Journal of Psychiatry*, **131**(12), 1338–1343 (1974).

Bethesda Conference Report. "Cardiac and Other Organ Transplantation in the Setting of Transplant Science as a National Effort." *American Journal of Cardiology*, **22**(6), 896–912 (1968).

Biörck, G. and G. Magnusson. "The Concept of Self as Experienced by Patients With a Transplanted Kidney." *Acta Medica Scandinavica*, **183**(3), 191–192 (1968).

Blachly, P. H. "Can Organ Transplantation Provide an Altruistic-Expiatory Alternative to Suicide?" Paper presented at Second Annual Conference of the American Association of Suicidology, March 29, 1969.

Black, Peter McL. "Criteria of Brain Death: Review and Comparison." *Postgraduate Medicine*, **57**(2), 69–74 (1975).

Blagg, C. R., M. Anderson, C. Shadle, G. Bilden, and S. Beer. "Rehabilitation of Patients Treated by Dialysis or Transplantation." Paper presented at the Third Annual Meeting of Clinical Dialysis and Transplant Forum, 1973, Washington, D.C.

Blatt, B. and W. T. Tsushima. "A Psychological Survey of Uremic Patients Being Considered for the Chronic Hemodialysis Program: Intellectual and Emotional Patterns in Uremic Patients." *Nephron*, **3**(4), 206–208 (1966).

Blau, Peter M. *Exchange and Power in Social Life.* New York: Wiley, 1964.

Blazer, Daniel G., William M. Petrie, and William P. Wilson. "The Treatment of Psychiatric Complications of Renal Transplant." Unpublished manuscript, Department of Psychiatry, Duke Medical Center, Durham, North Carolina.

Bleuler, Manfred. "The Offspring of Schizophrenics." *Schizophrenia Bulletin*, **1**(8), 93–107 (1974).

Bois, M. S., N. B. Barfield, C. E. Taylor, and C. D. Ross. "Nursing Care of Patients Having Kidney Transplants." *American Journal of Nursing*, **68**(6), 1238–1247 (1968).

Bonjean, Charles, Richard J. Hill, and S. Dale McLemore. *Sociological Measurement.* San Francisco: Chandler, 1967.

Bradburn, Norman M. *The Structure of Psychological Well-Being.* Chicago: Aldine, 1969.

——— and David Caplovitz. *Reports on Happiness.* Chicago: Aldine, 1965.

Brand, L. and N. I. Komorita. "Adapting to Long-Term Hemodialysis." *American Journal of Nursing*, **66**(8), 1778–1781 (1966).

Brewer, S. P. "Donors of Organs Seen as Victims." *New York Times*, April 19, p. 36 (1970).

Brim, Orville G., David C. Glass, David E. Lavin, and Norman Goodman. *Personality and Decision Processing.* Stanford: Stanford University Press, 1962.

Brown, H. W., J. F. Maher, L. Lapierre, F. H. Bledsoe, and G. E. Schreiner. "Clinical Problems Related to the Prolonged Artificial Maintenance of Life by Hemodialysis in

Chronic Renal Failure." *Transactions of American Society of Artificial Internal Organs*, **8**, 281–291 (1962).

Bullough, Bonnie. "The Medicare-Medicaid Amendments." *American Journal of Nursing*, **73**(11), 1926–1929 (1973).

Burns, Suzanne, and H. K. Johnson. "Rehabilitation Potential of a Dialysis Versus a Transplant Population." *Dialysis & Transplantation*, **5**(6), 54–56 (1976).

—— H. Keith Johnson, H. Earl Ginn, Phillip J. Walker, Paul Teschan, and Adelaide Hohanness. "A Study of the Rehabilitation of One Hundred-Two Patients on Chronic Hemodialysis," unpublished manuscript.

Burton, Benjamin T. "The Federal Role in Improving the Therapy of Uremia." *Transplantation Proceedings*, in press.

Calland, Chad H. "Iatro-genic Problems in End-Stage Renal Failure." *The New England Journal of Medicine*, **287**(7), 334–336 (1972).

Capron, Alexander M. "To Decide What Dead Means." *New York Times*, February 24, p. 6E (1974).

—— and Leon R. Kass. "A Statutory Definition of the Standards For Determining Human Death: An Appraisal and a Proposal." *University of Pennsylvania Law Review*, **121**(87), 87–118 (1972).

Castel, J. G. "Legal Aspects of Human Organ Transplantation in Canada." *Canadian Medical Association Journal*, **99**(11), 533–548 (1968).

—— "Medico-Legal Problems of Organ Transplantation." In John S. Najarian and Richard L. Simmons, Eds., *Transplantation*. Philadelphia: Lea & Febiger, 1972.

Castelnuovo-Tedesco, Pietro. "Organ Transplant, Body Image, Psychosis." *The Psychoanalytic Quarterly*, **42**(3), 349–363 (1973).

Chatterjee, Satya, John E. Payne, and Thomas V. Berne. "Difficulties in Obtaining Kidneys From Potential Postmortem Donors." *Journal of American Medical Association*, **232**(8), 822–824 (1975).

Christopherson, Lois K. and Thomas A. Ganda. "Patterns of Grief: End-Stage Renal Failure and Kidney Transplantation." *Transplantation Proceedings*, **5**(2), 1051–1057 (1973).

Chu, George. "Letter to Editor." *American Journal of Psychiatry*, **128**(4), 495–496 (1971).

Cialdini, Robert G., Betty Lee Darby, and Joyce E. Vincent. "Transgression and Altruism: A Case for Hedonism." *Journal of Experimental Social Psychology*, **9**(6), 502–516 (1973).

Cleveland, Sidney E. "Personality Characteristics, Body Image and Social Attitudes of Organ Transplant Donors versus Nondonors." *Psychosomatic Medicine*, **37**(4), 313–319 (1975).

—— and Dale L. Johnson. "Motivation and Readiness of Potential Human Tissue Donors and Nondonors." *Psychosomatic Medicine*, **32**(3), 225–231 (1970).

Coleman, J. S. *Equality of Educational Opportunity*. Washington, D.C.: U.S. Government Printing Office, 1966.

—— H. Menzel, and E. Katz. "Social Processes in Physicians' Adoption of a New Drug." *Journal of Chronic Diseases*, **9**(1), 1–19 (1959).

Collier, B. N., Jr. "Comparisons Between Adolescents With and Without Diabetes." *Personnel and Guidance Journal*, **47**(7), 679–684 (1969).

Colomb, G. and J. Hamburger, "Psychological and Moral Problems of Renal Transplantation." In H. S. Abram, Ed., *International Psychiatry Clinics: Psychological Aspects of Surgery*. Boston: Little, Brown, 1967.

Comty, Christina M., Arthur Leonard and Fred L. Shapiro. "Psychosocial Problems in Dialyzed Diabetic Patients." *Kidney International*, **6**(4), (Supplement No. 1), S–144–S–151 (1974).

Connally, Sue. "Homicide Victims—Dispute Arises on Transplants." *Dallas (Texas) News*, October 12 (1968).

Corday, E. "Definition of Death: A Double Standard." *Medical Tribune*, **11**, 13 (1970).

Coser, Lewis A. *The Functions of Social Conflict*. New York: Free Press, 1956.

Crain, Alan J., Marvin B. Sussman, and William B. Weil, Jr. "Family Interaction, Diabetes and Sibling Relationships." *International Journal of Social Psychiatry*, **12**(1), 35–43 (1966).

Cramond, W. A. "Renal Homotransplantation: Some Observations on Recipients and Donors." *British Journal of Psychiatry*, **113**(504), 1223–1230 (1967).

—— P. R. Knight, and J. R. Lawrence. "The Psychiatric Contribution to a Renal Unit Undertaking Chronic Haemodialysis and Renal Homotransplantation." *British Journal of Psychiatry*, **113**(504), 1201–1212 (1967).

Crane, Diana. Written communication, 1969.

—— *The Sanctity of Social Life: Physicians' Treatment of Critically Ill Patients*. New York: Russell Sage, 1975.

Crites, John. *Vocational Psychology*. New York: McGraw-Hill, 1969.

Crosbie, S. "The Administrator in the Organ Replacement Program." *Proceedings of the First International Symposium on Organ Transplantation in Human Beings*. Hanover, N. H.: Sandoz Pharmaceuticals, 1970.

Crosby, David L. and W. E. Waters. "Survey of Attitudes of Hospital Staff to Cadaveric Kidney Transplantation." *British Medical Journal*. **4**(5836), 346–348 (1972).

Cutter, Fred. "Some Psychological Problems in Hemodialysis." *Omega*, **1**(1), 37–47 (1970).

Cyert, R. B., H. A. Simon, and D. B. Trow. "Observations of a Business Decision." *Journal of Business*, **29**(4), 237–248 (1956).

Dahl, Robert A. "The Analysis of Influence in Local Communities." In Charles Adrian, Ed., *Social Science and Community Action*. East Lansing: Michigan State University, Institute of Community Development and Services, 1960.

Dansak, Daniel A. "Secondary Gain in Long-Term Hemodialysis Patients." *American Journal of Psychiatry*, **129**(3), 128–131 (1972).

Darley, John M. and Bibb Latané. "Norms and Normative Behavior: Field Studies of Social Interdependence." In J. Macaulay and L. Berkowitz, Eds., *Altruism and Helping Behavior: Social Psychological Studies of Some Antecedents and Consequences*. New York: Academic, 1970. Pp. 83–101.

Davis, Fred. *Passage Through Crisis*. Indianapolis: Bobbs-Merrill, 1963.

Dempsey, David. "Transplants are Common; Now It's the Organs that have become Rare." *The New York Times Magazine*, April 4, p. 83 (1974).

Densen, Paul. "Public Accountability and Reporting Systems in Medicare and Other Health Programs." *New England Journal of Medicine*, **289**(8), 401–406 (1973).

De Shazo, Claude V., Richard L. Simmons, Dorothy M. Bernstein, Maureen M. De Shazo, Justine Willmert, Carl M. Kjellstrand, and John S. Najarian. "Results of Renal Transplantation in 100 Children." *Surgery*, **76**(3), 461–468 (1974).

Deutsch, Cynthia P. and Judith A. Goldston. "Family Factors in Home Adjustment of the Severely Disabled." *Marriage and Family Living*, **22**(4), 312–316 (1960).

Douglas, Ruth A. "The Costs of Kidney Transplantation and Hemodialysis." In Felix T.

Rapaport, Ed., *A Second Look at Life: Transplantation and Dialysis Patients: Their Own Stories.* New York: Grune & Stratton, 1973. Pp. 75–78.

Duckeminier, J., Jr. and D. Sanders. "Organ Transplantation: A Proposal for Routine Salvaging of Cadaver Organs." *New England Journal of Medicine*, **279**(8), 413–419 (1968).

Duff, Raymond S. and August B. Hollingshead. *Sickness and Society.* New York: Harper & Row, 1968.

Durdin, Tillman. "Physicians Adopt Code on Death: Medical Assembly Acts Out of Concern over Transplants." *New York Times*, August 10, p. 25 (1968).

Dwarshuis, Louis. "Intellectual Assessment and Treatment, Prognosis in Hemodialysis Patients." Unpublished paper, VA Hospital, Hines, Illinois.

Eady, R. A. J. "Why I Have Not Had a Kidney Transplant After Nine and One-Half Years as a Hemodialysis Patient." In Felix T. Rapaport, Ed., *A Second Look at Life: Transplantation and Dialysis Patients: Their Own Stories.* New York: Grune & Stratton, 1973. Pp. 44–46.

Ebert, Ronald J. "Sequential Decision Making: An Aggregate Scheduling Methodology." *Psychometrika* **36**(3), 303–316 (1971).

Edwards, Charles C. Remarks made at the Regional Communications Seminar, New York, April 17, 1974.

Eichhorn, Robert L. and Ronald M. Andersen. "Changes in Personal Adjustment to Perceived and Medically Established Heart Disease: A Panel Study." *Journal of Health and Human Behavior*, **3**(3), 242–249 (1962).

Eisendrath, R. M. "The Role of Grief and Fear in the Death of Kidney Transplant Patients." *American Journal of Psychiatry*, **126**(3), 381–387 (1969).

——— R. D. Guttman, and J. E. Murray. "Psychological Considerations in the Selection of Kidney Transplant Donors." *Surgery, Gynecology, and Obstetrics*, **129**(2), 243–248 (1969).

Epstein, Nathan B. and William A. Westley. "Patterns of Intra-Familial Communication." In D. E. Cameron and M. Greenblatt, Eds., *Recent Advances in Neuro-Physiological Research, Psychiatric Research Report 11.* Washington, D. C.: American Psychiatric Association, 1959. Pp. 1–12.

Erikson, E. H. "The Problem of Ego-Identity." *Journal of American Psychoanalytic Association*, **4**(1), 53–121 (1956).

Etzioni, Amitai. *The Active Society: A Theory of Societal and Political Processes.* New York: Free Press, 1968.

——— "How Kidney Donations Can Be Increased." *Medical World News*, December 6, p. 80 (1974).

Farber, Bernard. "Effects of a Severely Mentally Retarded Child on Family Integration." *Monographs for the Society for Research in Child Development*, **24**(2), (1959).

——— "Family Organization and Crisis: Maintenance of Intergration in Families with a Severely Mentally Retarded Child." *Monographs for the Society for Research in Child Development*, **25**(1) (1960).

Farrell, Robert M., William T. Stubenbard, Robert R. Riggio, and Edward C. Muecke. "Living Renal Donors: Nephrectomy: Evaluation of 135 Cases." *The Journal of Urology*, **110**(6), 639–642 (1973).

Fellner, Carl H. and John R. Marshall. "Twelve Kidney Donors." *Journal of the American Medical Association*, **206**(12), 2703–2707 (1968).

——— and John Marshall. "Kidney Donors: The Myth of Informed Consent." *American Journal of Psychiatry*, **126**(9), 1245–1251 (1970).

—— and Shalom H. Schwartz. "Altruism in Disrepute: Medical vs. Public Attitudes Towards the Living Organ Donor." *New England Journal of Medicine*, **284**(11), 582–585 (1971).

Ferber, Robert. "Family Decision-Making and Economic Behavior." Paper delivered at Institute of Life Insurance Conference. Williamsburg, Virginia, 1971.

Ference, Thomas P. "Induced Strategies in Sequential Decision-Making." *Human Relations*, **25**(5), 377–389 (1972).

Ferris, G. N. "Psychiatric Aspects of Renal Transplantation: A Dialysis Symposium for Nurses." U.S. Dept. of HEW publication. Washington, D.C.: U.S. Government Printing Office, 1969.

Fine, R. N., B. M. Korsch, and H. Riddell. "Second Renal Transplants in Children." *Surgery*, **73**(1), 1–7 (1973).

Flanagan, T. A. and G. E. Murphy. *Archives of General Psychiatry*, **28**(5), 732–734 (1973).

Fost, Norman, "Children as Renal Donors." *New England Journal of Medicine*, **296** (February 17), 363–367 (1977).

Foster, F. Gordon, George L. Cohn, and F. Patric McKegney. "Psychobiologic Factors and Individual Hemodialysis—A Two Year Follow-up: Part I." *Psychosomatic Medicine*, **35**(1), 64–82 (1973).

Fox, Renée C. *Experiment Perilous.* Glencoe: Free Press, 1959.

—— "A Sociological Perspective on Organ Transplantation and Hemodialysis." *New York Academy of Sciences Annals*, **169**(Art. 2), 406–428 (1970).

—— and Judith P. Swazey. *The Courage to Fail: A Social View of Organ Transplants and Dialysis.* Chicago: University of Chicago Press, 1974.

Frederick, Richmond S., II. "Medical Jurisprudence—Determining the Time of Death of the Heart Transplant Donor." *North Carolina Law Review*, **51**(6), 172–184 (1972).

Freedman, Jonathan L. "Transgression, Compliance and Guilt." In J. Macaulay and L. Berkowitz, Eds., *Altruism and Helping Behavior: Social Psychological Studies of Some Antecedents and Consequences.* New York: Academic, 1970. Pp. 155–161.

Freidson, Eliot. "The Organization of Medical Practice." In H. Freeman, S. Levine, and G. Reeder, Eds., *Handbook of Medical Sociology*. Englewood Cliffs, N. J.: Prentice-Hall, 1963. P. 299.

—— and Buford Rhea. "Knowledge and Judgment in Professional Evaluations." *Administrative Science Quarterly*, **10**(1), 107–124 (1965).

Freyberger, H. "Six Years Experience as a Psychosomaticist in a Hemodialysis Unit." In J. Reusch, A. H. Schmale, Eds., *Psychotherapy and Psychosomatics.* Rochester, N. Y.: Karger, 1973. Pp. 226–232.

Fritz, Charles E. and Harry B. Williams. "The Human Being in Disasters: A Research Perspective." *Annals of the American Academy of Political and Social Sciences*, **309**(January), 42–51 (1957).

Frye, W. W. "The National Transplant Information Center" ("Current Opinion:" Guest Editorial). *Medical Tribune*, **10**(92), 19 (1969).

Gade, D. M. "Attitudes Towards Human Organ Transplantation—A Field Study of 119 People in the Greater Detroit Area." *Henry Ford Hospital Medical Journal*, **20**(1), 41–50 (1972).

Gallagher, Eugene B. and Maryrhea Morelock. "A Dialysis-Transplant Program and Its Growing Pains." *Medical Care*, **12**(6), 520–533 (1974).

Gallup Poll. *New York Times*, January 17, p. 18 (1968).

GAO (U.S. General Accounting Office). "Treatment of Chronic Kidney Failure: Dialysis, Transplant, Costs, and the Need for More Vigorous Efforts." A Report to the Congress by the Comptroller General of the United States, June 24, 1975.

Garmezy, Norman. "Children at Risk: The Search for the Antecedents of Schizophrenia. Part II: Ongoing Research Programs, Issues, and Intervention." *Schizophrenia Bulletin*, **1**(9), 55–125 (1974a).

——— "The Study of Competence in Children at Risk for Severe Psychopathology." In E. James Anthony and Cyrille Koupernik, Eds., *The Child In His Family: Children at Psychiatric Risk.* New York: Wiley, 1974b. Pp. 77–98.

——— with the collaboration of Sandra Streitman. "Children at Risk: The Search for the Antecedents of Schizophrenia. Part I. Conceptual Models and Research Methods." *Schizophrenia Bulletin*, **1**(8), 14–90 (1974c).

Gates, M. "A Comparative Study of Some Problems of Social and Emotional Adjustment of Crippled and Non-Crippled Girls and Boys." *Journal of Genetic Psychology*, **68**(Second Half), 219–244 (1946).

Gaylin, Willard. "Harvesting the Dead: The Potential For Recycling Human Bodies." *Harper's* **249**(1492), 23–30 (1974).

Ginzberg, Eli, Sol W. Ginsburg, Sidney Axelrad, and John L. Herma. *Occupational Choice: An Approach to a General Theory.* New York: Columbia University Press, 1951.

Glaser, G. "Psychotic Reactions Induced by Corticotrophin (ACTH) and Cortisone." *Psychosomatic Medicine*, **15**(4), 280–291 (1953).

Glassman, Barry M. and Allen Siegel. "Personality Correlates of Survival in a Long-Term Hemodialysis Program." *Archives of General Psychiatry*, **22**(6), 566–574 (1970).

Glick, Ira O., Robert S. Weiss, and C. Murray Parkes. *The First Year of Bereavement.* New York: Wiley Interscience, 1974.

Glueck, William F. "Decision Making: Organization Choice." *Personnel Psychology*, **27**(1), 77–93 (1974).

Goldberg, Richard. "Adjustment of Children with Invisible and Visible Handicaps." *Journal of Counselling Psychology*, **21**(5), 428–432 (1974).

Goldstein, A. and Marvin Reznikoff. "Suicide in Chronic Hemodialysis Patients from an External Locus of Control Framework." *American Journal of Psychiatry*, **127**(9), 1204–1207 (1971).

Gombos, E. A., T. H. Lee, M. R. Harton, and J. W. Cummings. "One Year's Experience With an Intermittent Dialysis Program." *Annals of Internal Medicine*, **61**(3), 462–469 (1964).

Gonzalez, T. M., R. C. Pabico, H. W. Brown, J. F. Maher, and G. E. Schreiner. "Further Experiences With the Use of Routine Intermittent Hemodialysis in Chronic Renal Failure." *Transactions of American Society for Artificial Internal Organs*, **9**, 11–20 (1963).

Goodey, J. and J. Kelly. "Social and Economic Effects of Regular Dialysis." *Lancet*, **2**(7506), 147–148 (1967).

Gordon, Gerald. *Role Theory and Illness: A Sociological Perspective.* New Haven: College and University Press, 1966.

Gottschalk, C. W. "Report of the Committee on Chronic Kidney Disease to the Bureau of U.S. Budget." September 1967.

Gouldner, Alvin W. "The Norm of Reciprocity: A Preliminary Statement." *American Sociological Review*, **25**(2), 161–178 (1960).

Gove, Walter R. and Jeannette F. Tudor. "Adult Sex Roles and Mental Illness." *American Journal of Sociology*, **78**(4), 812–835 (1973).

Graham, Victoria. "A Case of Life and Death: Epic Struggle May Bring a New Definition of Dying." *St Paul Sunday Pioneer Press*, December 2, p. 1 (1973).

Guetzkow, Harold. "Communications in Organization." In J. March, Ed., *Handbook of Organizations.* Chicago: Rand McNally, 1965. Pp. 534–573.

Hagberg, Bo. "A Prospective Study of Patients in Chronic Hemodialysis—III. Predictive Value of Intelligence, Cognitive Deficit and Ego Defence Structures in Rehabilitation." *Journal of Psychosomatic Research* **18**(3), 151–160 (1974).

Haggerty, Robert J., Klaus J. Roghmann, and Ivan B. Pless. *Child Health and The Community.* New York: Wiley, 1975.

Hamburger, J. and J. Crosnier. "Moral and Ethical Problems in Transplantation." In F. Rapaport and J. Dausset, Eds., *Human Transplantation.* New York: Grune & Stratton, 1968. Pp. 37–44.

Hansen, Donald and Reuben Hill. "Families Under Stress." In Harold T. Christensen, Ed., *Handbook of Marriage and the Family.* Chicago: Rand McNally, 1964. Pp. 782–822.

Hartke, Vance. *Congressional Record*—Senate, 22823, March 5, 1974.

Hayes, C. P., Jr. and J. C. Gunnels, Jr. "Selection of Recipients and Donors for Renal Transplantation." *Archives of Internal Medicine*, **123**(5), 521–530 (1969).

Herbich, Von J. "Rechtlicke Fragen Zur Organtransplantation" (Legal Issues of Organ Transplantation). *Wiener Klinische Wachenschrift* (Viennese Clinical Weekly Periodical), **84**(42/43), October 20, pp. 668–672 (1972).

Hertel, R. and J. P. Kemph. "Psychologic Effects of Kidney Transplantation." *Current Medical Digest*, **36**, 607 (1969).

HEW "HEW Interim Regulations on Payment for Treatment of Chronic Renal Disease." *Federal Register*, 17210–17212. July 1 (1973a).

——— (Department of Health, Education, and Welfare). "Final Policies—PL92–602, Section 2991. End-Stage Renal Disease Program of Medicare." April (1974).

——— "Proposed Rules, End-Stage Renal Disease—Conditions for Coverage." *Federal Register*, **40**(127), Part II, July 1 (1975).

——— "The Medicare End-Stage Renal Disease Program." PL 92–603, Section 2991, Policy Issues—ACTION" (memorandum). November 7, 1973b.

——— Part A, Intermediary Letter No. 73–25; Part B, Intermediary Letter No. 73–22. "Processing and Payment of Claims for Renal Dialysis and Transplant Services Performed for Eligible Medicare Beneficiaries after June 30, 1973." July (1973c).

Hickey, Kathleen. *Social Service Report.* Transplant Service, University of Minnesota Hospital, 1969.

Hill, Reuben. "Decision-Making and the Family Life Cycle." In E. Shanas and G. Streib, Eds., *Social Structure and the Family Generational Relations.* Englewood Cliffs, N.J.: Prentice-Hall, 1965. Pp. 113–145.

——— *Family Development in Three Generations.* Cambridge: Schenkman, 1970.

——— In collaboration with Elise Boulding, assisted by Lowell Dunigan and Rachel Ann Elder. *Families Under Stress: Adjustment to the Crisis of War Separation and Reunion.* New York: Harper, 1949.

Hirvas, Juhani, Mikael Enckell, Börje Kuhlback, and Amos Pasternack. *Acta Medica Scandinavica*, **200**(1, 2), 17–200 (1976).

Hollingshead, A. B. and F. C. Redlich. *Social Class and Mental Illness*. New York: Wiley, 1958.

Holsti, Ole R. "Crisis, Stress and Decision-Making." *International Social Science Journal*, **23**(1), 53–67 (1971).

Homans, George C. *Social Behavior: Its Elementary Forms*. New York: Harcourt, 1961.

Hughson, B. J., E. Anne Collier, J. Johnston, and D. J. Tiller. "Rehabilitation After Renal Transplantation." *Medical Journal of Australia*, **2**(20), 732–735 (1974).

Hyman, Herbert H., Ed. *The Politics of Health Care—Nine Case Studies of Innovative Planning in New York City*. New York: Praeger, 1973.

Idelson, Roberta K., Sydney H. Croog, and Sol Levine. "Changes in Self-Concept During the Year After a First Heart Attack: A Natural History Approach—Part I." *American Archives of Rehabilitation Therapy*, **22**(1), 10–21, (1974a).

——— Sydney H. Croog, and Sol Levine. "Changes in Self- Concept During the Year After a First Heart Attack: A Natural History Approach—Part II." *American Archives of Rehabilitation Therapy*, **22**(2), 25–31 (1974b).

Iglehart, John K. "Kidney Treatment Problem Readies HEW for National Health Insurance." *National Journal Reports*, **8**(2), 895–900 (1976).

Isen, Alice M. "Success, Failure, Attention, and Reaction to Others: The Warm Glow of Success." *Journal of Personality and Social Psychology*, **15**(4), 294–301 (1970).

Janis, Irving L. and Leon Mann. *Decison Making: A Psychological Analysis of Conflict, Choice, and Commitment*. New York: Free Press, in press.

Johnson, W. J., R. D. Wagoner, J. C. Hunt, G. J. Mueller, and G. A. Hallenbeck. "Long-Term Intermittent Hemodialysis for Chronic Renal Failure." *Mayo Clinic Proceedings*, **41**(2), 73–93 (1966).

Jones, Edward E. and Richard E. Nisbett. "The Actor and the Observer: Divergent Perceptions of the Causes of Behavior." In Edward E. Jones, David E. Kanouse, Harold H. Kelley, Richard E. Nisbett, Stuart Valins, and Bernard Weiner, Eds., *Attribution: Percieving the Causes of Behavior*. Morristown, N. J.: General Learning, 1971.

Kane, Stanley D. "Setting Precedents for Transplants." *Modern Medicine*, **41**(3), 84–85 (1973).

Kaplan De-Nour, A. and J. W. Czaczkes. "Emotional Problems and Reactions of the Medical Team on a Chronic Haemodialysis Unit." *Lancet*, **2**(7576), 987–991 (1968).

——— and J. W. Czaczkes. "Team-Patient Interaction in Chronic Hemodialysis Units." *Psychotherapy and Psychosomatics*, **24**(2–3), 132–136 (1974).

——— J. Shaltiel, and J. W. Czaczkes. "Emotional Reactions of Patients on Chronic Hemodialysis." *Psychosomatic Medicine*, **30**(5), 521–533 (1968).

Kass, L. R. "A Caveat on Transplants." *The Washington Post*, January 14, p. B1 (1968).

Katona, George. "Rational Behavior and Economic Behavior." *Psychology Review*, **60**(5), 307–319 (1953).

——— and Eva Mueller. "A Study of Purchase Decisions." In Lincoln Clark, Ed., *Consumer Behavior*. New York: New York University Press, 1954. Pp. 30–87.

Katz, A. and D. Proctor. "Social Psychological Characteristics of Patients Receiving Hemodialysis Treatment for Chronic Renal Failure: Report of Questionnaire Survey of Dialysis Centers and Patients During 1967." Washington, D. C.: U.S. Government Printing Office (July), 1969.

Katz, Jay and Alexander Morgan Capron. *Catastrophic Diseases: Who Decides What?* New York: Russell Sage Foundation, 1975.

Kemph, J. P. "Renal Failure, Artificial Kidney and Kidney Transplant." *American Journal of Psychiatry*, **122**(11), 1270–1274 (1966).

—— "Psychotherapy with Patients Receiving Kidney Transplant." *American Journal of Psychiatry*, **124**(5), 623–629 (1967).

—— E. A. Bermann, and H. P. Coppolillo. "Kidney Transplant and Shifts in Family Dynamics." *American Journal of Psychiatry*, **125**(11), 1485–1490 (1969).

Kendall, P. L. "The Relationships Between Medical Educators and Medical Practitioners." *Journal of Health and Human Behavior*, **6**(2), 79–82 (1965).

Kerr, D. S. "Provision of Services to Patients with Chronic Uremia" (editorial). *Kidney International*, **3**(4), 197–204 (1973).

Khan, Aman, M. A. Herndone, S. Y. Ahmadian. "Social and Emotional Adaptations of Children with Transplanted Kidneys and Chronic Hemodialysis." *American Journal of Psychiatry*, **127**(9), 1194–1198 (1971).

Kidney Disease Services, Facilities and Programs in the United States, Washington, D.C., U.S. Government Printing Office (Public Health Service Publication no. 1942), May 1969.

Kieren, Dianne, June Henton, and Ramona Marotz. *Hers and His: A Problem Solving Approach to Marriage.* Hinsdale, Ill.: Dryden, 1975.

King, S. H. "Social Psychological Factors in Illness." In H. Freeman, S. Levine, and L. Reeder, Eds., *Handbook of Medical Sociology*. Englewood, N. J.: Prentice-Hall, 1963. Chapter 3, 1st Edition.

Kjellstrand, Carl M., Richard L. Simmons, Frederick C. Goetz, Theodore J. Buselmeier, Jeffrey R. Shideman, Barry von Hartitzsch, and John S. Najarian. "Renal Transplantation in Patients With Insulin-Dependent Diabetes." *The Lancet*, **2**(7819), 4–8 (1973).

Klar, Ronald M. Remarks at the National Kidney Foundation Annual Meeting, Washington, D.C., November 16, 1973.

Klein, Susan D. "Chronic Kidney Disease: Impact on the Child and Family and Strategies for Coping." Unpublished doctoral dissertation, University of Minnesota, August, 1975.

—— and Roberta G. Simmons. "Chronic Disease and Childhood Development: Kidney Disease and Transplantation." *Research in Community and Mental Helath: An Annual Compilation of Research.* Greenwich, Conn.: JAI Press, in press.

Knowles, J. H. "Radiology: A Case Study on Technology and Manpower." *New England Journal of Medicine*, **280**(24), 1323–1329 (1969).

Kogan, Nathan and Michael A. Wallach. "Risk Taking as a Function of the Situation, the Person, and the Group." In *New Directions in Psychology III*. New York: Holt, Rinehart & Winston, 1967.

Kohn, Melvin. *Class and Conformity: A Study in Values.* Homewood, Ill.: Dorsey, 1969.

Kolff, W. J., S. Nakamoto, and J. P. Scudder. "Experiences with Long-Term Intermittent Dialysis." *Transactions of American Society of Artificial Internal Organs*, **8**, 292–299 (1962).

Korsch, Barbara. Oral communication, March 1970.

—— Vida Negrete, James E. Gardner, Carol L. Weinstock, Ann S. Mercer, Carl M. Grushkin, and Richard N. Fine. "Kidney Transplantation in Children: Psychosocial Follow-up Study on Child and Family." *The Journal of Pediatrics*, **83**(3), 399–408 (1973).

Kramer, Mark S., Diane Hudschek, Rasib M. Raja, and Jerry L. Rosenbaum. "For Rehabilitation—Dialysis or Transplantation?" *Dialysis and Transplantation*, **4**(5), 56–62 (1975).

Largiadèr, F. "Transplant Organ Procurement and Preservation." *Documenta Geigy Transplants: The Way Ahead*, by CIBA–GEIGY Limited, pp. 3–5 (1971).

Latané, Bibb and John M. Darley. "Social Determinants of Bystander Intervention in Emergencies." In J. Macaulay and L. Berkowitz, Eds., *Altruism and Helping Behavior: Social Psychological Studies of Some Antecedents and Consequences.* New York: Academic, 1970. Pp. 13–27.

Leavell, Jerome F. "Legal Problems in Organ Transplants." *Mississippi Law Journal*, **44**(5), 865–899 (1973).

Lecky, P. *Self-Consistency.* New York: Island, 1945.

Lederer, H. "How the Sick View Their World." In E. G. Jaco, Ed., *Patients, Physicians and Illness.* Glencoe, Illinois: Free Press, 1960. Chapter 26.

Lefebvre, Paul, J. C. Crombez, and Jacques LeBeuf. "Psychological Dimension and Psychopathological Potential of Acquiring a Kidney." *Canadian Psychiatric Association Journal*, **18**(6), 495–500 (1973).

Leik, Robert. "Critique and Discussion." In Joan Aldous, Thomas Condon, Reuben Hill, Murray Straus, and Irving Tallman, Eds., *Family Problem Solving: A Symposium on Theoretical, Methodological, and Substantive Concerns.* Hinsdale, Ill.: Dryden, 1971. Pp. 35–46.

Leopold, A. "Psychological Problems in Hemodialysis." *R.N.*, **31**(May), 42–45 (1968).

Levin, Carol. "Dialysis and Transplant—A Social Work Perspective." Presented at Children and Parents Under Stress, sponsored by the Children's Service of Langley Porter Neuropsychiatric Institute, San Francisco, May 28–30, 1975.

Levy, Norman B. "Sexual Adjustment to Maintenance Hemodialysis and Renal Transplantation: National Survey by Questionnaire: Preliminary Report." *Transactions of American Society of Artificial Internal Organs*, **19**, 138–143 (1973).

——— *Living or Dying.* Springfield, Ill.: Charles C. Thomas, 1974.

——— and Gary D. Wynbrandt. "The Quality of life on Maintenance Haemodialysis." *Lancet*, **9**(7920), 1328–1330 (1975).

Lewis, Melvin. "Kidney Donation by a 7-year-Old Identical Twin Child." *Journal of the American Academy of Child Psychiatry*, **13**(2), 221–245 (1974).

Lilly, John R., Geoffrey Giles, Richard Hurwitz, Gerhard Schroter, Hiroshi Takagi, Samuel Gray, Israel Penn, Charles G. Halgrinson, and Thomas E. Starzl. "Renal Homotransplantation in Pediatric Patients." *Pediatrics*, **47**(3), 548–557 (1971).

Lindemann, Erich. "Symptomatology and Management of Acute Grief." *American Journal of Psychiatry*, **101**(2), 141–148 (1944).

Lipowski, L. J. "Physical Illness, the Individual and the Coping Process." *Psychiatry in Medicine*, **1**(2), 91–102 (1970).

Litman, Theodor. "The Family as a Basic Unit in Health and Medical Care: A Social-Behavioral Overview." *Social Science and Medicine*, **8**(9/10), 495–519 (1974).

Little, A. D., Inc. "Financial Coverage for Victims of End-Stage Renal Failure." *Report*, April 21 (1969).

Livingston, G. Oral communication, March, 1970.

London, Perry. "The Rescuers: Motivational Hypotheses About Christians Who Saved Jews From the Nazis." In J. Macaulay and L. Berkowitz, Eds., *Altruism and Helping Behavior:*

Social Psychological Studies of Some Antecedents and Consequences. New York: Academic, 1970. Pp. 241–250.

Louisell, D. W. and L. Kilbrandon. "Ethical Problems in Medical Procedures" (General Discussion on R. Platt). In G. E. W. Wolstenholme and M. O'Connor, Eds., *Ethics in Medical Progress: With Special Reference to Transplantation* (Ciba Foundation symposium). Boston: Little, Brown, 1966. P. 161.

Lowi, Theodore. "American Business, Public Policy, and Political Theory." *World Politics*, **16**(4), 677–715 (1964).

Lowrie, Edmund G., J. Michael Lazarus, Altair J. Mocelin, George L. Bailey, Constantine L. Hampers, Richard E. Wilson, and John P. Merrill. "Survival of Patients Undergoing Chronic Hemodialysis and Renal Transplantation." *The New England Journal of Medicine*, **288**(17), 863–867 (1973).

Luce, Robert Duncan and Howard Raiffa. *Games and Decisions: Introduction and Critical Survey.* A Study of the Behavioral Models Project, Bureau of Applied Social Research, Columbia University. New York: Wiley, 1957.

Lunde, Donald T. "Psychiatric Complications of Heart Transplants." *American Journal of Psychiatry*, **126**(3), 369–373 (1969).

Lyons, Richard L. "Program to Aid Kidney Victims Faces Millions in Excess Costs." *New York Times*, January 11, p. 1 (1973).

Macaulay, J. and L. Berkowitz, Eds., *Altruism and Helping Behavior: Social Psychological Studies of Some Antecedents and Consequences.* New York: Academic, 1970.

MacDonald, J. "Nursing Care in Renal Transplantation." *Canadian Nurse*, **63**(10), 35–39 (1967).

MacNamara, M. "Psychosocial Problems in a Renal Unit." *British Journal of Psychiatry*, **113**(504), 1231–1236 (1967).

—— "The Family in Stress: Social Work Before and After Renal Homotransplantation." *Social Work* (New York), **14**(4), 89–97 (1969).

Malmquist, A. "A Prospective Study of Patients in Chronic Hemodialysis—I: Method and Characteristics of the Patient Group." *Journal of Psychosomatic Research*, **17**(5 & 6), 333–337 (1973).

—— and Bo Hagberg. "A Prospective Study of Patients in Chronic Hemodialysis—V. A Follow-up Study of Thirteen Patients in Home-Dialysis." *Journal of Psychosomatic Research*, **18**(5), 321–326 (1974).

Mangus, A. R. "Mental Health of Rural Children in Ohio." *Ohio Agricultural Experiment Station Research Bulletin*, **682** (1949).

Marmor, Theodore R. *The Politics of Medicare.* Chicago: Aldine, 1973.

Masland, Richard L. "When is a Person Dead?" *Resident and Staff Physician*, 21 (April), 49–52 (1975).

Matas, Arthur J., Richard L. Simmons, Theodore J. Buselmeier, Carl M. Kjellstrand, and John S. Najarian. "The Fate of Patients Surviving Three Years After Renal Transplantation." *Surgery*, **80**(3), 390–395 (1976).

Mattsson, Ake. "Long Term Physical Illness in Childhood—Challenge to Psychosocial Adaptation." *Pediatrics*, **50**(5), 801–811 (1972).

—— and Samuel Gross. "Adaptational and Defensive Behavior in Young Hemophiliacs and Their Parents." *American Journal of Psychiatry*, **122**, 1349–1356 (1966a).

——— and Samuel Gross. "Social and Behavioral Studies on Hemophiliac Children and Their Families." *Journal of Pediatrics*, **68**(6), 952–964 (1966b).

Matza, David. *Delinquency and Drift*. New York: Wiley, 1964.

Mauss, Marcell. *The Gift: Forms and Functions of Exchange in Archaic Societies*. New York: Norton, 1967.

McAnarney, Elizabeth R., I. Barry Pless, Betty Satterwhite, and Stanford B. Friedman. "Psychological Problems of Children with Chronic Juvenile Arthritis." *Pediatrics*, **53**(4), 523–528 (1974).

McCleery, Robert S., Louise T. Keelty, Russell E. Phillips, and Terrence M. Quirin. *One-Life—One Physician*. Washington, D.C.: Public Affairs Press, 1971.

McFadden, Joseph T. "The Donor and His Physician." *Surgery, Gynecology & Obstetrics*, **134**(6) 999–1000 (1972).

McGeown, M. G. "Ethics for the Use of Live Donors in Kidney Transplantation." *American Heart Journal*, **75**(5), 711–714 (1968).

McKegney, F. P. and P. Lange. "The Decision to No Longer Live on Chronic Hemodialysis." *American Journal of Psychiatry*, **128**(3), 267–274 (1971).

Meadow, Roy, J. Stewart Cameron, and Chisholm Ogg. "Regional Service for Acute and Chronic Dialysis of Children." *The Lancet*, **2**(7675), 707–709 (1970).

Meldrum, M. W., J. G. Wolfram, and M. E. Rubini. "The Impact of Chronic Hemodialysis Upon the Socio-Economics of A Veteran Patient Group." *Journal of Chronic Diseases*, **21**(1), 37–52 (1968).

Menzies, I. C. and W. K. Stewart. "Psychiatric Obervations on Patients Receiving Regular Dialysis Treatment." *British Medical Journal*, **1**(5591), 544–546 (1968).

Merrill, J. P. "Hemodialysis in the Home." *Journal of the American Medical Association*, **206**(1), 124 (1968a).

——— "Medical Management of the Transplant Patient." In F. T. Rapaport and J. D. Dausset, Eds., *Human Transplantation*. New York: Grune & Stratton, 1968b. Pp. 66–79.

Merton, R. K. *Social Theory and Social Structure*. Glencoe, Ill.: Free Press, 1957.

Metcalfe, Virginia. "Renal Disease Services Criteria and Standards." Monograph prepared for The Health Resources Administration, Department of Health, Education, and Welfare, Rockville, Md., January 1976.

Miller, Delbert C. and William H. Form. *Industrial Sociology: An Introduction to the Sociology of Work Relations*. New York: Harper & Brothers, 1951.

Minde, Klaus K., G. D. Hackett, D. Killou, and S. Silver. "How They Grow Up: 41 Physically Handicapped Children and Their Families." *American Journal of Psychiatry*, **128**(2), 1554–1560 (1972).

Mock, Clarence E. "Life Before and After Transplantation." In Felix T. Rapaport, Ed., *A Second Look At Life: Transplantation and Dialysis Patients: Their Own Stories*. New York: Grune & Stratton, 1973. Pp. 40–43.

Mondale, Walter. "Introduction of Joint Resolution to Establish a Commission on Health, Science and Society." *Congressional Record*, **114**(3), 2622 (1968).

Moore, Francis D., George E. Burch, Dwight E. Harken, H. J. C. Swan, Joseph E. Murray, and C. Walton Lillihei. "Cardiac and Other Organ Transplantation: In the Setting of Transplant Science and a National Effort." *Journal of the American Medical Association*, **206**(11), 2489–2500 (1968).

Moores, B., G. Clarke, B. R. Lewis, and N. P. Mallick. "Public Attitudes Towards Kidney Transplantation." *British Medical Journal*, **13**(March), 629–631 (1976).

Morgan, James N. "Some Pilot Studies of Communication and Consensus in the Family." *Public Opinion Quarterly*, **32**(1), 113–121 (1968).

Muller, P. H. "Legal Medicine and the Delimitation of Death." *World Medical Journal*, **14**(5), 140–142 (1967).

Munster, Andrew M., Rebecca E. Stengle, and M. Clinton Miller. "Community Attitudes to Renal Transplantation: A Statistical Survey." *The American Journal of Surgery*, **128**(3), 415–418 (1974).

Murphy, G. *Personality*. New York: Harper & Row, 1947.

Murphy, Lois. "Preventive Implications of Development in the Preschool Years." In Gerald Caplan, Ed., *Prevention of Mental Disorders in Children*. New York: Basic Books, 1961. Pp. 218–248.

Muslin, Hyman L. "Panel I—Psychiatric Problems in Extending Vital Capacity, Using Machines and Organ Replacements. The Emotional Response to the Kidney Transplant: The Process of Internalization." *Canadian Psychiatric Association Journal*, **17**(SS–II), SS–3–SS–8 (1972).

Najarian, J. S., R. L. Simmons, M. B. Talent, C. M. Kjellstrand, T. J. Buselmeier, R. L. Vernier, and A. F. Michael. "Renal Transplantation in Infants and Children." *Annals of Surgery*, **174**(4), 583–601 (1971).

National Heart Institute, *ad hoc* Task Force on Cardiac Replacement. Washington, D.C.: U.S. Government Printing Office, 1969.

National Kidney Foundation. "Position Paper – Guidelines for the Implication of Public Law 92–603, Title II, Section 2991 Concerned with Chronic Kidney Disease." April 1973.

Noe, N. H. and S. Ehrenfeld. "A Bayesian Sequential Multi-Decision Problem." *Management Science*, **20**(3), 274–281 (1973).

Nolen, William A. *A Surgeon's World*. Greenwich, Conn.: Fawcett Publications, 1970.

Norton, C. E. "Chronic Hemodialysis as a Medical and Social Experiment." *Annals of Internal Medicine*, **66**(6), 1267–1277 (1967).

Offord, D. R. and J. F. Aponte. "Distortion of Disability and Effects on Family Life." *Journal of the American Academy of Child Psychiatry*, **6**, 499–511 (1967).

Ogburn, W. F. *Social Change*. New York: Viking, 1922.

Olson, David and Carolyn Rabunsky. "Validity of Four Measures of Family Power." *Journal of Marriage and The Family*, **34**(2), 224–234 (1972).

Page, I. H. "The Ethics of Heart Transplantation: A Personal View." *Journal of the American Medical Association*, 207(1), 109–113 (1969).

Parets, A. "Emotional Reactions to Chronic Physical Illness: Implications for the Internist." *Medical Clinic of North America*, **51**(6), 1399–1408 (1967).

Parsons, Talcott and Renée C. Fox. "Illness Therapy and the Modern Urban American Family." In Seymour Martin Lipset and Neil J. Smelser, Eds., *Sociology, The Progress of a Decade*. Englewood Cliffs, N. J.: Prentice-Hall, 1961. Pp. 561–571.

Penn, Israel, Donald Bunch, David Olenik, and George Abouna. "Psychiatric Experiences with Patients Receiving Renal and Hepatic Transplants." *Seminars in Psychiatry*, **3**(1), 133–145 (1971).

——— Charles G. Halgrinson, D. Ogden, Thomas E. Starzl. "Use of Living Donors in Kidney Transplantation in Man." *Archives of Surgery*, **101**(2), 226–231 (1970).

Perez de Francisco, C., G. Huitron, S. Saltzman, and H. Villarreal. "Psychological Aspects of Kidney Transplantation." *Totus Homo*, **3**(3), 107–112 (1971).

Pierce, David M., Richard Freeman, Richard Lawton, and Margaret Fearing. "Longitudinal Stability of Psychological Status of Hemodialysis Patients." *Psychology—A Journal of Human Behavior*, **10**(2), 66–69 (1973a).

——— Richard Freeman, Richard Lawton, and Margaret Fearing. "Psychological Correlates of Chronic Hemodialysis Estimated by MMPI Scores." *Psychology—A Journal of Human Behavior*, **10**(2), 53–57 (1973b).

Pierce, Gene A. "The Administrator in an Organ Replacement Program." Presented at The First International Symposium on the Socio-Medical Aspects of Organ Transplantation in Human Beings, March 1970, Houston, Texas.

Pless, Ivan and Klaus Roghmann. "Chronic Illness and Its Consequences: Observations Based on Three Epidemiologic Surveys." *Journal of Pediatrics*, **79**(3), 351–359 (1971).

Pollard, William E. and Terence R. Mitchell. "A Decison Theory Analysis of Social Power." Technical Report 71–25, July, 1971. Organizational Research, Dept. of Psychology, University of Washington, Seattle, Washington.

Prial, Frank J. "Bill is Proposed on Transplants." *New York Times*, March 11, p. 22 (1975).

Puscheck, Herbert C. and James H. Greene. "Sequential Decision Making in a Conflict Environment." *Human Factors*, **14**(6), 561–571 (1972).

Rados, David L. "Selection and Evaluation of Alternatives in Repetitive Decision Making." *Administrative Science Quarterly*, 17(2), 1–11 (1972).

Rae, A. I., T. A. Marr, R. E. Steury, L. A. Gothberg, and R. C. Davidson. "Hemodialysis in the Home: Its Integration Into General Medical Practice." *Journal of the American Medical Association*, **206**(1), 92–96 (1968).

Raible, Jane A. "System for Increasing Organ Donation" (letter to the editor). *The New England Journal of Medicine*, **292**(5), 271 (1975).

Rapaport, Felix T. *A Second Look at Life: Transplantation and Dialysis Patients: Their Own Stories*. New York: Grune & Stratton, 1973.

Rapoport, Amnon and Graham J. Burkheimer. "Models for Preferred Decision Making." *Journal of Mathematical Psychology*, **8**(4), 508–538 (1971).

Reichsman, Franz and Norman B. Levy. "Problems in Adaptation to Maintenance Hemodialysis. A Four-Year Study of 25 Patients." In Norman B. Levy, Ed., *Living or Dying: Adaptation to Hemodialysis*. Springfield, Ill.: Charles C. Thomas, 1974. Pp. 30–49.

Reinhard, H. C. "The Administrative Aspects of Organ Transplantation." Paper presented at First International Symposium on the Socio-Medical Aspects of Organ Transplantation in Human Beings, Houston, Texas, March 1970.

Renal Physicians Association. "Position Paper 1." *Dialysis & Transplantation*, **3**(2), 45–46 (1974).

Retan, J. W. and H. Y. Lewis. "Repeated Dialysis of Indigent Patients for Chronic Renal Failure." *Annals of Internal Medicine*, **64**(2), 284–292 (1966).

Rettig, Richard A. "Valuing Lives: The Policy Debate on Patient Care Financing for Victims of End-Stage Renal Disease." *The Rand Paper Series*, P–5672, March 1976.

——— and Thomas C. Webster. "Implementation of the End-Stage Renal Disease Program: A Mixed Pattern of Subsidizing and Regulating and Delivery of Medical Services." Paper presented at American Political Science Association Meetings, San Francisco, September, 1975.

Richardson, Stephen A., Albert H. Hastorf, Norman Goodman, and Sanford M. Dornbusch. "Cultural Uniformity in Reaction to Physicial Disabilities." *American Sociological Review*, **26**(2), 241–247 (1961).

Riley, C. M. "Thoughts About Kidney Transplantation in Children." *Journal of Pediatrics*, **65**(5), 797–800 (1964).

Riteris, J. M. "The Basis for Ethical Decisions on Clinical Transplantation as Viewed by a Transplant Recipient." In Felix T. Rapaport, Ed., *A Second Look At Life: Transplantation and Dialysis Patients: Their Own Stories.* New York: Grune & Stratton, 1973. Pp. 71–74.

Rosenberg, Florence R. and Roberta G. Simmons. "Sex Differences in the Self-Concept in Adolescence." *Sex Roles: A Journal of Research*, **1**(2), 147–159 (1975).

Rosenberg, Morris. *Society and The Adolescent Self-Image.* Princeton, N. J.: Princeton University Press, 1965.

——— and Roberta G. Simmons. *Black and White Self-Esteem: The Urban School Child.* Washington, D.C.: American Sociological Association, Arnold and Caroline Rose Monograph Series, 1972.

Rosenblatt, D. And E. A. Suchman. "Blue Collar Attitudes and Information Toward Health and Illness." In A. Shostak and W. Gomberg, Eds., *Blue Collar World.* Englewood Cliffs, N.J.: Prentice-Hall, 1964. P. 324.

Rosenstock, Irwin. "Decision-Making by Individuals." Health Education Monograph, Number 11 (1961).

Rosenthal, D. *Genetic Theory and Abnormal Behavior.* New York: McGraw-Hill, 1972.

Rubini, M. E. and R. Goldman. "Chronic Renal Disease." *California Medicine,* **108**(2), 90–95 (1968).

Ruesch, Jurgen. *Disturbed Communication.* New York: Norton, 1957.

Rybak, Leonard P. "Liver Transplants for the Chronic Alcoholic" (Correspondence section). *The New England Journal of Medicine*, **290**(6), 346 (1974).

Sadler, Alfred M., Jr., Blair L. Sadler, and George E. Schreiner. "A Uniform Card for Organ and Tissue Donation." *Modern Medicine*, **37**(26), 20 (1969a).

——— Blair L. Sadler, and E. Blyth Stason. "Transplantation and the Law: Progress Toward Uniformity." *New England Journal of Medicine*, **282**(13), 717–723 (1970).

——— Blair L. Sadler, E. Blyth Stason, and Delford L. Stickel. "Transplantation: A Case for Consent." *New England Journal of Medicine*, 280(16), 862–867 (1969b).

Sadler, H. Harrison, Leslie Davison, Charles Carroll, and Samuel L. Kountz. "The Living, Genetically Unrelated, Kidney Donor." In P. Castelnuovo-Tedesco, Ed., *Psychiatric Aspects of Organ Transplantation.* New York: Grune & Stratton, 1971. Pp. 86–101.

Salaman, J. R. "Death After Kidney Transplantation." *British Medical Journal*, **3**(5933), 736–737 (1974).

Salisbury, R. E. "Behavioral Responses of a Nine-Year-Old Child With Chronic Dialysis." *Journal of American Academy of Child Psychiatry*, **7**, 282–289 (1968).

Salk, Lee, Margaret Hilgartner, and Belle Granick. "Psycho-Social Impact of Hemophilia on the Patient and His Family." *Social Science and Medicine*, **6**(4), 491–505 (1972).

Sampson, Tom F. "Level of Adjustment In One or More Year Post-Transplant and In-Center Dialysis Patients." Presented at the 81st Annual American Psychological Association Convention, Montreal, Quebec, Canada, August, 1973.

——— "The Child in Renal Failure." *Journal of the American Academy of Child Psychiatry*, **14**(3), 462–476 (1975).

Sand, P., G. Livingston, and R. G. Wright. "Assessment of Candidates for Hemodialysis." *Annals of Internal Medicine*, **64**(3), 602–610 (1966).

Santiago-Delphin, E. A., R. L. Simmons, R. G. Simmons, T. J. Tierney, D. Bernstein, C. M. Kjellstrand, T. J. Buselmeier, and J. S. Najarian. "Medico Legal Management of the Juvenile Kidney Donor." *Transplantation Proceedings*, **6**(4), 441–445 (1974).

Savage, J. "Organ Transplantation with an Incompetent Donor: Kentucky Resolves the Dilemma of Strunk vs. Strunk." *Kentucky Law Journal*, **58**(2), 129–160 (1969).

Scharer, K. "Incidence and Causes of Chronic Renal Failure in Childhood." *Proceedings of the European Dialysis and Transplant Association*, **8**, 211–217 (1971).

Schmeck, Harold A., Jr. "Transplantation of Organs and Attitudes: The Public's Attitude Toward Clinical Transplantation." *Transplantation Proceedings*, **1**(1, Part II), 670–674 (1969).

——— "Forty-two States Ease Laws on Transplants." *New York Times*, April 13, p. 30 (1970).

———"Brain Death: When Does Life Cease?" *New York Times*, June 4, p. E7 (1972).

Schowalter, John E. "Multiple Organ Transplantation and the Creation of Surgical Siblings." *Pediatrics*, **46**(4), 576–580 (1970).

Schreiner, G. E. "Mental and Personality Changes in the Uremic Syndrone." *Medical Annals of the District of Columbia*, **28**(6), 316–323 (1959).

——— "Problems of Ethics in Relation to Haemodialysis and Transplantation." In G. E. W. Wolstenholme and M. O'Connor, Eds., *Ethics in Medical Progress: With Special Reference to Transplantation*, Ciba Foundation Symposium. Boston: Little, Brown, 1966. Pp. 126–133.

——— and J. F. Maher. "Hemodialysis for Chronic Renal Failure, III: Medical, Moral and Ethical, and Socio-Economic Problems." *Annals of Internal Medicine*, **62**(3), 551–557 (1965).

Schwartz, Shalom H. "Elicitation of Moral Obligation and Self-Sacrificing Behavior: An Experimental Study of Volunteering to be a Bone Marrow Donor." *Journal of Personality and Social Psychology*, **15**(4), 283–293 (1970a).

——— "Moral Decision Making and Behavior." In J. Macaulay and L. Berkowitz, Eds., *Altruism and Helping Behavior: Social Psychological Studies of Some Antecedents and Consequences.* New York: Academic, 1970b. Pp. 127–141.

——— "The Justice of Need and the Activation of Humanitarian Norms." *Journal of Social Issues*, **31**(3), 111–136 (1975).

——— "Normative Influences on Altruism." In *Advances in Experimental Social Psychology: Vol. 10.* New York: Academic, in press.

Scribner, Belding H. "Introduction." In Norman B. Levy, Ed., *Living or Dying: Adaptation to Hemodialysis.* Springfield, Ill.: Charles C. Thomas, 1974. Pp. xi–xii.

——— E. B. Fergus, S. T. Boen, and E. D. Thomas. "Some Therapeutic Approaches to Chronic Renal Insufficiency." *Annual Review of Medicine*, **16**, 285–300 (1965).

Shambaugh, P. W., C. L. Hampers, G. L. Bailey, D. Snyder, and J. P. Merrill. "Hemodialysis in the Home: Emotional Impact on the Spouse." *Transactions of the American Society for Artificial Internal Organs*, **13**, 41–45 (1967).

Shapiro, Fred L. "Chronic Hemodialysis—An Overview." Unpublished manuscript.

——— Arthur Leonard, and Christina M. Comty. "Mortality, Morbidity and Rehabilitation Results in Regularly Dialyzed Patients With Diabetes Mellitus." *Kidney International*, **6**(4), Supplement No. 1, S–8–S–14 (1974).

Shea, E. J., D. F. Bogdan, R. B. Freeman, and G. E. Schreiner. "Hemodialysis for Chronic Renal Failure. IV. Psychological Considerations." *Annals of Internal Medicine*, **62**(3), 558–563 (1965).

Shelley, E. G. "Ethical Guidelines for Organ Transplantation." *Journal of the American Medical Association*, **205**(6), 341–342 (1968).

Short, M. J. and R. J. Alexander. "Psychiatric Considerations for Center and Home Hemodialysis." *Southern Medical Journal*, **62**(December), 1476–1479 (1969).

——— and N. L. Harris. "Psychiatric Observations of Renal Homotransplantations." *Southern Medical Journal*, **62**(December), 1479–1482 (1969).

Silverman, Charlotte. *The Epidemiology of Depression*. Baltimore: John Hopkins Press, 1968.

Silverman, Daniel, M. G. Saunders, R. S. Schwab, and R. S. Masland. "Cerebral Death and the Electroencephalogram. Report of the *ad hoc* Committee of the American Electroencephalographic Society on EEG Criteria for Determination of Cerebral Death." *Journal of the American Medical Association*, **209**(10), 1505–1510 (1969).

Simmons, R. L., E. J. Thompson, C. M. Kjellstrand, E. J. Yunis, R. M. Condie, S. M. Mauer, T. J. Buselmeier and J. S. Najarian. "Parent-to-Child and Child-to-Parent Kidney Transplants: Experience with 101 Transplants at One Centre." *The Lancet*, February 14, 321–331 (1976).

——— E. J. Thompson, E. J. Yunis, H. Noreen, C. M. Kjellstrand, D. S. Fryd, R. M. Condie, S. M. Mauer, T. J. Buselmeier and J. S. Najarian. "115 Patients with First Cadaver Kidney Transplants Followed Two to Seven and a Half Years: A Multifactorial Analysis." *The American Journal of Medicine*, **62**(February), 234–241 (1977a).

——— E. J. Van Hook, E. J. Yunis, H. Noreen, C. M. Kjellstrand, R. M. Condie, S. M. Mauer, T. J. Buselmeier and J. S. Najarian. "100 Sibling Kidney Transplants Followed Two to Seven and a Half Years: A Multifactorial Analysis." *Annals of Surgery*, **185**(2), 196–204 (1977b).

Simmons, Roberta G., John Bruce, Rita Bienvenue, and Julie Fulton. "Who Signs an Organ Donor-Card: Traditionalism versus Transplantation." *Journal of Chronic Diseases*, **27**(9/10), 491–502 (1974).

——— and Julie Fulton. "Ethical Issues in Kidney Transplantation." In Claude A. Frazier, Ed., *Is It Moral to Modify Man*. Springfield, Ill.: Charles C. Thomas, 1973. Chapter 11. Pp. 171–188.

——— Julie Fulton, and Robert Fulton. "The Prospective Organ Transplant Donor: Problems and Prospects of Medical Innovation." *Omega*, **3**(4), 319–339 (1972).

——— Kathleen Hickey, Carl M. Kjellstrand, and Richard L. Simmons. "Donors and Non-Donors: The Role of the Family and the Physician in Kidney Transplantation." *Seminars in Psychiatry*, **3**(1), 102–115 (1971a).

——— Kathy Hickey, Carl M. Kjellstrand, and Richard L. Simmons. "Family Tension in the Search for a Kidney Donor." *The Journal of the American Medical Association*, **215**(6), 909–912 (1971b).

——— and Susan D. Klein. "Family Non-Communication: Search for Kidney Donors." *American Journal of Psychiatry*, **129**(6), 63–68 (1972).

——— Susan Klein, and Kenneth Thorton. "The Family Member's Decision to be a Kidney Transplant Donor." *Journal of Comparative Family Studies*. Special issue on the family in health and illness, **4**(1), 88–115 (1973a).

——— and Florence Rosenberg. "Sex, Sex-Roles, and Self-Image." *Journal of Youth and Adolescence*, **4**(3), 229–258 (1975).

——— Florence Rosenberg, and Morris Rosenberg. "Disturbance in the Self-Image at Adolescence." *American Sociological Review*, **38**(5), 553–568 (1973b).

——— and Kathleen J. Schilling. "Rehabilitation: Diabetic vs. Non-Diabetic Transplants." *Transplantation Proceedings*, **7**(1), Supplement 1, 719–722 (1975).

——— and Kathleen J. Schilling. "The Social and Psychological Rehabilitation of the Diabetic Transplant Patient." *Kidney International*, **6**(4), Supplement 1, S–152–S–158 (1974).

——— and Richard L. Simmons. "Organ Transplantation: A Societal Problem." *Social Problems*, **19**(1), 36–57 (1971).

——— and Richard L. Simmons. "Sociological and Psychological Aspects of Transplantation." In J. S. Najarian and R. L. Simmons, Eds., *Transplantation*. Philadelphia: Lea & Febiger, 1972. Chapter 9.

Simon, Herbert A. *Administrative Behavior*, 2nd Ed. New York: Macmillan, 1957.

Sisson, Roger L. "How Did We Ever Make Decisions Before the Systems Approach?" *Socio-Economic Planning Sciences*, **6**(6), 523–529 (1972).

Smith, R. B., K. Walton, E. L. Lewis, G. D. Perdue, and G. Hemdon, Jr. "Operative Morbidity Among 40 Living Kidney Donors." *Journal of Surgical Research*, **12**(3), 199–203 (1972).

Snortland, Neil E. and John E. Stanga. "Neutral Principles and Decision-Making Theory: An Alternative to Incrementalism." *The George Washington Law Review*, **41**(5), 1006–1032 (1973).

Soelberg, Peer O. "Unprogrammed Decision Making." *Industrial Management Review*, **8**(2), 19–29, (1967).

Somers, Anne R. "Catastrophic Health Insurance? A Catastrophe!" *Medical Economics*, May 10, pp. 213–214 (1971).

——— and Herman M. Somers. "The Organization and Financing of Health Care: Issues and Direction for the Future." *American Journal of Orthopsychiatry*, **42**(1), 119–136 (1972).

Spanos, P. K., R. L. Simmons, R. G. Simmons, M. Goldberg, and J. S. Najarian. "The Aging Related Kidney Donor: Prognosis for Donor, Recipient and Kidney." Abstracts of the Sixth Annual Meeting of The American Society of Nephrology, 1973.

——— R. L. Simmons, E. Lampe, L. C. Rattazzi, C. M. Kjellstrand, F. C. Goetz, and J. S. Najarian. "Complications of Related Kidney Donation." *Surgery*, **76**(5), 741–747 (1974).

Starzl, T. E. In discussion on J. E. Murray, "Organ Transplantation: The Practical Possibilities." In G. E. W. Wolstenholme and M. O'Connor, Eds., *Ethics in Medical Progress: With Special Reference to Transplantation*. Ciba Foundation Symposium. Boston: Little, Brown, 1966a. P. 76.

——— "The Role of Organ Transplantation in Pediatrics." *Pediatric Clinics of North America*, **13**(2), 381–422 (1966b).

Stickel, D. L. "Ethical and Moral Aspects of Transplantation." *Monographs of Surgical Science*, **3**(4), 267–301 (1966).

Stuart, Frank P. "Progress in Legal Definition of Brain Death and Consent to Remove Cadaver Organs." *Surgery*, **81**(1), 68–73 (1977).

Suchman, E. A. "Sociomedical Variations Among Ethnic Groups." *American Journal of Sociology*, **70**(3), 319–331 (1964).

Sudnow, D. *Passing On, The Social Organization of Dying*. Englewood Cliffs, N.J.: Prentice-Hall, 1967.

Sullivan, Michael F. "The Dialysis Patient and Attitudes Toward Work." *Psychiatry in Medicine*, **4**(2), 213–219 (1973).

Sultz, Harry A., Edward R. Schlessinger, William E. Mosher, and Joseph G. Feldman. *Long Term Childhood Illness.* Pittsburgh: University of Pittsburgh Press, 1972.

Swenson, Wendell M., John S. Pearson, David Osborne. *An MMPI Sourcebook—Basic Items, Scale and Pattern Data on 50,000 Medical Patients.* Minneapolis: University of Minnesota Press, 1973.

Tallman, Irving. "The Family as a Small Problem Solving Group." *Journal of Marriage and the Family*, **32**(1), 94–104 (1970).

Taylor, Donald. "Decision-Making and Problem Solving." In James March, Ed., *Handbook of Organizations.* Chicago: Rand McNally, 1965. Pp. 48–86.

Taylor, Lee. *Occupational Sociology.* New York: Oxford Press, 1968.

Thomas, Lewis. "Guessing and Knowing: Reflections on the Science and Technology of Medicine." *Saturday Review*, p. 54, January (1973).

Titmuss, Richard M. *The Gift Relationship: From Human Blood to Social Policy.* New York: Pantheon Books, 1971.

Tomkins, Richard M. "Evaluating National Health Insurance Legislation: A Summary Review." *Hospital Administration*, **19**(3), 74–84 (1974).

Trimakas, Kestutis A. and Robert C. Nicolay. "Self-Concept and Altruism in Old Age." *Journal of Gerontology*, **29**(4), 434–439 (1974).

Turner, Ralph H. *Family Interaction.* New York: Wiley, 1970.

Tyler, H. R. "Neurological Complications of Dialysis, Transplantation and Other Forms of Treatment in Chronic Uremia." *Neurology*, **15**(12), 1081–1088 (1965).

Van Till-d'Aulnis de Bourouill, Adrienne. "How Dead Can You Be?" *Medicine, Science and the Law*, **15**(2), 133–147 (1975).

Vaux, K. "A Year of Heart Transplants. An Ethical Valuation." *Postgraduate Medicine*, **45**(1), 201–205 (1969).

Viederman, Milton. "The Search for Meaning in Renal Transplantation." *Psychiatry*, **37**(3), 283–290 (1974).

Visscher, M. B. "Assisting Survival." *Minnesota Medicine*, **53**(6), 626–627 (1970).

Waller, Willard. *The Family: A Dynamic Interpretation*. New York: Cordon, 1938.

Wasmuth, C. E. *Law and the Surgical Team*. Baltimore: William & Wilkins, 1969.

Wells, L. E. and G. Marwell. *Self-Esteem: Its Conceptualization and Measurement*. Beverly Hills, Calif.: Sage Publications, Inc., 1976.

West, Darrell. "The World Is a Beautiful Place." In Felix T. Rapaport, Ed., *A Second Look At Life: Transplantation and Dialysis Patients: Their Own Stories*. New York: Grune & Stratton, 1973. Pp. 12–13.

Whatley, Lydia W. "Home and In-Center Hemodialysis Patients." *Dialysis and Transplantation*, **4**(4), 18–27 (1975).

White, D. J. *Decision Theory*. Chicago: Aldine, 1970.

Wylie, R. C. *The Self-Concept*. Lincoln: University of Nebraska Press, 1961.

Wilkins, Margaret B. "Funding for End-Stage Renal Patients." In G. L. Bailey, Ed., *Hemodialysis Principles and Practice*. New York: Academic, 1972.

Williams, G. M., H. M. Lee, and D. M. Hume. "Renal Transplants in Children." *Transplant Proceedings*, **1**(1, Part I), 262–266 (1969).

Wilson, W. P., D. L. Stickel, C. P. Hayes, Jr., and N. L. Harris. "Psychiatric Considerations of Renal Transplantation." *Archives of Internal Medicine*, **122**(6), 502–506 (1968).

Wolstenholme, G. E. W. and M. O'Connor. *Ethics in Medical Progress: With Special Reference to Transplantation*. Ciba Foundation Symposium. Boston: Little, Brown, 1966.

Wright, B. *Physical-Disability—Psychological Approach*. New York: Harper & Row, 1960.

Wright, I. S. "A New Challenge to Ethical Codes: Heart Transplant." *Journal of Religion and Health*, **8**(3), 226–241 (1969).

Wright, R. G., P. Sand, and G. Livingston. "Psychological Stress During Hemodialysis for Chronic Renal Failure." *Annals of Internal Medicine*, **64**(3), 611–621 (1966).

Zeckhauser, Richard. "Procedures for Valuing Lives." *Public Policy*, **23**(Fall), 447–448 (1975).

Zuk, G. H. "The Religious Factor and the Role of Guilt in Parental Acceptance of the Retarded Child." *American Journal of Mental Deficiency*, **64**(1), 139–147 (1959).

GLOSSARY

A-Match A transplant between siblings who share all the identifiable transplantation antigens in common. Because of such strong immunologic similarities, the rate of transplant success exceeds 90%.

Antilymphoblast globulin (ALG) An immunosuppressive product used to reduce the rejection of a foreign graft. It is a purified product of horse serum that has the capacity to destroy those cells in man responsible for rejection.

Arterial-sclerotic heart disease Hardening of the arteries.

Cadaver list A list of patients who need kidney transplants who are waiting for kidney donations from recently dead, in fact, brain-dead persons. Such kidney transplant patients usually do not have relatives who can donate kidneys.

Cardiac arrhythmias Irregularity; loss of rhythm; denoting especially an irregularity of the heartbeat.

Creatinine A waste product of protein metabolism normally excreted in the urine. An elevated creatinine level in the blood is a sign of poor kidney function and in transplant patients, a sign of kidney rejection.

Cross-matching The process of testing serum of the recipient and potential kidney donor to see if the recipient already has preexisting immunity to the donor. If so, the donor cannot be used.

Cushingoid Puffy, moonface, and rotund figure, produced as a side-effect of steroid medications given to posttransplant patients to prevent immunological rejection.

Diabetes A disorder of carbohydrate metabolism resulting from inadequate production or utilization of the hormone insulin. Long-term complications include cardiovascular disease, blindness, involvement of the nervous system, and kidney disease—diabetic glomerulosclerosis.

Dialysis (hemodialysis) Treatment using the artificial kidney machine. The patient is connected by tubes to the machine through which his blood flows. Waste products are removed and the blood is returned to him. Used when patient's own kidneys are incapable of removing waste products from blood.

Embolus A plug, composed of a detached clot, mass of bacteria, or other foreign body, obstructing a blood vessel.

End-stage renal disease The stage of kidney impairment that is virtually always irreversible and permanent and requires dialysis or kidney transplantation to ameliorate uremic symptoms and maintain life. The patient's kidneys are incapable of removing waste products from the blood, and without treatment there will be fatal disturbances of the body's chemical balance.

Glomerulonephritis A group of kidney diseases characterized by inflamation of the glomeruli (a tuft of capillaries in the kidney).

Graft Transplanted organ.

Hematocrit Ratio of volume of red blood cells to volume of whole blood. Anemia is reflected in a reduced hematocrit reading.

Imuran An immunosuppressive drug used to help prevent rejection of the transplanted kidney.

Immunological rejection Attempted or actual destruction of transplanted kidney by the body's immunological system. The body's immunological system attempts to destroy all foreign tissues or organisms.

Immunosuppression Drug therapy given to patients to make their bodies less capable of the immunological reaction that might destroy the new transplanted organ. The body also becomes less capable of fighting disease-bearing organisms when these drugs are given.

Malignancy Cancer.

Mitral insufficiency A defect in the function of one of the heart valves.

Nephrectomy The surgical removal of the kidney.

Nephrologist A physician who treats patients with kidney disease.

Neuropathy Impairment of nerve function, which may occur as a result of kidney disease or diabetes. It may affect both motor and sensory nerves, sensory changes occurring first with numbness in the extremities. It may be only partially reversible in uremic patients.

Pediatric Pertaining to children.

Prednisone A steroid drug used to prevent the transplanted kidney from being immunologically rejected; often causes various side effects.

Pyelonephritis Bacterial infection of the kidney.

Renal Pertaining to the kidney.

Thrombophlebitis Inflammation of a vein with secondary thrombus (clot) formation.

Tissue typing The process of testing serum of the recipient and potential kidney donor to determine the degree of compatibility. This includes the cross-match tests and tests to determine the degree to which the donor and recipient share transplantation antigens. The more antigens of a certain type they share, the better the "match." If the match is a perfect, or "A" match, the transplanted kidney is not likely to be immunologically rejected. Although the evidence is not completely firm for other levels of matching and typing, transplant centers generally give preference to better matches and more shared antigens for transplantation to minimize the possibility of immunological rejection. In addition, the donor and recipient must be of compatible blood types (A, B, O) as in the case of blood donation.

Transplant A surgical procedure and its results, involving the placement of an organ from one human being (donor) into another human being (recipient) so that it performs its normal functions in the recipient.

Uremia Severe kidney disease.

Uremic Suffering from severe kidney disease.

Vascular system The circulatory system, which includes the heart, blood vessels, and lymphatic system.

Ventricular tachycardia Relating to or suffering from rapid action of the ventricles of the heart

INDEX